Negotiating the Pandemic

I0042081

This book centers on negotiations around cultural, governmental, and individual constructions of COVID-19. It considers how the coronavirus pandemic has been negotiated in different cultures and countries, with the final part of the volume focusing on South Asia and Pakistan in particular. The chapters include autoethnographic accounts and ethnographic explorations that reflect upon experiences of living with the pandemic and its implications for all areas of life. The book explicates people's dealings with COVID-19 at various levels, situates the spread of rumors, conspiracy theories, and new social rituals within micro- and/or macro-contexts, and describes the interplay between the virus and various institutionalized forms of inequalities and structural vulnerabilities. Bringing together a variety of perspectives, the volume relates to the past, describes the Covidian present, and offers futuristic implications. It enlists distinct imaginaries based on current understandings of an extraordinary challenge that holds significant importance for our human future.

Inayat Ali, PhD, is a Research Fellow in the Department of Social and Cultural Anthropology at University of Vienna, Austria. He is a medical anthropologist whose research focuses on infectious diseases, vaccination, COVID-19, maternal health, syndemics, structured disparities, geopolitics, and biopolitics. He is one of the founding members of the South Asia Anthropology Forum (SAAF), and the Principal Investigator (PI) of a project: *Exploring and Understanding the Impacts of COVID-19: A Qualitative Inquiry*, approved by the National Bioethics Committee of Pakistan. Also, he has led research on COVID-19 in Sri Lanka, Bangladesh, and Nigeria. He has authored numerous peer and non-peer-reviewed articles.

Robbie Davis-Floyd, PhD, is an Adjunct Professor in the Department of Anthropology at Rice University, USA, and specializes in medical and interpretive anthropology and the anthropology of reproduction. She is an international speaker and is author of multiple articles and encyclopedia entries and two books, and lead or co-editor of 18 volumes. Her latest book is the co-authored *Ritual: What It Is, How It Works, and Why* (2022).

Routledge Studies in Health and Medical Anthropology

Locating Zika
Social Change and Governance in an Age of Mosquito Pandemics
Edited By Kevin Bardosh

Affective Health and Masculinities in South Africa
An Ethnography of (In)vulnerability
Hans Reihling

Wandering the Wards
An Ethnography of Hospital Care and its Consequences for People Living
with Dementia
Katie Featherstone, Andy Northcott

Actively Dying
The Creation of Muslim Identities through End-of-Life Care in the
United States
Cortney Hughes Rinker

amaXhosa Circumcision
Stories of Manhood and Mental Health
Lauraine M. H. Vivian

Treating Heroin Addiction in Norway
The Pharmaceutical Other
Aleksandra Bartoszko

Childlessness in Bangladesh
Intersectionality, Suffering and Resilience
Papreen Nahar

Negotiating the Pandemic
Cultural, National, and Individual Constructions of COVID-19
Edited by Inayat Ali and Robbie Davis-Floyd

Negotiating the Pandemic
Cultural, National, and Individual Constructions of COVID-19

Edited by Inayat Ali and
Robbie Davis-Floyd

Routledge
Taylor & Francis Group
LONDON AND NEW YORK

An electronic version of this book is freely available, thanks
to the support of libraries working with Knowledge Unlatched
(KU). KU is a collaborative initiative designed to make
high quality books Open Access for the public good. The
Open Access ISBN for this book is 9781003187462. More
information about the initiative and links to the Open Access
version can be found at www.knowledgeunlatched.org.

First published 2022
by Routledge
4 Park Square, Milton Park, Abingdon, Oxon OX14 4RN

and by Routledge
605 Third Avenue, New York, NY 10158

Routledge is an imprint of the Taylor & Francis Group, an informa business

British Library Cataloguing-in-Publication Data
A catalogue record for this book is available from the British Library

Library of Congress Cataloging-in-Publication Data
A catalog record has been requested for this book

ISBN: 978-1-032-02840-8 (hbk)
ISBN: 978-1-032-03473-7 (pbk)
ISBN: 978-1-003-18746-2 (ebk)

DOI: 10.4324/9781003187462

Typeset in Sabon
by Newgen Publishing UK

Inayat Ali
I dedicate this book to four generations of my extended family—my uncles, aunts, and cousins, and especially to my heroes—my mother, Aman Rani, my grandfather, Aba Allah Dad Khan Gopang, my father, Aba Hyder Bukhsh (famously known as Bakhat Ali), and my uncle Baba Khuda Bukhsh—and to my inspirations: Shagufta, Uzma, Saman, Shabaz, Miskeen, Abbas, Najaf, Reema (deceased—a great soul who had wanted to become a doctor), Mansoor, Savera, Tahira (& Co.), and Malhar, better known as Shayaan Haider-Ali.

Robbie Davis-Floyd
I dedicate this book to the thousands of community midwives in the United States and other countries who have so bravely risen to the challenges of attending far more births than usual during this pandemic as birthgiving families flee hospital contagion and potential separation from their support people and from their newborns in favor of birth at home or in freestanding birth centers.

Inayat Ali and Robbie Davis-Floyd
Together we dedicate this book to the entire human family, particularly to those who have most suffered from the effects of the coronavirus pandemic, and to those who will act on the lessons learned about the importance of worldwide pandemic preparedness, and thus will help all future generations to grow up in a world that is pandemic-free. More pandemics are inevitable—it is how quickly, effectively, and culturally appropriately we deal with them that will count.

Contents

List of Figures   xi
List of Tables   xii
Notes on Contributors   xiii

Introduction: Constructing and Negotiating COVID-19   1
INAYAT ALI AND ROBBIE DAVIS-FLOYD

PART I
Autoethnographic Reflections on Negotiating the Coronavirus
Pandemic   11

1   My Great-Grandmother, Malinowski, and My "Self":
    An Autoethnographic Account of Negotiating the
    COVID-19 Pandemic   13
    INAYAT ALI

2   Negotiating COVID-19 in the Media: Autoethnographic
    Reflections on Sweden and International Reporting   27
    RACHEL IRWIN

3   Loss and Longing for the Field During COVID-19 in
    Australia, and Finding It Again Because "*Ngukurr* Is
    Everywhere"   42
    KATE SENIOR, RICHARD CHENHALL, AND FRANCES EDMONDS

PART II
**Conceptualizing and Negotiating the Pandemic Across
Professions, Cultures, and Countries**   59

  4 "As Soon as People See You Cough, They Say You Have
    the Disease": Negotiating COVID-Related Stigma and
    Health-Seeking Behaviors in Kenya   61
    VIOLET BARASA

  5 How US Maternity Care Providers Conceptualize
    COVID-19 and Negotiate Practice Changes: The
    Tensions Between Organizational Protocols and
    Childbearers' Needs   76
    KIM GUTSCHOW AND ROBBIE DAVIS-FLOYD

  6 Health Literacy and Information Fatigue: Understanding
    People's Beliefs and Behaviors as They Negotiate
    COVID-19 in Germany   94
    MAYARÍ HENGSTERMANN

  7 "Flexible Lockdown" in Switzerland: Individual
    Responsibility and the Daily Navigation of Risk and
    Protection   110
    NOLWENN BÜHLER, MELODY PRALONG, CÉLIA BURNAND,
    CLOÉ RAWLINSON, SEMIRA GONSETH NUSSLÉ, VALÉRIE D'ACREMONT,
    MURIELLE BOCHUD, AND PATRICK BODENMANN

  8 Practicing Resilience while Negotiating the
    Pandemic: The Experiences of People with Rare Diseases
    in Poland   125
    KATARZYNA E. KRÓL AND MAŁGORZATA RAJTAR

  9 Negotiating COVID-19 in Russia on the Eve of the
    Introduction of Social Restrictions   139
    TATIANA O. NOVIKOVA, DMITRY G. PIROGOV,
    TATYANA V. MALIKOVA, AND GEORGIY A. MURZA-DER

 10 The Quest for a Cure for COVID-19: Controversies
    and Negotiations Around Biomedical Treatments and
    Traditional Asian Medicines   155
    DANUTA PENKALA-GAWĘCKA

11 How Do Small-to-Medium Enterprises (SMEs)
Negotiate the COVID-19 Pandemic in Indonesia?   172
SANTIRIANINGRUM SOEBANDHI, KRISTININGSIH,
AND IRA DARMAWANTI

PART III
**Culturally Constructing and Negotiating COVID-19
in South Asia**   189

12 Sri Lankans' Negotiations Around COVID-19: Can a
Culture Control a Viral Outbreak?   191
THARAKA ANANDA AND INAYAT ALI

13 Negotiating COVID-19 in Bhutan: Successfully Aligning
Science, Politics, Culture, and Religion in a Unique
Public Health Strategy   205
MARY GRACE A. PELAYO, IAN CHRISTOPHER N. ROCHA, AND
JIGME YOEZER

14 Negotiating India During the COVID-19 Crisis: Issues
and Challenges   216
SUMAN CHAKRABARTY

15 Contesting COVID-19 in Bangladesh: Government
Responses and Local Perceptions   232
INAYAT ALI AND SUDIPTA DAS GUPTA

PART IV
**Negotiating COVID-19 in Pakistan: Cultural Conceptions
and Pandemic Responses**   253

16 Social Constructions of the Concept of COVID-19 in
Pakistan: An Anthropological Investigation   255
SARA AKRAM AND RAO NADEEM ALAM

17 Local Perceptions of COVID-19 in Pakistan's Sindh
Province: Political Game, Supernatural Test, or Western
Conspiracy?   270
INAYAT ALI, SALMA SADIQUE, AND SHAHBAZ ALI

18 Negotiating Online Shopping Behaviors after the
COVID-19 Outbreak in Pakistan   281
TAYYABA RAFIQUE MAKHDOOM, SANAULLAH JAMALI,
AND MARIA TUFAIL MEMON

19 How Students Negotiated a University Closure: The
Impacts of "Covistress" on Undergraduate Students of
the University of Sindh During Online Education   299
ABDUL RAZAQUE CHANNA AND UMBREEN SOOMRO

Conclusions: Global Negotiations Around COVID-19   312
INAYAT ALI AND ROBBIE DAVIS-FLOYD

Index   332

Figures

3.1 Karen Rogers exploring the Feather Flowers at the Koori Heritage Trust. Photograph by Kate Senior   53

3.2 Daphne Daniels and Kate Senior exploring the Copley Archive. Photograph by Paige Wright, University of Newcastle Library   55

4.1 An Infrared Thermometer Showing the Presence of Fever   67

6.1 The Campaign Poster. The literal translation of the heading is "The middle finger for everyone without a mask. We adhere to the corona rules." Public domain   101

15.1 Vaccinating Their Children   244

15.2 Knowledge about the COVID-19 Vaccine   245

18.1 Platforms Used for Online Shopping   292

18.2 Payment Methods   292

18.3 Influencing Factors in Purchasing Decisions   292

18.4 Preferring Physical Stores Over Online Shopping   293

18.5 Products Shopped for the Most Online   294

18.6 E-browsing and Impulse Buying   294

Tables

9.1   Respondents' Awareness of COVID-19 and Evaluation
of Subjective Knowledge of and Satisfaction with Their
Knowledge about COVID-19   142
9.2   COVID-19 Information Exchange, %   144
9.3   Daily Routine Changes, %   145
9.4   Subjective Willingness to Follow Social Restrictions (M)   149
9.5   The Possible Negative Effects of COVID-19   150
9.6   The Possible Positive Effects of COVID-19   152
11.1   Summary of Interviews on the Conditions of SMEs during
the COVID-19 Pandemic   177
11.2   Summary of the Interview Results about SMEs' Business
Adaptations   178
11.3   Summary of the Interview Results Regarding SMEs'
Expectations   179
12.1   Cumulative COVID-19 Cases and Deaths per Million   194
15.1   Attitudes towards the COVID-19 Vaccine   245
16.1   Socio-economic Characteristics of Respondents   257
16.2   Opinions about the Coronavirus   258
16.3   Cultural Activities   260
16.4   Mask Wearing and Physical Distancing   263
18.1   Demographic Factors and Their Effects on Online
Shopping   287
18.2   Earning Situations and Their Effects on Online Shopping   289
18.3   Earning Situations and Propensity to Shop Online
in Future   291

Contributors

Sara Akram is a PhD candidate at Sun Yat-Sen University of China. Her major fields of research interest are gender; class-based social patterning; health priorities in various ethnic groups; and specific health-seeking behaviors in Pakistani culture.

Rao Nadeem Alam has a PhD in social anthropology from the University of Vienna, Austria. He is often engaged in research on social issues of contemporary society. His interests are health, religion, Indigenous communities, and visual anthropology.

Inayat Ali, PhD, is a Research Fellow in the Department of Social and Cultural Anthropology, University of Vienna, Austria. Being a medical anthropologist, his focus is on infectious diseases, vaccination, COVID-19, maternal health, syndemics, structured disparities, geopolitics, and biopolitics. He is one of the founding members of the South Asia Anthropology Forum (SAAF). Also, he is the Principal Investigator (PI) of a project: *Exploring and Understanding the Impacts of COVID-19: A Qualitative Inquiry*, approved by the National Bioethics Committee of Pakistan. Also, he has led research on COVID-19 in Sri Lanka, Bangladesh, and Nigeria. He has authored numerous peer and non-peer-reviewed articles.

Shahbaz Ali, MPhil, is Project Coordinator at Sindh Institute of Ophthalmology & Visual Sciences (SIOVS) Hyderabad, Pakistan. He specialized in medical anthropology and focuses on infectious diseases; local perceptions; public health; global health; and systematic disparities.

Tharaka Ananda is Lecturer in Anthropology in the Department of Anthropology, University of Sri Jayewardenepura, Sri Lanka. She is one of the founding members of the South Asia Anthropology Forum (SAAF).

Violet Barasa is a medical anthropologist based in London, UK. She is a senior tutor at the Institute of Development Studies at the University of Sussex, UK.

Murielle Bochud is Full Professor of Public Health at the Faculty of Biology and Medicine of the University of Lausanne, Switzerland.

Patrick Bodenmann is Associate Professor and head of the Department of Vulnerabilities and Social Medicine at the University Center for Primary Care and Public Health (Unisanté), Lausanne, Switzerland.

Nolwenn Bühler is an anthropologist of biomedicine and health with a background in nursing. She currently works as an SNSF senior researcher at the University of Lausanne, Switzerland, and as a research manager at the University Center for Primary Care and Public Health (Unisanté), Lausanne, Switzerland.

Célia Burnand is a sociologist who works as a research fellow at the University Center for Primary Care and Public Health (Unisanté), Lausanne, Switzerland, in the SérocoViD project, a SARS-CoV-2 Seroprevalence study.

Suman Chakrabarty is Assistant Professor (Stage III) and Head of the Department of Anthropology, Mrinalini Datta Mahavidyapith, India. He is one of the founding members of the South Asia Anthropology Forum (SAAF).

Abdul Razaque Channa is a Mittal Research Affiliate at the Lakshmi and Family South Asia Institute at Harvard University, USA, and Assistant Professor of Anthropology at the University of Sindh, Jamshoro, Pakistan.

Richard Chenhall is Professor of Medical Anthropology in the Melbourne School of Population and Global Health at the University of Melbourne, Australia.

Valérie D'Acremont is a physician and epidemiologist specializing in infectious and tropical diseases, responsible for digital and global health at the University Center for Primary Care and Public Health (Unisanté), Lausanne, Switzerland, and a professor at the University of Lausanne, as well as a research group leader at SwissTPH, Basel.

Ira Darmawanti is a lecturer and researcher at the Universitas Negeri Surabaya, Indonesia, in the Department of Psychology, and is currently taking her Doctorate Program in the Department of Education, University of Vienna, Austria.

Sudipta Das Gupta is an anthropologist by training who graduated from the Department of Anthropology, Shahjalal University of Science and Technology, Sylhet, Bangladesh. He also works in the field of Public Health and has worked with some of the most renowned research organizations in Bangladesh.

Robbie Davis-Floyd is Adjunct Professor, Department of Anthropology, Rice University, Fellow, Society for Applied Anthropology, and Senior Advisor to the Council on Anthropology and Reproduction. She is also a cultural/ medical anthropologist specializing in the anthropology of reproduction.

Frances Edmonds is Senior Research Fellow in the School of Culture and Communication, University of Melbourne, working on the Australian Research Council Indigenous Discovery Project (2001000420) "Storytelling and the Living Archive of Aboriginal Knowledge."

Kim Gutschow is Senior Lecturer in Anthropology and Religion at Williams College, USA, where she is affiliated with Public Health, Science & Technology Studies, Asian Studies, Women's, Gender, & Sexuality Studies, Environmental Studies, and Asian Studies.

Mayarí Hengstermann is a Co-PI at the Centre of Health Studies (CES) from the Universidad del Valle de Guatemala (UVG).

Rachel Irwin is a researcher in ethnology at the Department of Arts and Cultural Sciences, Lund University, Sweden.

Sanaullah Jamali is pursuing his PhD Degree in Mathematics and has been serving as an Assistant Professor at Sindh University Laar Campus, Badin, Pakistan.

Katarzyna E. Król is a doctoral student at the Graduate School for Social Research, Poland, and a member of the Rare Disease Social Research Center in the Institute of Philosophy and Sociology at the Polish Academy of Sciences.

Kristiningsih is a lecturer and researcher in the field of marketing management and strategic management at Universitas Wijaya Kusuma, Surabaya, Indonesia.

Tayyaba Rafique Makhdoom has been teaching at Sindh University Laar Campus, Badin, Pakistan for 12 years.

Tatyana V. Malikova is Associate Professor at Saint-Petersburg State Pediatric Medical University, Russia.

Maria Tufail Memon is a research scholar currently doing her PhD at the University of Sindh Jamshoro, Pakistan.

Georgiy A. Murza-Der is Senior Lecturer at Saint-Petersburg State Pediatric Medical University, Russia.

Tatiana O. Novikova is Associate Professor at Saint-Petersburg State Pediatric Medical University, Russia

Semira Gonseth Nusslé is an executive at the University Center for Primary Care and Public Health (Unisanté), Lausanne, Switzerland. She is a medical doctor specializing in prevention and a researcher in epidemiology, with a focus in epigenetics. She is a co-investigator of the Swiss Health Study, a

Swiss population-based pilot study, and of the COVID-19 seroprevalence study in the Canton of Vaud, SérocoViD.

Mary Grace A. Pelayo is a health social scientist, researcher, and community trainer in the Philippines.

Danuta Penkala-Gawęcka is Profesor Emerita at the Institute of Anthropology and Ethnology, Adam Mickiewicz University in Poznań, Poland.

Dmitry G. Pirogov is Associate Professor at Saint-Petersburg State Pediatric Medical University, Russia. He is also a researcher on the project "Social Net Program to Involve PLHIV to the System of Medical Service."

Melody Pralong is a PhD candidate in the Department of Social Medicine and Vulnerabilities at the University Center for Primary Care and Public Health (Unisanté), Lausanne, Switzerland. She is an anthropologist working as a junior researcher at the University of Lausanne, at Unisanté, and at CHUV.

Małgorzata Rajtar is Associate Professor and Head of the Rare Disease Social Research Center in the Institute of Philosophy and Sociology at the Polish Academy of Sciences.

Cloé Rawlinson is a psychologist in the Department of Social Medicine and Vulnerabilities, at the University Center for Primary Care and Public Health (Unisanté), Lausanne, Switzerland.

Ian Christopher N. Rocha is a health social scientist, global health researcher, and healthcare professional in the Philippines.

Salma Sadique is Assistant Professor of Medical Anthropology at the Community Health Sciences, Peoples University of Medical & Health Science for Women Nawabshah, Shaheed Benazirabad, Sindh, Pakistan. Her research interests includes COVID-19, vaccination, gender, structural violence, and public health.

Kate Senior is Associate Professor of Anthropology in the School of Humanities and Social Science at the University of Newcastle, Australia.

Santirianingrum Soebandhi is a lecturer and researcher at Universitas Wijaya Kusuma Surabaya, Indonesia.

Umbreen Soomro is Lecturer in the Department of Anthropology and Archaeology, University of Sindh, Jamshoro, Pakistan.

Jigme Yoezer is a medical doctor at a tertiary care hospital in southern Bhutan.

Introduction

Constructing and Negotiating COVID-19

Inayat Ali and Robbie Davis-Floyd

> "To negotiate" is "to deal or bargain with another or others"; "to manage, transact, or conduct"; "to move through, around, or over in a satisfactory manner."
>
> (dictionary.com)

Negotiation characterizes much of our lives. We humans constantly negotiate with ourselves, within our communities, and among regions and countries as we navigate our lifeworlds. And, for the past two years, we have been "negotiating COVID-19" at all these levels. Scholars too have been negotiating COVID-19 in their research, writings, and personal lives. Never before has there been such a rapid explosion of social science research on a given topic; thus we have also witnessed a "publication pandemic." This literature explosion encouraged us to bring some of this work together in one volume. Our chapters pay close attention to all of these different types of negotiations around COVID-19, and to its multiple and varied cultural perceptions and constructions.

First recognized and reported in Wuhan, a city of China's Hubei Province on December 31, 2019, the disease caused by the novel coronavirus, COVID-19, has challenged the entire world. On January 30, 2020, the World Health Organization (WHO) officially announced COVID-19 as the sixth public health emergency requiring worldwide attention. This announcement followed the criteria used for H1N1 (2009); polio (2014); Ebola in West Africa (2014); Zika (2016); and Ebola in the Democratic Republic of Congo (2019). (WHO did not include the Great Influenza pandemic of 1918–1919, as WHO was founded in 1948.) Finally, on March 11, 2020, WHO designated the novel coronavirus outbreak a "pandemic" (ibid.). The potential threat of the coronavirus was identified as early as 1965, and after almost 60 years, this virus caused a pandemic. As it spread, at first many, including the WHO, called it a "pneumonia of unidentified source," then "novel coronavirus," and "coronavirus 2," because the "new" virus resembles the previous coronaviruses that caused Severe Acute Respiratory Syndrome (SARS) and Middle Eastern Respiratory Syndrome (MERS). Then the coronavirus became officially

DOI: 10.4324/9781003187462-1

known as SARS-CoV-2. "Co" has been taken from "corona" (used because under the microscope, the virus looks like a crown); "V" from virus; and "2" stands for the virus's second strain. WHO officially named the disease this virus causes "COVID-19" on February 11, 2020, borrowing "CO" from coronavirus, "VI" from virus, "D" from disease, and 19 from 2019, the year of the disease's origin. Thereafter, two variants have also been named with the Greek Alphabet letters: Delta and Omicron. By December 2021, it is the latter variant that, after originating in Africa, is spreading around the world. This naming is a laudable effort of the World Health Organization to reduce the chances of intra-country stigmatization. These two variants are not discussed in our chapters, as they were written before these variants appeared.

Although the potentially severe longer-term consequences of this pandemic are yet to come, its shorter-term consequences over the first year and a half of its global spread need to be recognized and are reported for multiple cultures and countries in this book. One tiny, microscopic virus has significantly affected our socio-cultural patterns, (geo-)political systems, economic policies, and daily behaviors and practices. During its first months of global spread in 2020, it rapidly shaped various "new normals" at individual, community, national, and international levels, including different ways of greeting; mask wearing in public; isolation and quarantine—either self-generated or government-required; and "social distancing"—better termed "physical distancing," as humans are inherently social creatures who need social interaction (see Ali and Davis-Floyd 2020). On an international scale, new apparatuses have been implemented to create "new untouchables" (Inayat Ali nd) and close borders while declaring some countries and populations as at elevated risk of viral transmission, and national and global economies have been adversely affected.

Thus, as lead editor Inayat Ali (2021) has pointed out, in addition to causing a medical pandemic, SARS-CoV-2 has caused multiple other pandemics. In addition to the "publication pandemic" mentioned above, these include an economic pandemic, a social pandemic, a structural pandemic, an emotional/psychological pandemic, and a political pandemic (Ali 2021). To these we add here the "infodemic" and "the misinformation pandemic," which stem from the overwhelming amounts of information and misinformation spread daily through multiple sources, especially various types of media. Many of our chapter authors note that mainstream media reports on the pandemic and social media debates often fuel uncertainty and fear that contribute to the circulation of rumors and conspiracy theories (see below).

Dealing with these multiple pandemics has widely involved the processes of negotiations, contestations, and constructions of COVID-19. The differing perspectives and interplays among numerous COVID-19-related "realities" have revealed (in)visible contestations temporally and spatially, and thus have opened a vast arena to be explored by social scientists, as we noted above. As our title indicates, this book centers on how the pandemic is culturally constructed and negotiated by individuals, societies, governments, and international organizations—while considering that political and economic systems also have "cultures." Studying these diverse circumstances as they are, in what we are terming *Covidian anthropology* (for which we have coined the term *coronaviral* spread, as opposed to simply viral spread, and two of our chapter authors—Abdul Razaque Channa and Umbreen Soomro—have coined the term *Covistress* to index the increased stress levels caused by the pandemic), our authors employ various analytical entry points to comprehend the dynamics of dealing with the virus and to situate it within specific contexts. Based on original ethnographic or autoethnographic often virtual research from different cultures and countries—including Pakistan, Austria, Sweden, Australia, Kenya, the United States, Germany, Switzerland, Poland, Russia, Indonesia, Sri Lanka, Bhutan, India, and Bangladesh—the chapters in this volume address unsettling questions and related seminal explorations of the impacts of COVID-19; how various stakeholders (ranging from local to global) negotiate these impacts, and what factors (such as politics, mistrust, and structured disparities) lie behind these contestations. These include explorations and analyses of:

- personal experiences, emotions, and navigations during the pandemic;
- anthropologists as "context-brokers" (as opposed to "culture brokers");
- the "end of fieldwork" and longings for the field created by the sudden inaccessibility of many anthropologists' geographical regions of research;
- utilizing "cyber-ethnography" in creative and innovative ways;
- sources of mis- and dis-information and information (lack of) awareness, and how "health literacy" plays a significant role in the use of available data to acquire (too much) information and justify specific behaviors that involve not following preventive measures;
- changes in healthcare-seeking behaviors: many people in low- and high-resource countries alike are denied healthcare facility entry due to short-staffing or to staff fears of contagion, and many in all countries have become more reliant on home- or self-care and/or alternative therapies such as naturopathy, homeopathy, and Chinese and Tibetan medicines;
- how biomedicine, even in a state of emergency, resists other knowledge systems and guards its epistemic borders;
- how, in some countries such as India, China, Sri Lanka, and Bhutan, as a result of biomedicine's inability to find a cure for COVID-19, biomedical and traditional medical practitioners have been working together in truly complementary ways; and thus how, just as traditional medicines have been called "alternative" and "complementary" to biomedicine, so biomedicine can be thought of as "alternative" and "complementary" to traditional medicinal systems;

- changes in maternity care provision in the USA as providers negotiate COVID-19 and its effects on pregnant women and newborns, which were completely unknown at the beginning of the pandemic and had to be figured out over time, resulting in rapid and confusing ongoing changes in protocols and practices that negatively affected childbearing experiences;
- stigmatization and social ostracizing or active punishment of those infected—or believed to be infected;
- difficulties in testing and tracking the disease in various countries;
- official government responses and policies vs. individual and community beliefs and behaviors;
- obfuscating messages sent by governments and healthcare authorities in many countries that confused people to the extent that they often did and do not bother to follow these constantly changing messages and policies, in what one of our chapter authors, Mayarí Hengstermann, has called *the prevention paradox*;
- the vulnerability of people with rare metabolic diseases and how the "chronic living" they have become accustomed to may actually make them more prepared than others to practice COVID-19 prevention measures;
- the development of "barrier gestures" in Switzerland—boundaries, both material and symbolic, that are made and negotiated in practice;
- specific traits in Sri Lankan Buddhist culture and in the Buddhist culture of Bhutan that have enabled those countries to cope well with the virus and to prevent or fully stop its spread;
- specific national policies in India that have done just the opposite;
- adjustments in small-to-medium businesses in Indonesia as they adapt to online sales;
- local perceptions of COVID as encoded in narratives;
- rumors and conspiracy theories around COVID-19 as meaningful ways to understand both structural and interpersonal forces that operate in the backdrop of health behaviors;
- the impact of the closure of a university on student mental health;
- vaccine uptake and vaccine refusal in many countries that may prevent the development of "herd immunity";
- the possibly irreversible life changes that may make us rethink "normal daily life" both now and in the future.

A Brief Overview of This Volume

This volume is organized into four parts, all of which are focused on negotiations around cultural, governmental, and individual constructions of COVID-19. Part I contains autoethnographic accounts from Austria, Sweden, and Australia, in which anthropologists describe their constructions of and negotiations with COVID in their lived experiences, perceptions, and practices relating to the pandemic. In the Austrian context, book editor Inayat Ali describes his conversations and negotiations with himself during self-quarantine in Vienna due to a probable COVID-19 infection. For Sweden, Swedish citizen Rachel Irwin describes her dismay at her country's stigmatization in the international media for its "open"—as opposed to "locked down"—policies and what she was able to do about it. And for Australia, Kate Senior, Richard Chenall, and Fran Edmonds describe what it is like to be cut off from a field you have been working in for over 30 years and how they coped with their "loss and longing" for that field by rediscovering it, right where they were.

Part II illustrates detailed perspectives on how the pandemic has been culturally and governmentally constructed and negotiated in different cultures, professions, and countries, including Kenya, the United States, Germany, Switzerland, Poland, Russia, and Indonesia. Our Kenya chapter deals with how stigma has created panic and affected the provision of health care when biomedical personnel refuse to attend patients with high temperatures, and community members publicly lynched one man who was considered to be a "super-spreader"—even though he did not have the disease. The USA chapter describes maternity care practitioners' complex negotiations around COVID-19 with themselves and their childbearing patients. The chapter on Germany explores health literacy and its lack, and how the plethora of "too much" information can confuse people and leave gaps in which misinformation and mistrust can spread—an example of the "prevention paradox." Our Swiss chapter describes how "barrier gestures"—*gestes-barrière*—are constructed and negotiated by individuals and COVID+ people to protect themselves and their families. The chapter on Poland centers on the resilience shown by people with rare diseases as they negotiate the impacts of the pandemic on their ability to access needed health care, and on their pre-pandemic preparation for—and thus easy acceptance of—the government-imposed preventive measures. Our Russia chapter analyzes public awareness of and negotiations around people's self-reflective readiness to cope with social restrictions and the multiple roles of information in dealing with COVID-19. Our chapter on the quest for a cure for COVID-19 investigates biomedical research on possibly curative drugs, and describes how many people turn to traditional Chinese and Tibetan medicines, which have been officially accepted in some countries for COVID-19 treatment—sometimes in conjunction with biomedical treatments. This chapter also highlights the role of mediatization in the spread of (mis)information about the pandemic in close connection with "biocommunicability," and illustrates different ways of production, circulation, and reception of health knowledge that generate uncertainty and fear. Regarding the "economic pandemic" mentioned above, our chapter on Indonesia investigates the impacts of COVID-19 on small-to-medium businesses, which constitute the backbone of Indonesia's economy, and how these businesses have negotiated and mitigated these impacts via switching to online marketing and sales.

Part III focuses on South Asia, with chapters from Sri Lanka, Bhutan, India, and Bangladesh that center around cultural and national constructions of and negotiations around COVID-19, showing how the cultures of Bhutan and Sri Lanka have facilitated stopping viral spread, while many higher-resource countries have not. And our chapter on India describes negotiations around the pandemic at national and state levels, and among various ethnic groups and "Scheduled Tribes." Our chapter on Bangladesh addresses how laypeople have perceived COVID-19: what factors have driven them to follow or not follow preventive measures; how they perceive the government's efforts to contain the virus and COVID-19 vaccination; and when and how they think the pandemic might end, if ever.

Part IV takes one country—Ali's native Pakistan—as a case study revealing the dynamic interplay between local and national perceptions and practices, such as the development of new cultural rituals resulting from the pandemic. Two chapters in Part IV highlight the effects of the pandemic on Pakistan's small-to-medium businesses and on its underdeveloped education system. The other two chapters in Part IV investigate the rumors and conspiracy theories that Pakistanis, especially those living in rural areas, have created around COVID-19, focusing on what these rumors and conspiracy theories reveal about local people's perceptions of this disease. These perceptions include such deep distrust of their government and of the "Western world" that many rural Pakistanis do not even believe the disease is real, considering it instead as a government tool employed to gain more foreign funding and to control its populace via travel restrictions and other means—or as a "Western plot" against Muslims. In our Conclusions, we summarize the main findings of the studies on which our chapters are based.

Rumors, Conspiracy Theories, and Stigmas Related to COVID-19 around the World

Rumors and conspiracy theories have had such tremendous impacts on people's perceptions and behaviors around the coronavirus pandemic that they are addressed in almost all of our chapters.[1] Thus below, based on the work of Islam and colleagues (2020), as background and context for our chapters, we provide the global context for the breadth of the rumors, conspiracy theories, and stigmatizations surrounding COVID-19. After identifying over 2,300 reports on media and social media in 25 languages in 87 countries, Islam and colleagues (2020) gathered the following 56 different local narratives—rumors, conspiracy theories, and narratives showing stigma.

Rumors

- "Novel coronavirus is in the cloud."
- "Coronavirus is a snake flu."

- "Pet animals are the sources of coronavirus."
- "Novel coronavirus strain is a type of rabies."
- "Coronavirus outbreak [is] in the livestock."
- "Poultry eggs are contaminated with coronavirus."
- "Cookies, rice, and Chinese red bull were contaminated with the virus."
- "Eating bat soup is the source of the (COVID-19) outbreak."
- "COVID-19 [is] found in orange[s]."
- "Coronavirus [comes] from imported goods."
- "Mobile phone can transmit coronavirus."
- "Notes [currency] are sources of coronavirus."
- "Common cold had been renamed as coronavirus."

Rumor[s] about Treatment, Prevention, and Control

- "Eating garlic can cure coronavirus."
- "Drinking bleach may kill the virus."
- "Drinking alcohol may kill the virus."
- "Gargling vinegar and rose water or vinegar and salt may kill the virus in [the] throat."
- "Drinking cow urine and cow dung can cure coronavirus."
- "[Colloidal] Silver [(cAg)] solution [works] for coronavirus treatment."
- "Wearing warm socks, mustard patches, and spreading goose fat on one's chest as treatment."
- "Keeping throat moist, avoid spicy food and taking vitamin C may prevent the disease."
- "Avoiding cold or preserved food and drinks, such as ice cream and milkshakes, may prevent infection."
- "Spraying chlorine all over your body can prevent coronavirus infection."
- "Sesame oil can prevent coronavirus infection."
- "Granite bath can prevent coronavirus infection."
- "Sea lettuce can prevent coronavirus infection."
- "Vitamin C intake can prevent coronavirus infection."
- "Vitamin D can prevent coronavirus infection."
- "Eating Centella asiatica may prevent coronavirus infection."
- "Drinks containing mint or white willow, and spices like saffron, turmeric, and cinnamon would strengthen the lungs and the immune system against the virus."
- "Rinse mouths with saltwater solution to prevent infection from the new virus outbreak."
- "Do not hold your thirst because once your membrane in your throat is dried, the virus will invade into your body within 10 minutes."
- "Applying petroleum jelly around your nostrils will protect against dangerous air pollutants."
- "[Use a] do-it-yourself coronavirus detection test."

- "Cannabis boosts immunity against the novel coronavirus."
- "Frequent[ly] washing clothes can reduce transmission."

Conspiracy Theories

- "Novel coronavirus is engineered, laboratory-generated virus either accidentally or deliberately released in the area of the Wuhan seafood and animal market."
- "COVID-2019 outbreak was planned."
- "It's a bio-weapon funded by the Bill & Melinda Gates foundation to further vaccine sales."
- "Biological weapon manufactured by CIA."
- "President Donald Trump targeted the city with coronavirus to damage its culture and honor in Iran."
- "The virus is an attempt to wage 'economic' war on China."
- "America's Jews are driving America's wars."
- "Zionists are against regional security."
- "This outbreak is medical terrorism."
- "United States and Israel [are] behind the creation and spread of the deadly coronaviruses, [which are] part of an economic and psychological war against China."
- "This outbreak is a population control scheme."
- "Tom Cotton claimed that COVID-19 was manufactured in [a] Chinese bio-laboratory."
- "Rush Limbaugh opining that whole COVID-19 is a conspiracy against Trump to [keep him from winning the] election. He purported it as a worse flu."
- "New coronavirus vaccines already exist." [This is now true, but was not at the time during which Islam and colleagues (2020) were gathering this data.]
- "Pneumonia vaccines are effective against the Wuhan coronavirus."
- "Israel has sent a vaccine to Wuhan city for patients infected with coronavirus."

Stigmas

- "I am not a virus: French Asians angered by racism."
- "Chinese are uncivilized."
- "Chinese are bioterrorists."
- "A French newspaper with headline 'Yellow Alert' tagged an Asian woman image wearing mask."
- "Chinese are dropping their coronavirus."
- "Every disease ever has come from China."
- "Chinese dietary habits caused COVID-19."
- "Keep your virus, dirty Chinese."

Our chapter authors identify many of these in their respective countries, from low resource to high, and search for their deeper meanings and sources. Clearly, this long list indicates the global need for increased population-wide health literacy, as explicated by Mayarí Hengstermann in Chapter 6, and for anthropological involvement in that endeavor, as indicated in most of our chapters and as further discussed in our Conclusions.

In Summation

Overall, this book explicates people's negotiations with COVID-19 at multiple levels—individual and across cultures and countries, situates the spread of rumors, conspiracy theories, and new social rituals within micro- and/or macro-contexts, and describes the interplay between viral contagion and various institutionalized forms of inequalities and structural vulnerabilities. Bringing together various intriguing perspectives, this book relates to the past, describes and analyzes the Covidian present, and offers futuristic implications for pandemic negotiations. Its chapters enlist distinct imaginaries based on current understandings of an extraordinary challenge that holds significant importance for our human future, as what we learn from the coronavirus pandemic—*if* we learn from it—can help us all to be more prepared for pandemics yet to come, as we also further address in our Conclusions, where we summarize key findings from our chapters.

Due to its cross-cultural local, regional, national, and global contexts, this book will be relevant to multiple audiences around the world, including social scientists, medical anthropologists, medical sociologists, bioethicists, public health officials, policymakers, governmental and non-governmental organizations, and managers who lead the development, implementation, and delivery of emergency medicine. Students of anthropology, sociology, psychology, education, public health, and global health will find this book both informative and intriguing. Thus far, though multiple articles have addressed various aspects of the pandemic, there is no actual academic book that has thoroughly addressed this pandemic while it is still ongoing, as it may well be in many countries for years to come (see Conclusions). We trust that this book will help to fill that gap and will serve as a stimulus for further research, especially during the post-pandemic phase.

Note

1 We have rephrased the title of this list, and there are no bullets in the original; we have added these to make this list easily readable.

References

Ali, I. 2021. Rituals of containment: Many pandemics, body politics, and social dramas during COVID-19 in Pakistan. *Frontiers in Sociology* 6: 83. https://doi.org/10.3389/fsoc.2021.648149

Islam, M.S., Sarkar, T., Khan, S.H., Mostofa Kamal, A-H., Murshid Hasan, S.M., et al. 2020. COVID-19-related infodemic and its impact on public health: A global social media analysis. *American Journal of Tropical Medicine and Hygiene* 103(4): 1621–1629. https://doi.org/10.4269/ajtmh.20-0812

Part I

Autoethnographic Reflections on Negotiating the Coronavirus Pandemic

1 My Great-Grandmother, Malinowski, and My "Self"

An Autoethnographic Account of Negotiating the COVID-19 Pandemic

Inayat Ali

Introduction

In this chapter, I provide an autoethnographic account of living in and living with the pandemic, in which I also reflect on what I had learned about anthropology and how I had learned it. Within the arena of what my co-editor Robbie Davis-Floyd and I are calling "Covidian anthropology," I situate my first-hand experiences of this pandemic and how I negotiated them and related them to anthropological theories, methods, and existing inequalities. After becoming presumably infected by the coronavirus, herein I reflect on the transformations in my personality that resulted both from my anthropological work and from my experiences of COVID-19.

During my voluntary yet enforced months of isolation, when danger seemed to lurk everywhere, and after becoming extremely ill, I continuously thought, read, followed news reports, and wrote. Putting myself in self-quarantine in one room for 15 consecutive days, I spent time communicating and negotiating with myself in an effort to better understand my "self." The inspiration for dissecting myself came from the book *Soul Mountain*, written by Gao Xingjian in 2000, for which he won the Nobel Prize for Literature. In his own self-dissection, Xingjian (2000) responds to the "devastation of the self" due to the Cultural Revolution in China that led him to choose to be a political refugee. As I describe in this chapter, to effectively communicate with myself to deal with anxiety and loneliness, and to keep life interesting, I dissected myself into the singular pronouns "I" and "me," and used "You" to communicate closely with myself, to critically reflect on the COVID-19 situation as it personally affected me, and to examine my relationship with anthropology—my chosen field.

Moreover, while I was alone in that room, I longed to go *somewhere*. In my imaginaries, the two best places for me to go were the Trobriand Islands, an archipelago of Papua New Guinea, Melanesia, where famed early anthropologist Bronislaw Malinowski conducted his original ethnographic fieldwork during the First World War, and Mars. I really wanted to see these places, both for personal and for academic inspiration. Yet both were

DOI: 10.4324/9781003187462-3

impossible to reach. This chapter will dissect my personal imaginaries during the pandemic, seek to autoethnographically explore my negotiations with it and myself, and will analyze what I have learned in relation to certain fundamental anthropological theories and methods.

Literature Review: Autoethnography Revisited

The debate about "objectivity" and "subjectivity" in the social sciences has long remained a prime area of academic inquiry (Foucault 1970; Diesing 1972; Longino 1990; Hastrup and Hervik 2003).[1] Is it acceptable for anthropologists to write about their subjective experiences and present themselves as sources of data, or must we focus on "objective" knowledge about others? This "crisis of representation" in the 1980s paved the way for autoethnography to present the self as a site of study (Campbell 2016). Thus Reed-Danahay (1997: 1) views that this was the beginning of a "renewed interest in personal narrative, in life history, and autobiography." Crawley (2012) noted that "auto" ethnography has its roots in the ethnographic tradition, as Karl Heider (1975) used it for the first time in regard to "the natives'" ability to offer insights about their personal experiences and emotions; Heider considered such insights to be autoethnographic.

Autoethnography, formerly considered too "subjective," has now become an accepted source of first-hand data (Chang 2016) and is also considered to be pivotal for extending sociocultural understandings (Sparkes 2000; Wall 2008). Autoethnography centers the scholar's emotions and requires a great deal of self-reflexivity (Styhre and Tienari 2014) to comprehend the links between "self" and "society," and it rejects the positions of positivism about reliability and validity (ibid.; Campbell 2016). In other words, autoethnography considers the researcher as an individual who is also a member of society. In her article "Personal Narratives as Sociology," Barbara Laslett (1999: 392) described the individual/social relationship as a new window on theoretical debates in the social sciences, as self-accounts vividly highlight "micro-macro linkages; structure, agency and their intersections; social reproduction and social change." Thus, focusing on the researcher's lived experiences and emotions has received satisfactory agreement across academic circles (Ellingson and Ellis 2008). For Reed-Danahay (1997: 4), as a postmodernist lens, autoethnography "involves a rewriting of the self and the social."

Wall (2008: 39) deconstructs the term auto + ethno + graphy, stating that each part represents a strand focusing on "self," "sociocultural connection," and "the application of the research process," respectively. Reed-Danahay (1997: 2) and Crawley (2012) note that there are several strands of autoethnography, yet two appear to be major types: "evocative" and "analytic" (Denshire and Lee 2013). Some of the most famous works in evocative autoethnography include Ellis (1997, 1999) and Behar (2014);

in analytic autoethnography such works include Anderson (2006), Denzin (2006), and Vryan (2006).[2]

Emphasizing narrative presentations, evocative autoethnography focuses on telling "embodied stories about self and other, including the author's emotions," while seeking to evoke "emotional conversations with readers" (Bochner and Ellis 2016: 39–40). In contrast, analytic autoethnography views a researcher as: "(1) a full member in the research group or setting; (2) visible as such a member in published texts; and (3) committed to developing theoretical understandings of broader social phenomena" (Anderson 2006: 373).

This chapter is simultaneously both *evocative* and *analytical*. I see it as a synthesis of both approaches, as I tell embodied stories about myself while also seeking to evoke emotional "conversations" with my readers. And I analyze these stories via Geertzian "thick description" in order to develop "theoretical understandings of broader social phenomena" while recalling my past emotions (as did Mcgreehan [2017]), and also living in the present, challenging moment.

"You" and "I" Converse: Living with COVID-19

"Hello! How do you live during the days of COVID-19—these testing, challenging, frightening and overwhelming times?" "You" asked "I."

"Well! I really don't know, I have mixed feelings, after consuming news reports all the time, living inside the room, coughing, sneezing, high temperature, away from my family, productive, alone, exploring," I replied to You.

"Could you please elaborate on that a bit further?" You asked.

I replied, "Okay! I will tell you the entire story. Please bear with me! At the end of February, my housemate, whom I will call Jacob, became very ill with apparent 'flu,' fever, and cough, and we called in a doctor on an emergency basis because Jacob was unable to walk. The doctor diagnosed a common flu and recommended medication accordingly. It is important to mention that Jacob took quite a long time to recover. In the early days of March 2020, I too became seriously ill with the same symptoms. The intensity of the symptoms increased gradually. I became worried about my situation, in part due to Jacob's long illness and because we were all becoming aware of COVID-19 as a global pandemic. After I got sick, the dustbin in my room was full of tissues and masks that I consumed. Jacob was constantly telling me about the growing rates of COVID-19 infection in Vienna, including a few of his classmates. This news only increased my worries. I did not even want to tell my family about my aggravating situation, mainly due to not wanting to worry them. I understood that even if I did tell them, there was nothing they could do, as they were in Pakistan and I was in Austria."

While nodding his head and taking deep breaths at my request, You said to I, "Please continue."

I responded, "One evening, my situation was so critical that I was unable to speak due to constant coughing. Many serious thoughts were dominating my mind. Jacob suggested that I should see a doctor, saying, 'Perhaps it is COVID-19.' In the evening, we decided to go to a hospital. Jacob asked, 'Can you please walk?' Although I felt really unable to walk, due to an intense fever, repetitive sneezing, and cough, I said that I was fine and could walk to the bus stop, to avoid more worries for him. The bus stop was around one kilometer away from the hostel where we lived. With Jacob's help, we reached it. Because it was going to take 10 minutes for the next bus to arrive, and that bus was not going directly to the hospital, and also because I was reluctant to travel by bus as I was continually sneezing and coughing that could make other passengers worried, Jacob booked a car via the Ober online taxi service; the price would be one Euro. After five minutes, a black Mercedes stopped to pick us up. When we entered the car from the back door, the driver looked at me in surprise, as I was wearing a mask—something that most Viennese were not yet doing. I observed that he felt a fear of infection. Our journey to the hospital began."

You interrupted, "It seems an overwhelming story. Please continue."

I said, "My roommate thought he was bringing me to the nearby hospital. Although he had only been in Vienna for a few weeks, I trusted that he knew where we were going. My roommate gave the hospital's address to the driver to put into google maps. The approximate time to reach the hospital was around 14 minutes. However, the drive took around 40 minutes, as the hospital was not in the city center but on its periphery. The driver seemed angry due to not finding the hospital and receiving only one Euro, which was already paid online. This long journey disturbed me too, as I was trying very hard not to sneeze in the car. Somehow, I also felt bad that I had not asked Jacob about the hospital prior to the journey. The driver dropped us off when the google map showed that the hospital was only a few meters away, although we could not see it. I was happy to leave the car and feel the fresh air on my face. When we started searching for the hospital, it took us around 20 minutes to reach a place showing some hospital signs. But it turned out to be a psychiatric hospital, and I told Jacob that we were at the wrong place. I did not want him to feel bad, because he showed great concern. I asked him to go back to our hostel because I was feeling so weak. Since an Ober would take too long to come, we took a bus to reach a tram stop and then back to our hostel. When I entered the bus, the driver was constantly looking at me in his rearview mirror because I was fully masked."

You showed his great concern, "Interesting indeed...what happened afterward?"

I continued, "Back at the hostel, I threw myself on my bed. I was too exhausted to do anything else. My roommate was eager to take me to a closer hospital, but I rejected that option without telling him that I now felt weaker and more exhausted. I preferred to call a doctor. My roommate called an emergency doctor, who said he would be here within half an hour."

You promptly inquired, "Did a doctor then visit you? What did s/he say? What treatment did the doctor recommend?"

I shared the tale further, "Yes, a team of two male medical personnel—one doctor and his assistant—visited me almost after half an hour. They checked my temperature, tongue and lungs. Thereafter, the doctor said, 'Since you have neither been to China nor to Italy, you do not have a COVID-19 infection, but the common flu,' and recommended some medication.

It made me happy that I was not infected by COVID-19—although I now think that doctor was wrong—which, starting in December 2019, had turned into a global pandemic. In a matter of 100 days—by March 2020, when I got sick—the virus had infected around 2 million people worldwide and killed 120,000. Everything is interrupted: offices, institutions, shops, and houses. Perhaps these are the times to live in new forms of 'caves' but with modern technologies inside: television, mobile phones, Internet, light, laptops.

After spending more than a month with restrictions, dangers, fears, uncertainties, and chaos, I started to think that people might turn mainly into two forms: (1) a highly focused and wise person—a new Buddha; (2) a highly shattered person—an anti-Buddha. I am uncertain which I would turn into, as living in this new form of 'caves' is still not over. Nonetheless, one thing that is already clear is that that I am too tired to consume 'news' anymore, so I am watching old movies that contrast with this modern world. I am too exhausted to cook, so I am merely making efforts to fill my stomach but certainly with healthy food, such as fruits and fresh juices."

You, while nodding his head, said, "That *is* rather interesting—most especially your concept of the 'new Buddha' and the 'anti-Buddha.' Please tell me more about what you mean by these concepts."

I responded, "Well! What I mean by 'new Buddha' could entail almost everyone sitting in self-quarantine—either infected or due to fear of being infected or of infecting others. This has given us an opportunity to gather our thoughts, re-examine our priorities, and spend time with *self*. Spending time with 'self' could potentially enable us to find within ourselves a sense of peace and cosmic connection, and, once our quarantines are over, to use that sense of peace and connection in positive ways for our selves, for our families, for our societies, for our countries, and for the world: precisely, we could become better, more enlightened human beings. This would entail the possibility of great personal and societal transformation. But living with *self* is not that easy. That missing link between *social* and *self* during quarantine can affect our mental health positively—in the ways I have just mentioned— or adversely. Adverse effects could include the possibility that after this phase of self-quarantine, many will be so traumatized and shattered that they lose focus, find no sense of peace and interconnection, and as a result they can negatively affect their *self*, family, society, and humanity in general. This is what I mean by 'anti-Buddha.' "

You said, "That is quite fascinating. We could certainly benefit from a society full of 'new Buddhas.' Please keep on sharing your experiences and thoughts."

So I continued, "This self-isolation and self-quarantine have helped me to write several articles on this disease and its local and global impacts. And this state has opened numerous other hidden treasures for me. Now, for instance, I can understand why, during my upbringing, we were repeatedly told not to eat food with the left hand because we used that hand to wash ourselves after defecation. Since we did not have soap, the left hand especially contained germs. My great-grandmother, although entirely uneducated in the modern sense, was brilliant and wise. She knew already what science was proving." And now I can comprehend why my great-grandmother used to say:

> Son! If you wear your shoes in bed, then this is disrespect of the bed. Once the bed is humiliated, then *Ballā* [a local term that is used especially for all species of snakes and for all kinds of trouble] is allowed to climb on it and bite and kill people. Otherwise, they are not allowed to climb.

Grandma's story was inscribed on our minds. I don't think that I ever violated this norm. If someone else broke this rule, we would teach that person about the deadly consequences. We were extremely scared of snakes.

"But now I can relate and decipher that story very well—I can layer in what Geertz (1973) called "thick description." It was not the physical or real form of Ballā that could climb on the bed, but the metaphorical one—in the form of the viruses and bacteria carried on shoes, which were the abodes of these potentially deadly microorganisms. Grandma did not know anything about these microscopic beings, yet she understood the danger of wearing shoes in bed. Those shoes could bring a metaphorical Ballā to our beds and then make us sick."

Papua New Guinea, or Mars?

You continuously listened to I with full attention because I was situating our childhood teachings into our current circumstances. Hence, You inquired, "Please tell me more about what's happening around you, and how are your making sense of everything?"

So I continued, "This self-isolation is both challenging and productive. I have been thinking about things I have never thought about before. For example, I have been thinking where is the safest place to go, where the virus is not present, or at least not much."

You asked, "Oh! I see—then where do you think to go?"

I exclaimed, "Well! The first idea that popped into my mind was the planet Mars. This is because, for the last couple of years, I have been fascinated with Mars and wish to go there. I have been watching numerous documentaries, movies, listening to lectures, and reading books about it. During the night, I look at the sky and try to imagine how these other planets would be. I am sure that one day, human beings will 'colonize' these planets, too. Why am I saying that? For sure, our minds respond to accumulated societal memories. And my mind is full of these stories about the colonizers, who spared almost no place on Mother Earth from colonization. So I'm sure such colonizers will also seek to do the same on other planets, once the technology is available. Nonetheless, despite my wish to go to Mars, I obviously can't get there, nor could I stay alive there."

You said, with a smile on his face, "That is really interesting. I can understand how it feels when you aspire to do something but can't make that aspiration come true. So, where else might you go?"

I, with deep sighs, continued, "Owing to these impossibilities, I thought, 'Okay! Where is the safest place on Mother Earth, where the virus has not yet broken out or is causing little harm?' "

"What did you find, then?" You asked.

I responded, "I scrolled around the website of Johns Hopkins University, which since the beginning of the COVID-19 outbreak had been constantly updating the number of infections and deaths. On that website, I found 12 countries with single-digit cases: Gambia and Nicaragua with 9 cases each; the Holy See (Vatican) with 8; Mauritania with 7; Western Sahara with 6; Bhutan and Burundi with 5; São Tomé and Principe, South Sudan, and Timor-Leste with 4; Papua New Guinea with 2; and the last one is Yemen with 1 case."

You: "So, you found 12 options. Aren't they too many?"

I said, "Yes, they are many. And I will tell you one funny thing."

You asked eagerly, "What thing?"

I: "I must accept that although I am very much interested to go to Mars and know a bit about that planet, I do not know about all these countries: this is the first time I have read the names Holy See, Mauritania, São Tomé and Principe—which is the name of one country—and Timor-Leste. This shows how disconnected even an educated person can be, even though we are all interconnected, whether we realize it or not."

"So, now where to go?" You asked.

"Well! Yemen has only one case. And, during my upbringing, I have heard many good stories about the Yemeni people, and especially about the precious stones, such as 'Yemeni *Aqeeq*' that is used to wear as a ring-stone. Maybe, better to go there," I answered.

You responded, "No, no, no! Come on! Have you lost your mind? Although there is only a single case reported so far, that is likely due to a dearth of testing facilities. Plus, it is a highly suicidal idea to go to Yemen. Don't you remember what has been happening in that country? Don't you remember that for ages, the country has been a battleground?"

I inquired, "For ages? What do you mean? Please be specific and don't exaggerate."

You responded, "Okay, okay! What I meant by 'for ages' is that this entire region has remained a battleground for centuries. And since 2015, there has been a Saudi-led intervention in Yemen by a group called the Arab Coalition. Including Saudi Arabia, ten countries from West Asia and Africa are part of this intervention. This intervention started in response to calls from the internationally recognized pro-Saudi president of Yemen, Abdrabbuh Mansur Hadi, to seek military support when the Houthi movement ousted him due to economic and political grievances and inequalities, and he fled to Saudi Arabia. Because of this dangerous situation, I am stopping you from even thinking of going there. A virus may spare you due to your good immune system, but not a bullet. Did you hear me?" You asked I.

I felt scared, "Oh My God! Then it is really dangerous to go there. Okay, thanks for educating me. I am deleting this option."

You said, "Now that's solid, logical thinking. This thought is good for your survival."

I shared with You, "Out of these 12 countries, where the virus is still in single digits, I liked Yemen and then Papua New Guinea."

"Oh, I see! Then why don't you think about Papua New Guinea?" You asked I.

You further continued, "For your information, you already have enough knowledge about this country. You have read about it. Don't you remember about Bronislaw Malinowski—the Polish anthropologist who pioneered participant observation? He traveled to Papua New Guinea a century ago, in 1914. At that time, this country was called merely Papua. He conducted long-term fieldwork there on Mailu Island and afterward in the Trobriand Islands. This was the fieldwork that made him famous and taught many others how to really be anthropologists," You reminded I.

I responded to You, "Oh! Thanks a lot for reminding me about all this. Please keep talking. I am really enjoying this conversation."

You continued, "It's great to hear that you're enjoying this late-night conversation! Okay, I was telling you about Malinowski. Based on that fieldwork, he authored the famous book, *Argonauts of the Western Pacific,* published in 1922. In this book, he elaborated on the 'Kula Ring.' After asking himself, 'Why would men risk life and limb to travel across huge expanses of dangerous ocean to give away what appear to be worthless trinkets?' Malinowski carefully traced the network of exchanges of bracelets and necklaces across the Trobriand Islands and concluded that these items are part of an exchange system (the Kula Ring), and that this entire exchange system is linked to political authority. Do you remember anything about that?"

I responded, "Yes, I remember. The first time I heard about Malinowski, the Kula Ring, and Papua New Guinea was in spring 2005—that was when I started studying anthropology. It was quite hard for me, as a native Sindhi speaker (from Pakistan's Sindh Province), to pronounce his name correctly. Please keep communicating—this is refreshing!"

You seemed in a talkative mood, so he continued, "Perfect! In his book, Malinowski (2002 [1922]: 64) wrote about the role of the ethnographer." You got that book off of our shelf and read:

> Yet it must be remembered that what appears to us an extensive, complicated, and yet well-ordered institution is the outcome of so many doings and pursuits, carried on by savages [sic], who have no laws or aims or charters definitely laid down. They have no knowledge of the total outline of any of their social structure. They know their own motives, know the purpose of individual actions and the rules which apply to them, but how, out of these, the whole collective institution shapes, this is beyond their mental range. Not even the most intelligent native has any clear idea of the Kula as a big, organized social construction, still less of its sociological function and implications...The integration of all the details observed, the achievement of a sociological synthesis of all the various, relevant symptoms, is the task of the Ethnographer... the Ethnographer has to construct the picture of the big institution, very much as the physicist constructs his theory from the experimental data, which always have been within reach of everyone, but needed a consistent interpretation.

You continued, "Please remember! He pioneered the approach of participant observation, in which he describes how to *become* a 'native' while conducting ethnographic fieldwork. This work not only gave Malinowski a doctorate but also British citizenship in 1933. More importantly, this fieldwork in Papua New Guinea led him to conceive the theory of *functionalism* in contrast to Radcliffe-Brown's [a famous British anthropologist] theory of *structural-functionalism*. By 'functionalism,' Malinowski meant that culture functions to fulfill the needs of society. When the needs of individuals, who comprise society, are fulfilled, then society's needs are fulfilled. Later, he challenged the Oedipus complex theory pioneered by Sigmund Freud."

"Sorry to interrupt you," I said, as I wanted to make a point.

"No problem!" said You. "Please talk. I have already talked a lot."

I shared, "Thanks indeed! There was a time when I was very much inclined towards this theory of Malinowski. It impressed me and strengthened my thoughts about the power of an individual. I used to believe that the individual is more potent than society. You remember the Weberian concept—that individuals create the norms and values of a society. After their creation, those abstract rules become robust and control individual behavior. Yet individuals still can break and remake them. I think Malinowski shared that idea, do you know what I mean?"

You responded while having a cup of tea, "Yes, I do follow you! Please keep sharing."

I, in continuation of the previous point, stated, "So, I was telling you how impressed I was to read him. However, my thoughts are changed now—or at least modified to a great extent. After reading enough critical literature—especially Karl Marx's *False Consciousness* [see Lukács 1971 (1920)], Michel Foucault's [2008] *Biopolitics*, Paul Farmer's [1996] *Structural Violence*, and Arthur Kleinman and colleague's [1997] *Social Suffering*, I believe that structures are more powerful than many individuals, except a few. That means these structures serve specific individuals, who are more robust than those structures because they help to create them. These individuals remain invisible agents. And we often talk about the structures without identifying any individual agency for their existence. Perhaps Malinowski's theory of functionalism is truly relevant to these selective individuals, who are above all others—social structures fulfill the needs of these individuals. Like Malinowski's tracing of the Kula Ring, if we trace what I am terming a *structural ring*, then it becomes clear that all the resources are part of a structured system of exchange (the structural ring)—this whole exchange system is linked to political authority and power," do you understand what I mean?"

You nodded, "Oh! Yes, I do understand and second you."

I now wanted to stop talking to listen to You, so I said, "Thanks very much! I will stop this discussion here and come to the main questions. So, we were discussing about going to Papua New Guinea during this COVID-19 pandemic. You were sharing something about it. I give you the floor."

You replied, "Many thanks! Papua New Guinea is a nice country to go to. However, you are missing many important things due to your curiosity to explore unfamiliar places, especially Papua owing to your academic attachment. But you are naïve. Should I tell you what the current situation in that country is?"

I eagerly said, "Oh! Yes, please do educate me."

You stated, "Although there are merely two cases so far in New Guinea, the country is already overwhelmed."

"Overwhelmed?" I interrupted You.

You responded, "Yes, overwhelmed. The country's healthcare system is already shattered. The nurses are forced to wear rice packets in place of gloves due to a dearth and unavailability. They are using detergents to disinfect the places."

I interrupted You, "Seriously? This is frightening then."

You kept sharing his point: "That is a fact, which is why I was saying that you are naïve. The country has a fragile healthcare system: for a population of 8.78 million, there is a total of 500 doctors, 4,000 nurses, 5,000 beds, and only 14 ventilators."

I, with a frightened face, "What did you just say? 14?"

You continued, "Yes, only 14 ventilators. Hence, imagine the uncertainty, danger, and fear in the Papua. If high-income countries like the United States of America, the United Kingdom, Italy, Spain, France, Switzerland—perhaps all of Europe—are overwhelmed, what destruction can this virus cause in a country like Papua or Yemen?"

I replied, "I indeed was unaware of the situation. After listening to you, my theoretical distancing from Malinowski is further increased. Your points make me think that structures are indeed more powerful than individuals. These structures have created a great and unbearable divide. Due to structural disparities, some individuals have accumulated almost the entire wealth of their countries and of the world. The UN report on inequality mentions that 20% of the population holds 80% of its wealth. According to the UN's (2005, 1)"Report on the Word Social Situation: The Inequality Predicament," 1 billion people living in the "developed" countries own 80% of the gross domestic product (GDP), while the remaining over 5 billion people have only 20% of the GDP. Owing to these disparities, now Papua's healthcare system is among the weakest—that is why such colossal dangers are looming there."

You said to I, "Oh! Interesting. So, you do know some facts and figures about the inequalities."

I replied, "Yes, I know a bit about these phenomena. I already told you that the critical anthropology literature has opened my eyes and mind. On the one hand, this literature has offered me 'new eyes,' and on the other hand, it has inflicted pain on me—because now I can easily see the inequalities. We—You and I—grew up with them always in the background in our small village in Sindh Province in Pakistan, but at the time, we could not see them—it was just the way things were."

You then suggested, "Since you know all these things, I would suggest you please don't plan to go elsewhere. No place is safe, including Yemen, Papua, and our childhood home in Sindh. If you really want to survive, don't go anywhere, just spend your time here in our apartment. No place is safer than where we are now."

I responded, "Thank you so very much! This is a great and practical suggestion that will work for you and me and everybody. It was lovely talking to you. Please take incredibly diligent care of yourself."

You, in return, wished I well, saying, "Indeed! It was a pleasure talking to you. I enjoyed the entire communication—that was fun and worthy. Please, you, too, take excellent care of yourself during these testing times. Goodbye, until we decide to converse again."

Then I and You remained in self-isolation, reading and experiencing the Covidian situation from inside the four walls of our room. Our daily routine consisted of eating, listening to the news, reading literature, continually checking the WHO and the Johns Hopkins University's websites to watch the escalation of COVID-19 infections and deaths, researching, and writing, both scientifically and creatively. During this one month, we wrote dozens of articles, some of which have been published (Ali 2020a, b, c, d, e; Ali and Davis-Floyd 2020; Ali, Sadique, and Ali 2020). Eventually, we started going outside for short walks, which sparked us to think about those millions of people, particularly women in many countries, such as Afghanistan, who spend entire days, weeks, months, and years inside their homes.

Additionally, these short walks provided us with insights into what was going on outside. How were people making sense of the pandemic? How were they coping? For example, we (I and You) saw that people were wearing masks, keeping physical distance, changing their paths if they saw someone coming towards them. Although COVID-19 had massively impacted their lives, the people we saw were healthy—this was the most pleasant news we received during those extraordinary times. And You and I remain aware that, although vaccines are now being rapidly distributed, many may refuse them, and COVID-19 is likely to remain with and around us for a very long time.

Conclusion

Synthesizing *evocative* and *analytical* autoethnographic approaches, I have presented embodied stories about myself, (hopefully) evoked "conversations" with my readers, and analyzed these stories via Geertzian "thick description" to create theoretical understandings of broader social phenomena. This autoethnography has been an attempt to illustrate some of the coping mechanisms I developed to both survive and thrive—at least intellectually—during my long (to me) period of self-isolation in my small room in a Viennese hostel. I never found out whether I actually did or did not have COVID-19. I am simply grateful to have survived and to be able to share these self-reflections with you. I hope that my coping strategies of self-dissection and self-analysis may be useful to other researchers, and may add something of value to the growing body of autoethnographic literature, and that they clearly illustrate how I personally negotiated COVID-19 and the self-isolation it required.

Notes

1 Some parts of this section are derived from Ali 2021.
2 For a third strand, "performance" autoethnography, see Spry (2016, 2001).

References

Ali, I. 2020a. Anthropology in emergencies: The roles of anthropologists during the COVID-19 pandemic. *Practicing Anthropology* 42(3): 16–22. doi.org/10.17730/0888-4552.42.3.4

Ali, I. 2020b.The COVID-19 pandemic: Making sense of rumor and fear. *Medical Anthropology* 39(5): 376–379. doi:10.1080/01459740.2020.1745481

Ali, I. 2020c. COVID-19: Are we ready for the second wave? *Disaster Medicine and Public Health Preparedness* 14(5): e16–e18. doi: 10.1017/dmp.2020.149

Ali, I. 2020d. Impact of COVID-19 on vaccination programs: Adverse or positive? *Human Vaccines and Immunotherapeutics*: 1–7. doi: 10.1080/21645515.2020.1787065

Ali, I. 2020e. Impacts of rumors and conspiracy theories surrounding COVID-19 on preparedness programs. *Disaster Medicine and Public Health Preparedness*: 1–6. doi: 10.1017/dmp.2020.149

Ali, I. 2021. *A Critical Autoethnography of Living in Pre- and Post-Refugee Vienna: Changes, Experiences and Coping Mechanisms*. Unpublished ms.

Ali, I., and R. Davis-Floyd. 2020. The interplay of words and politics during COVID-19: Contextualizing the universal pandemic vocabulary. *Practicing Anthropology* 42(4): 20–24. doi:10.17730/0888-4552.42.4.20

Ali, I., S. Sadique, and S. Ali. 2020. COVID-19 significantly affects maternal health: A rapid-response investigation from Pakistan. *Frontiers in Global Women's Health* 1. doi:10.3389/fgwh.2020.591809

Anderson, L. 2006. Analytic autoethnography. *Journal of Contemporary Ethnography* 35 (4): 373–395.

Behar, R. 2014. *The Vulnerable Observer: Anthropology that Breaks Your Heart*. Boston, MA: Beacon Press.

Bochner, A., and C. Ellis. 2016. *Evocative Autoethnography: Writing Lives and Telling Stories*. London: Routledge.

Campbell, E. 2016. Exploring autoethnography as a method and methodology in legal education research. *Asian Journal of Legal Education* 3(1): 95–105.

Chang, H. 2016. Autoethnography in health research: Growing pains? *Qualitative Health Research* 26(4): 443–451.

Crawley, S.L. 2012. "Autoethnography as Feminist Self-Interview." In J.F. Gubrium, J.A. Holstein, A.B. Marvasti, and K.D. McKinney (eds.), *The SAGE Handbook of Interview Research: The Complexity of the Craft*, 143–160. London: Sage.

Denshire, S., and A. Lee. 2013. Conceptualizing autoethnography as assemblage: Accounts of occupational therapy practice. *International Journal of Qualitative Methods* 12(1): 221–236.

Denzin, N.K. 2006. Analytic autoethnography, or déjà vu all over again. *Journal of Contemporary Ethnography* 35(4): 419–428.

Diesing, P. 1972. Subjectivity and objectivity in the social sciences. *Philosophy of the Social Sciences* 2(1): 147–165. doi: 10.1177/004839317200200111

Ellingson, L.L., and C. Ellis. 2008. "Authoethnography as Constructionist Project." In J.A. Holstein and J.F. Gubrium (eds.), *Handbook of Constructionist Research*, 445–460. New York: Guilford Press.

Ellis, C. 1997. "Evocative Autoethnography: Writing Emotionally About Our Lives." In W.G. Tierney and Y.S. Lincoln (eds.), *Representation and the Text: Re-framing the Narrative Voice*, 115–142. Albany, NY: State University of New York.

Ellis, C. 1999. Heartful autoethnography. *Qualitative Health Research* 9(5): 669–683.

Farmer, P. 1996. On suffering and structural violence: A view from below. *Daedalus* 125(1): 261–283.

Foucault, M. 1970. *The Order of Things: An Archaeology of the Human Sciences*. Translated by A. Sheridan. New York: Pantheon. Original edition, 1966.

Foucault, M. 2008. *The Birth of Biopolitics: Lectures at the Collège de France, 1978–1979*. Translated by G. Burchell. New York: Springer.

Gao, X. 2000. *Soul Mountain*. Translated by M. Lee. Sydney: HarperCollins.

Geertz, C. 1973. "Thick Description: Toward an Interpretive Theory of Culture." In C. Geertz (ed.), *The Interpretation of Cultures: Selected Essays*, 3–30. New York: Basic Books.

Hastrup, K., and P. Hervik. 2003. *Social Experience and Anthropological Knowledge*. London: Routledge.

Heider, K.G. 1975. What do people do? Dani auto-ethnography. *Journal of Anthropological Research* 31(1): 3–17.

Kleinman, A., V. Das, and M. Lock (eds.) 1997. *Social Suffering*. Berkeley, CA: University of California Press.

Laslett, B. 1999. Personal narratives as sociology. *Contemporary Sociology* 28(4): 391–401.

Longino, H.E. 1990. *Science as Social Knowledge: Values and Objectivity in Scientific Inquiry*. Princeton, NJ: Princeton University Press.

Lukács, G. 1971 [1920]. *History and Class Consciousness: Studies in Marxist Dialectics*. Cambridge, MA: MIT Press.

Mcgreehan, D. 2017. "Lost in Hope: (De)constructing Hope in 'Missing Person' Discourses." In S.L. Pensoneau-Conway, T.E. Adams, and D.M. Bolen (eds.), *Doing Autoethnography*, 115–126. Boston, MA: Sense Publishers.

Malinowski, B. 2002 [1922]. *Argonauts of the Western Pacific: An Account of Native Enterprise and Adventure in the Archipelagoes of Melanesian* New Guinea. London: Routledge.

Reed-Danahay, D. 1997. *Auto/ethnography: Rewriting the Self and the Social, Explorations in Anthropology*. Oxford: Berg.

Sparkes, A.C. 2000. Autoethnography and narratives of self: Reflections on criteria in action. *Sociology of Sport Journal* 17(1): 21–43.

Spry, T. 2001. Performing autoethnography: An embodied methodological praxis. *Qualitative Inquiry* 7(6): 706–732.

Spry, T. 2016. *Body, Paper, Stage: Writing and Performing Autoethnography*. London: Routledge.

Styhre, A., and J. Tienari. 2014. Men in context: Privilege and reflexivity in academia. *Equality, Diversity and Inclusion: An International Journal* 33(5): 442–450.

United Nations (UN). 2005. *Report on the World Social Situation 2005: The Inequality Predicament*. New York: United Nations Publications.

Vryan, K.D. 2006. Expanding analytic autoethnography and enhancing its potential. *Journal of Contemporary Ethnography* 35(4): 405–409.

Wall, S. 2008. Easier said than done: Writing an autoethnography. *International Journal of Qualitative Methods* 7(1): 38–53.

2 Negotiating COVID-19 in the Media

Autoethnographic Reflections on Sweden and International Reporting

Rachel Irwin

Introduction: Stereotypical Views of Sweden and the Swedes

In November 2020, US talk show host and comedian Stephen Colbert ran a segment on The Late Show about Sweden and COVID-19 with the title: "Herd Immunity Isn't the Only Thing Sweden Got Horribly Wrong." Colbert began the segment by describing how Scott Atlas, then an advisor on the White House Coronavirus Task Force, was pushing for a herd immunity strategy in the USA. He then turned his attention across the Atlantic, saying, "One place that resisted lockdowns and decided to give herd immunity a whirl was Sweden ... I have to tell you, regardless of what Atlas says, the results have not been good."

Colbert cited a November 2020 article from *Business Insider* that claimed, "Sweden's per capital death rate from the coronavirus is one of the highest in the world" and referred to the country's "Let them catch it" policy. He did not mention that *Business Insider* was actually citing out-of-date mortality data from May 2020. Instead, he went on to say: "We should not be taking medical advice from Sweden, as Atlas seems to be doing. They seem smart over there, but they're mostly just tall and blonde."

In the course of the segment, he also worked in a series of Swedish-related jokes about Death (the character from Ingmar Bergman's film *The Seventh Seal*), the music group ABBA,[1] the crime series *Wallander*, *Midsommar* (the holiday), IKEA, lingonberries, herring, Beowulf, maternity leave, black liquorice, meatballs, the Skarsgård acting family, the Swedish Chef from The Muppet Show, and, finally, the Swedish Bikini Team, a made-up gag used in Old Milwaukee Beer advertisements in the 1990s.

This Late Show segment was perhaps the most egregious, but also representative, example of how the international media portrayed Sweden during the COVID-19 pandemic. It was factually incorrect and rested, not on Sweden as it really is, but on the tired stereotypes noted above. And the segment was not even really about Sweden; rather Sweden was used to criticize American domestic politics, specifically the role of Scott Atlas in the Trump administration's handling of the pandemic.

DOI: 10.4324/9781003187462-4

In this chapter, I reflect upon my experiences as an anthropologist studying the international media's portrayal of Sweden and COVID-19 (Irwin 2020a, b, c). I started this research from a personal place: what I was reading in the international media did not match my daily life in Sweden. While my experience of COVID-19 is not the only "truth," I was frustrated by the international media's portrayal of my country. I was also emotionally unprepared for the vitriol directed at Sweden in social media and online comments.

I first discuss broadly the challenges and opportunities for anthropologically engaging with the news media during a pandemic. I then turn to the Swedish experience, describing how the country was portrayed as reckless and irresponsible and the ways in which Swedish culture was used and misused to explain its handling of the pandemic. Finally, I discuss my own frustrations and experiences with the research relied on by the media, and conclude with reflections on how anthropologists and other researchers could and should engage with the media.

Anthropologists, the News, and Studying "Now"

Anthropologists rely on news sources, to "set the scene," to corroborate facts, and to describe dominant discourses. In recent years, anthropologists have also turned to the study of the media itself (Peake 2020). The news is the "one popular genre that claims to describe reality for the public" (Bird 2010: 5) but it is not neutral. It is a cultural practice that offers a "slice of reality entrenched with the values and biases of those who produce it" (Sussel 1992: 1). Because of these inherent questions of power and legitimacy, anthropology has a responsibility to better understand how media is consumed, produced, and circulates knowledge (Briggs and Nichter 2009).

Writing specifically of COVID-19, Roland Bal and colleagues (2020) set out a research agenda for health policy analysis, and that also offers inspiration for the social sciences in general. As the first global pandemic in the age of social media, these authors argue that more attention is needed not only to the interactions among different types of media, but also to the ways in which the media influence policy-making and behavior. They further note that what would previously have been "backroom" discussions over evidence among scientists from different backgrounds now play out in the media. The media also *construct expertise* through giving platforms to certain experts while ignoring others.

This COVID-19 media environment has been chaotic. Although not specifically about Sweden, a letter in the *British Medical Journal* characterized this overall media environment:

> Sadly, there has been a trend towards "tabloid journalism," with emotive language, misleading soundbites, and cherry-picked citations. Only a handful of this editorial's references are peer reviewed research;

half are newspaper articles, personal opinions, and blogs. In this era
of worldwide connectivity, it is all too easy for personal opinion to be
referenced, re-cited, and repeated as gospel.

(Slingo 2020)

Slingo's statement is similar to what anthropologist Carlo Caduff (2020: 486)
has described, criticizing the ways in which:

> Under-scrutinized science, lack of data, speculative evidence, strong
> opinions, deliberate misinformation, exaggerated mortality rates, the
> 24/7 news media attention, and the rapid spread of dramatic stories on
> social media have led to poor political choices and major public anxiety.

I entered this chaotic fieldsite in March 2020, when it became apparent
that the international media's portrayal of the Swedish experience bore
little resemblance to my daily life. I read English-language outlets with a
significant international audience. I also followed Swedish news and Twitter
feeds in both languages. I watched press conferences from the World Health
Organization (WHO) and the Swedish Public Health Agency, and followed
various links that took me all over the Internet. By the end of April 2021,
I had collected 828 screenshots, mostly of Twitter posts, and 1,755 articles
from English and Swedish-language press. I had a 33-page field note
document (8,000 words) with links and transcriptions of news. I also kept
a diary as part of the Corona Diaries Project, organized by the German
medical anthropology journal *Curare*.

Like many other academics, at the beginning of the pandemic I was
busy moving my courses online and reorganizing my ongoing research
so that I could work from home; I was also coming to terms with the
general emotional unease of living in the pandemic. Simultaneously, I was
engaging with online media for up to 10 hours a day. As previously noted,
I was unprepared for the amount of hate and toxicity directed at Sweden,
particularly in social media and in online comments. Handling this almost
endless amount of (mis)information took an emotional toll—I found myself
having physical reactions, even waking up shaking. After the first month
of the pandemic, I had to gradually taper off my engagement, still paying
attention and being in the field, but not so intensely.

Temporality

This intensity of rapid research relates to a second challenge: temporality.
Since I often take a historical perspective in my research, I am used to
studying public health debates years after they have taken place, often using
archival sources. I can sit in an archive in peace and quiet, and systematically
go through documents and news articles. Studying a fieldsite based on a
24-hours-a-day news cycle is very different. Practically, reading an online

newspaper in real-time offers a visual experience: one can see comments, links, and accompanying photographs. In contrast, the use of a media database to retrieve articles typically presents plain text only. Similarly, many news sites had live updates—important materials that are not necessarily indexed in media databases.

Looking more broadly, a future historian might ask, "What was the beginning of the pandemic like?" People will remember that there was a lot of discussion about the Swedish approach, but they may not necessarily remember the complexity of public discourse in the initial months of the pandemic. Writing of side effects from the H1N1 vaccine in 2009 six years later, ethnologist Birgitta Lundgren (2016: 1114) noted:

> It is my impression from talking about the issue of the side effect in public gatherings, conferences etc., that the six years that have passed have erased much of the memories of the pandemic ("Yes, I remember now, we had a pandemic") and the knowledge of the side effects. What remains is often a blurred sense that "something went wrong."

The temporality of rapid, real-time ethnography allows for a depth that post-event research does not allow, but it misses the wider understanding-at-a-distance that future research on COVID-19 will have. At the time I was writing, I did not yet know how or when the pandemic might end, nor did I have the analytical or emotional distance that future generations of researchers will have. If I had written this chapter even 12 months after the pandemic, I would have been able to interview the key players—civil servants, politicians, and healthcare staff. Eventually I would have had access to archival materials, which are usually embargoed for 20 or 25 years, depending on the archive. I would have access to the post-pandemic evaluations of the government. Instead, I could only record the quick, almost instantaneous reactions and analyses.

Online, but Also in Real Life

A third challenge is the relationship between online and offline worlds, which highlights the importance of long-term fieldwork. Costello and colleagues (2017) have argued that passive approaches to Internet ethnography miss out on opportunities found in participatory approaches. There are also related, albeit slightly different, challenges with rapid ethnography. That is, good ethnography should be long-term, involving "sustained immersion" in a society or culture in order to produce a deep understanding and "sensitivity to context" (Hammersly 2006; Ingold 2014: 384; Vougioukalou et al. 2019: 20). Clearly, rapid ethnographies of media environments—particularly during a crisis—would be enhanced by long-term fieldwork and holistic approaches. A pandemic response touches on culture, economics, law, history and other aspects of society, highlighting the limits of a micro-ethnographic approach, and cannot be fully analyzed without a broader approach.

My broader familiarity with the field comes in part from my prior research on Swedish domestic and foreign policy (Irwin 2019a, b). It also comes from my position as a dual Swedish-US national who lived in the UK for almost a decade. Many of the media outlets and social media posts I read came from the USA and the UK, and I was able to contextualize the political slants and cultural references in the material. Simultaneously, I had first-hand experience of daily life in Sweden during the pandemic, both on- and offline. I had Zoom meetings with colleagues. I went to local shops and made small talk, and I had conversations with my neighbors by shouting from the balcony of my apartment. Later, as the weather improved, we could socialize, with 2 meters distance, in the garden. While I do not explicitly draw upon these interactions, they impacted how I analyzed the media debates and understood the Swedish experience. I also learnt a lot about Sweden during this time; because of my contextual understanding, I knew *how* to learn and had an internal framework for judging what information was reliable and what was not. Unfortunately, as I discuss in the following section, many media pundits did not.

Critiquing "The Swedish Experiment"

Sweden's anti-lockdown experiment flopped. Now it faces a wave of pandemic pain.

(*Washington Post*, 1 December 2020)

The international media highlighted Sweden as having an "open society" relative to most other high-income countries, in that, for example, most restaurants and shops stayed open and there were few compulsory restrictions on individual movement. Some of the reporting was balanced and factual, but much of it was highly editorialized: many outlets framed Sweden as deviant for not "shutting down," even though many of the same media outlets that criticized China's draconian measures in Wuhan later criticized Sweden's "lax" approach (see Caduff 2020). Others, primarily the more politically conservative outlets in the USA and the UK, lauded Sweden's approach as preserving civil liberties. Misinformation, and even disinformation, characterized much of this polarized coverage (Irwin 2020a).

The initial critiques largely came from within the country. Some scientists and clinicians wrote opinion pieces in Swedish newspapers criticizing the government's and authorities' handling of the pandemic. Many raised a number of serious questions around the various policy measures, testing and tracing capacities, and the disadvantages and advantages of mathematical modelling; most ultimately called for more of a lockdown approach. However, some were part of a loosely organized group that launched an active disinformation campaign, writing opinion pieces in international newspapers and repeatedly calling for the state epidemiologist to be tried for crimes against humanity (*The Local* 2021). Many of the critics repeatedly claimed that Sweden had a "herd immunity strategy" without offering any evidence for that claim. This idea, as later incorrectly characterized in a *New York Times* editorial, was that the Swedish strategy "apparently relies on 'herd immunity,' in which a critical mass of infection occurs in lower-risk populations that ultimately thwarts transmission" (Bremmer et al. 2020). That is, the logic behind the herd immunity rumor was that Sweden was staying open to let the virus spread through the population.

The international media quickly picked up on the domestic criticism and reported it as gospel, rather than contextualizing or questioning it; the criticism then became amplified through news and social media and spread through various online media. Journalists and various experts with no connection to the country passed judgment on its response in quotes, articles and newspaper commentaries, and at times on social media. The basic criticisms were that by "refusing" to lock down, Sweden had acted irresponsibly and cost lives in the pursuit of herd immunity. Others went as far as to assert that "there is a clear element of eugenics in the proposals to pursue herd immunity as a strategy against the pandemic" (Laterza and Romer 2020).

However, Sweden did not have a "herd immunity" strategy. Part of the reason for a seemingly voluntary approach to restrictions was that most types of societal closures are somewhat incompatible with Swedish law. The right to freely move throughout the country is enshrined in the Constitution, curfews are basically illegal, and other laws make it difficult to close commercial facilities, to provide just a few examples. Although temporary pandemic laws were passed to provide the government with more options for lockdown-like measures, these still needed to be compatible with Constitutional rights. Beyond the legal frameworks, representatives from the public health agency repeatedly stressed that they were taking a wider public health approach, cognizant of the expected and unexpected consequences of lockdown. They were also concerned about sustainability: maintaining a lockdown for one week is one thing, but holding it until after the pandemic was over would be very difficult—as has been the case in many other countries.

In actuality, Sweden did implement many restrictions, including compulsory limits on the number of people at public events and in commercial spaces. Although many other preventive measures took the form of "voluntary" recommendations, they were nevertheless governed by social norms, with the threat of "social punishment" for not following them (Irwin 2020b; see Lundgren on H1N1 in Sweden). For instance, ethnologist Katarzyna Herd has compared social norms around COVID-19 in Sweden with "witch hunts," recounting the words of an acquaintance who told her: "Every time you take the bus to work, you're killing a grandmother" (Herd, cited in Johansson 2020). This statement suggests the importance of

Sweden's Covidian social norms, along with fear, in ensuring adherence to recommendations for physical distancing, working from home, and reducing social contacts.

Multiple misleading and sensationalized news articles circulated on social media, including Twitter. In these posts, the government and authorities were accused of not taking the virus seriously, engaging in a "giant experiment," and "gaslighting" (psychologically manipulating) the Swedish people. Representatives of the Public Health Agency were referred to as "instruments of Satan." Swedes themselves were described as "arrogant," "stupid," "reckless," "national chauvinists," and "cult members," and there were references to the horror film *Midsommer*, implying that Swedes were happy to kill off the elderly.

Some of those posting were individuals who clearly had no first-hand knowledge of the country. For example, one Twitter user had to ask what "week 25" meant on a graph from the Swedish Public Health Agency. This user clearly did not know that it is common in Sweden and other Nordic countries to number the weeks of the year. In another instance, on June 21, 2020, a series of Twitter posts from four separate users speculated about why Sweden had not posted new death and infection statistics, implying that cases were so bad that the government was trying to cover them up. The real reason was that it was the *Midsommar* holiday weekend when the whole country shuts down.

That lay individuals critique a country on social media is not such a problem, but some of those active on Twitter were public figures. In August 2020, Nobel Laureate Paul Krugman tweeted, "The new Eurostat numbers say that Sweden and Denmark have had identical economic performance … . So all Sweden got from its herd immunity strategy was a bunch of dead Swedes." Helen Clark, a former Prime Minister of New Zealand, compared the Swedish state epidemiologist Anders Tegnell to Donald Trump. Two weeks later, Clark was named the co-chair of a WHO panel reviewing the WHO's and governments' handling of the pandemic. In a December 3, 2020 Twitter post, Andy Slavitt, an advisor to President Biden, implied that the Swedish state epidemiologist deserved comparison to the Nazis, writing:

> Scott Atlas's brother-by-another-mother, Anders Tegnell, who masterminded the "just ignore it" strategy in Sweden, is also out. Again—only so long can your strategy kill people before you either get fired or compared to the Nazis. Or both.

Needless to say, Twitter is not the most appropriate forum for the complex task of health policy evaluation. The comparison of cross-country data is challenging, owing to differences in case definitions, testing rates, and myriad other contextual factors. Moreover, different countries put in different measures at different times, and adherence to these measures is not always captured in follow-up evaluations.

Even if we pretend that the data is comparable, then a year into the pandemic, Sweden's "performance" had been inconclusive: according to Johns Hopkins University, Sweden had the 32nd highest death toll in the world per capita. This was far above its neighboring countries of Denmark and Norway, but lower than many other European countries, including Belgium, the Czech Republic, France, Spain, Slovakia and the UK—all of whom imposed more compulsory restrictions than Sweden. By the measure of "excess mortality"—the number of deaths from all causes over what would be "expected" under normal circumstances—Sweden was below the European average in 2020, as measured by the European Statistical Office (Eurostat). Thus these data alone cannot be used to definitively "prove" the success or failure of lockdown measures and, in any case, these data do show that many of the criticisms of Sweden's "open approach" were unjustified.

Nevertheless, and despite the pitfalls of cross-country comparisons and the lack of conclusive results, many global health influencers took to Twitter to judge the Swedish approach. These were often university professors at prestigious universities in the UK and USA who are active in social media and in the news. Their posts and news reports called Sweden a "cautionary tale" and a "gamble," "Darwinian," and rested on the (incorrect) belief that Sweden had a herd immunity strategy. One well-known American professor joked on Twitter that it seemed as if everyone needed to have an opinion about Sweden—and went on to give one. Within this global media environment, there was a sense that Sweden was fair game for criticism, and no actual experience with the country was needed to participate.

From Culture to Context

The notion of Swedish "culture" regularly played a role in the media environment. Official approaches to COVID-19 were often framed in relation to not only epidemiological, clinical and quantitative demographic data, but also to an explicitly and implicitly defined sense of "Swedishness" and what it means to be a "good citizen." Focus was placed on the notions of moral common sense and decency (*folkvett*) and of solidarity, which has long provided a foundation for public health work (Lundgren 2016; Irwin 2020b). There were also cultural codes for how to interpret the word "recommendation." That is, as already alluded to, rather than being "lax," voluntary recommendations from the authorities were better understood as compulsory, but not legally binding (Irwin 2020b).

Attention to culture is important, not least because of the leitmotiv running through medical anthropology that national and international health policies ignore local experiences and contexts. But at the same time, as mentioned above, the conceptualizations of "Swedishness" often focused on superficial and stereotypical markers of identity, not only in the international but also in the national press. At best, Swedes were described as trusting in their government and "inclined to follow recommendations."

At worst, this was interpreted to mean that Swedes were sheep who blindly followed their leaders. The media also highlighted the alleged "exotic" practices of the Swedes: a news item about one person getting a tattoo of the state epidemiologist garnered disproportional attention in the news; many social media users saw this as proof of "cult-like" behavior.

Part of the problem with cultural explanations is that how anthropologists debate the concept of "culture" is different than what is meant in the news, in casual conversation, or in other disciplines. In the past, anthropologists were often called in to be "culture-brokers" for governments and other agencies to explain why the groups in question acted a certain way. This is an outdated model because in it, "culture" was often reduced to "superstitions" or "ignorance" and framed as an obstacle to public health interventions; this model also often ignored wider structural issues affecting health (Stellmach et al. 2018). However, while anthropology as a discipline has moved on, others with whom we interact have not.

Another problem is that "Swedishness," or Swedish norms and values, are inherently contested. As with any national identity, norms and values change over time, are often partially based on myths, and tend to be defined in relation to the politics of the time (Johansson 2004; Almqvist and Glans 2004). For example, over the past decade, Swedish values have often been misused to criticize immigration and Islam. In this vein, anthropologists Sylva Frisk and Maris Boyd Gillette (2019) have discussed how the burka was constructed as a "problem" in relation to Swedish norms and values. Indeed, as right-wing and far-right political movements have tried to define Swedish norms and values in juxtaposition to immigration, others have countered this with their own definitions of Swedishness, based on tolerance and openness.

A third problem with culture-as-explanation is that Swedes are not a homogenous group; thus it is ridiculous to speak of "the Swedes" as thinking one thing or another or behaving in a certain way. There are different ways of experiencing life in Sweden, depending on age, social class, background, religion, gender, region, and myriad overlapping categories of identity. Over the course of the pandemic, my own thoughts on "culture" evolved, and I eventually came to the conclusion that *culture* is too damaged as a concept to be useful, whereas *context* was easier to discuss. Certainly, there is a habitus of "being Swedish": there are cultural codes and repertoires and ways of going about daily life and perceiving the world that are shared by most Swedes (Irwin 2020a; Frykman 2004). These contextual factors are important; but it is less important to define "Swedishness"—a Sisyphean task—and more meaningful to examine how it defined, by whom, and for what purpose.

My Frustrations in Engaging with the Media

I became incredibly frustrated by the media coverage for multiple reasons— as the daughter of a journalist, as an anthropologist, and as a Swede. My mother had been as a journalist, and I spent my earliest years following her around as she worked on stories. I grew up believing that I could trust the news and that articles had been fact-checked. Instead, I was seeing misinformation and even disinformation in highly respected outlets such as the *Washington Post*, the *New York Times*, and National Public Radio. There was plenty to critique about the Swedish handling of the pandemic, such as high numbers of deaths in elderly care homes or class and ethnic disparities in death rates, without exaggerating or outright lying.

I also felt frustration as an anthropologist whose research focuses on the relationships among society, culture, and health policy, in both Swedish and global contexts. I was disturbed by the simplistic assumption that the Swedish "strategy" could be explained by outdated or superficial markers of Swedish identity. Beyond this, there was an assumption in English-language media that "the Nordic countries are all the same" and thus comparisons among them are automatically valid. I was also frustrated by the simplicity with which health policy analysis was portrayed in the media. Researchers who should have known better were perpetuating rumors or even falsehoods, cherry-picking data, and making conclusive statements often based on a poor understanding of Swedish public administration and politics, or on the idea that Stockholm represented the whole country.

As a Swede, I felt frustration at how the media declared our lives to be "normal," and the notion that Sweden "did nothing" was offensive, not least to people who had lost jobs due to the voluntary preventive measures and restrictions that were rendered compulsory by social norms; this was particularly acute in the hospitality sector when people drastically cut down on travel and restaurant visits during the spring of 2020. While from an outside perspective, our daily lives may have seemed "normal" in comparison to other countries, in fact we made many changes in order to adhere to the recommendations and restrictions. The media pointed to "crowded" shopping centers, but I was reading about how shops in those same malls were going out of business due to lack of customers.

This is not to suggest that everyone followed recommendations all of the time. As in other countries, adherence to the recommendations waxed and waned as the pandemic wore on. But mobile phone data, surveys, and ongoing qualitative research regularly demonstrated the great extent to which people had adapted to the pandemic and were following the recommendations to maintain physical distance, reduce social contacts, and work from home (FoHM 2021; Orbe 2020). In most cases, the Public Health Agency did not recommend masks in community settings. This is partly because the WHO did not change its guidance until June 2020 to recommend masks when physical distancing was unfeasible, partly because the evidence base for mask wearing in community settings was not that strong at the time, and partly because there were concerns about enough personal protective equipment (PPE) for health and other essential workers—especially during the so-called "first wave." In addition, the Public Health Agency expressed concerns that if mask wearing were normalized, people would socialize more in indoor spaces, work at the office, or crowd public transport. Context is also important here: there are 10 million people in a country the size of California. Obviously, population density differs greatly across the country, but there are many places where physical distancing is relatively easy to maintain.

During autumn 2020, mask wearing organically became more common overall and was often required for visits to healthcare providers. In the winter of 2021, it was officially recommended for use on public transport during rush hour (nationally) or all the time (in some regions). Overall, primary focus was instead placed on physical distancing and reducing social contacts, but the lack of population-wide mask wearing became yet another touchpoint for criticizing Sweden's COVID-19 response.

To channel my frustrations over the media coverage, I began to document my own experiences in relation to the international reporting and social media chatter. I also began to engage with national and international media through writing opinion pieces myself, fact-checking other articles, and giving interviews. It was empowering to realize that I could be part of the conversation, and I met a number of lovely national and international journalists. Yet this engagement also led to further frustrations and concerns.[2]

One frustration was what I refer to as "Swede-splaining," a portmanteau of the words "Swede" and "explaining." In one example, an Autumn 2020 article in a well-respected US news outlet quoted a professor in the USA as saying that Sweden had done "virtually nothing," that it had "made a point of refusing to [lock down]" and had "ignored everything for so long." I contacted that journalist and explained that while we took a more voluntary approach than other countries, we had done a lot to combat the virus. His response was that, while they had considered not running the quotes, it was the professor's opinion, not fact. The journalist also said that the professor's "take on Sweden" was not "completely disconnected from reality."

In another example, in September 2020, a Pulitzer Prize-winning journalist authored a piece in a well-respected new outlet, writing that Sweden had "established a policy of deliberately allowing the virus to spread in a fruitless quest for 'herd immunity.' " When I sent a reply, the journalist responded by explaining my own country's "herd immunity strategy" to me. In both cases, I was left feeling angry that a journalist in the USA was Swede-splaining my country's responses and describing my daily life to me, a Swede.

Another source of frustration, or rather discomfort, was the polarization in the media. I gave one interview in which I felt that the journalist was pushing me into declaring the "Swedish strategy" either a success or failure. My answer was non-committal, suggesting that some things had worked well, others not so well, and that we did not have enough data yet to fully evaluate the various policies in the country. Perhaps I misinterpreted the response over the Zoom connection, but the journalist almost seemed disappointed that I had not provided a more polarized response.

The media reporting was also split along political lines in English-speaking contexts. Right-wing and libertarian groups, particularly in the USA and the UK, lauded Sweden for staying open in comparison to implementing lockdowns. As a Twitter user noted: "the COVID-19 response was unwarranted and hysterical. It has greatly curtailed human freedom and given way too much power to governments around the world. Sweden was sensible there."

As seen in the TV piece by Stephen Colbert, some left-wing pundits labeled Sweden as "bad" because the right liked its approach, neglecting to mention that the right's interpretation of the Swedish approach was somewhat flawed. This was one of the most bizarre aspects of the pandemic: normally the left-wing English-language media highlights the benefits of the Swedish welfare state, whereas the right-wing media uses the country to warn about the dangers of immigration (Rapacioli 2018). In my diary, I wrote: "When [a far-right news site known for disinformation] has some of the most accurate reporting, there is a problem. Sometimes the left loves us, usually the right hates us, but now the right likes us? What is going on?" (May 25–31, 2020).

Partly because my research was about how the news media had maligned Sweden based on faulty information, and also because I used examples from outlets disparagingly referred to as "mainstream" media by the right, I was asked several times to give interviews to or write in right-wing media. My own political leanings are pretty far to the left, even by Swedish standards, so this felt strange to me. One newspaper I wrote for was right-leaning, but was also an established and respected outlet. While I would not normally be a reader, I felt comfortable writing for that newspaper. But there was another other media request from a far-right outlet that I really struggled over. Ultimately, I decided it was better to talk to "the other side" than to avoid them, but I made sure to be extremely careful with my phrasing and word choice, trying to anticipate how they could misinterpret my comments. In the end, I was happy with how I was quoted.

Conclusions: Anthropological Engagements with the Media

As anthropologists, we engage with the media in three main ways. First, we often use it to set the scene and to provide facts and context for our ethnographic findings. Unfortunately, the portrayal and misuse of Sweden in the media offer good reminders to be careful when using news articles. This is particularly the case when we are new to a fieldsite and do not yet have the experience to assess claims to truth. It is also the case during an ongoing crisis, where the reporting may be more prone to sensationalism and exaggeration.

Second, an increasing number of us formally analyze framings, debates, discourses, interactions, and communities within the wider media environment, encompassing a range of forums, from "traditional" online newspapers to various social media platforms. Personally, I was exhausted by the sheer amount and boundless nature of this fieldsite, and I was also affected by the toxic nature of some of the posts. As researchers, we should be cognizant of the mental health risks of online research and feel comfortable stepping back from it when needed.

Third, we participate in the media. It is important for us as anthropologists to speak within the limits of our understanding, which also highlights the need for long-term ethnographic engagement with a setting. Bluntly put, it is irresponsible to make authoritative statements about a context you do not understand. I recognize that researchers in precarious employment may have no other choice than to take a consultancy or short-term ethnographic assignment that, in turn, may lead to a publication that is less informed than it should be. However, the ways in which high-level public figures and global health influencers, speaking from positions of power, defined, represented, and critiqued Sweden policies and even "the Swedes" were irresponsible.

Overall, it is clear that if anthropologists do not engage with media, then others—some of whom speak with authority in the absence of experience—will define, use, and abuse the concept of culture. Certainly, the anthropologist as culture-broker is an outdated model, but we do have a responsibility to be context-brokers.

Acknowledgments

I presented an earlier version of this chapter at the 2020 Autumn meeting of *Dokumentation av samtida Sverige* (DOSS), a network of Swedish museums and other cultural institutions. I am appreciative of the feedback and comments from this networking meeting. The research for this chapter was funded by the Swedish Research Council, Grant #2018–05266.

Notes

1 ABBA is a world-famous Swedish pop group formed in Stockholm in 1972 by Agnetha Fältskog, Björn Ulvaeus, Benny Andersson, and Anni-Frid Lyngstad.
2 In this section, I have anonymized details of names and articles to protect the integrity of those cited. See also Chapter 4 of the Swedish Research Council's guide Good Research Practice (2017).

References

Almqvist, K., and Glans, K., eds. 2004. *The Swedish Success Story?* Stockholm: Axel and Margaret Ax:son Johnson Foundation.
Bal, R., de Graff, B., van de Bovenkamp, H., and Wallenburg, I. 2020. Practicing Corona—Towards a research agenda of health policies. *Health Policy* 124(7): 671–673. https://doi.org/10.1016/j.healthpol.2020.05.010
Bird, S.E. 2010. Anthropological engagement with news media. Why now? *Anthropology News*. April: (5): 9.

Bremmer, I., Kupcham, C., and Rosenstein, S. 2020. Coronavirus and the Sweden myth. May 4. *The New York Times*. www.nytimes.com/2020/05/04/opinion/ coronavirus-sweden-herd-immunity.html, accessed April 28, 2021.

Briggs, C.L., and Nichter, M. 2009. Biocommunicability and the biopolitics of pandemic threats. *Medical Anthropology* 28(3): 189–198. doi:10.1080/ 01459740903070410

Caduff, C. 2020. What went wrong: Corona and the world after the full stop. *Medical Anthropology Quarterly* 34(4): 467–487. doi:10.1111/maq.12599

Colbert, S. 2020. Herd Immunity Isn't The Only Thing Sweden Got Horribly Wrong. The Late Show with Stephen Colbert. November 17. www.youtube.com/ watch?v=aQ77auKIIAY, accessed April 28, 2021.

Costello, L., Wallace, R., and McDermott, M-L. 2017. Netnography: Range of practices, misperceptions, and missed opportunities. *International Journal of Qualitative Methods* 16(1). https://doi.org/10.1177%2F1609406917700647

FoMH. 2021. Rapport om rörelse-och resemått, vecka 16 2021. [Report about movement and travel, week 16 2021]. Stockholm: Folkhälsomyndigheten [Public Health Agency of Sweden]. www.folkhalsomyndigheten.se/smittskydd- beredskap/utbrott/aktuella-utbrott/covid-19/statistik-och-analyser/analys-och- prognoser/veckorapport-om-rorelsedata/, accessed May 4, 2021.

Frisk, S., and Gillette, M.B. 2017. Sweden's burka ban: Policy proposal, problematisations, and the production of Swedishness. *NORA—Nordic Journal of Feminist and Gender Research*. 27(4): 271–284 https://doi.org/10.1080/ 08038740.2019.1668847

Frykman, J. 2004. Swedish mentality: Between modernity and cultural nationalism. In Almqvist, Kurt and Glans, Kay, eds. 2004. *The Swedish Success Story?* Stockholm: Axel and Margaret Ax:son Johnson Foundation. 121–132.

Hammersley, M. 2006. Ethnography: Problems and prospects. *Ethnography and Education* 1(1): 3–14. doi: 10.1080/17457820500512697

Ingold, T. 2014. That's enough about ethnography! *Hau: Journal of Ethnographic Theory* 4(1): 383–395. doi: 10.14318/hau4.1.021

Irwin, R. 2019a. Lessons from Sweden's feminist foreign policy for global health. *The Lancet* 393(10171): e27–e28.

Irwin, R. 2019b. Sweden's engagement in global health: A historical review. *Globalization and Health* 15: 79.

Irwin, R. 2020a. Misinformation and de-contextualization: International media reporting on Sweden and COVID-19. *Globalization and Health* 16(62). https:// doi.org/10.1186/s12992-020-00588-x

Irwin, R. 2020b. A wink and a recommendation: Thick description in the Covid-19 pandemic. *MAQ Blog*. https://medanthroquarterly.org/rapid-response/2020/ 05/a-wink-and-a-recommendation-thick-description-in-the-covid/, accessed April 28, 2021.

Irwin, R. 2020c. The "Swedish Experiment." *Medical Anthropology at UCL Blog*. https://medanthucl.com/2020/04/06/the-swedish-experiment/, accessed April 28, 2021.

Johansson, R. 2004. "The Construction of Swedishness." In Almqvist, Kurt and Glans, Kay, eds., *The Swedish Success Story?* Stockholm: Axel and Margaret Ax:son Johnson Foundation, 109–120.

Johansson, Y. 2020. Vem blir du under coronahotet—den som bedriver häxjakt eller den som gör gott? [Who are you during the corona threat—do you organise

witch hunt or do you do good?] *Sydsvenskan*. April 5, 2020. www.sydsvenskan.
se/2020-04-05/vem-blir-du-under-coronahotet-den-som-bedriver-haxjakt-eller,
accessed April 28, 2021.

Laterza, V., and Romer, L.P. 2020. Coronavirus, herd immunity and the eugenics
of the market. April 14. *Al-Jazzera*. www.aljazeera.com/indepth/opinion/
coronavirus-herd-immunity-eugenics-market-200414104531234.html, accessed
July 16, 2020.

The Local. 2021. "Threat to democracy?" Why an online campaign group criticising
Sweden's coronavirus strategy has caused a stir. February 11. www.thelocal.
se/20210211/threat-to-democracy-why-an-online-campaign-group-criticising-
swedens-coronavirus-strategy-has-caused-a-stir/, accessed April 28, 2021.

Lundgren, B. 2016. Solidarity at the Needle Point—the Intersection of Compassion
and Containment during the A(H1N1) Pandemic in Sweden 2009. *Sociology and
Anthropology* 4(12): 1108–1116.

Orbe, J. 2020. Resultat "coronabarometern" 21 mars – 5/6 april 2020.[Results from
"corona barometer"] Stockholm: Kantar Sifo & MSB. www.msb.se/siteassets/
dokument/aktuellt/nyheter/corona-covid19/msb-resultat-coronaundersokning-
200406.pdf, accessed May 4, 2021

Peake, B. 2020. B. Media anthropology: Meaning, embodiment, infrastructure and
activism. In *Perspectives: An Open Introduction to Cultural Anthropology, 2nd
edition*. https://courses.lumenlearning.com/suny-culturalanthropology/chapter/
media/, accessed July 16, 2020.

Rapacioli, P. 2018. *Good Sweden, Bad Sweden*. Stockholm: Volante.

Slingo, M. 2020. Covid-19: Now is not the time to judge the UK's response. *BMJ*
369: m2448. http://dx.doi.org/10.1136/bmj.m2448

Stellmach, D., Beshar, I., Bedford, J., du Cros, P., and Stringer, B. 2018. Anthropology
in public health emergencies: What is anthropology good for? *BMJ Global Health*
3: e000534. http://dx.doi.org/10.1136/bmjgh-2017-000534

Sussel, R. 1992. *News of an Epidemic: Exploring the Discourse of 'Deviance' in
the Construction of AIDS. Thesis in the Department of Communication Studies*.
Montreal: Concordia University.

Vougioukalou, S., Boaz, A., Gager, M., and Locock, L. 2019. The contribution
of ethnography to the evaluation of quality improvement in hospital settings:
reflections on observing co-design in intensive care units and lung cancer
pathways in the UK. *Anthropology & Medicine*. 26(1): 18–32. doi: 10.1080/
13648470.2018.1507104

Washington Post. 2020. Sweden's anti-lockdown experiment flopped. Now it faces a
wave of pandemic pain. *The Washington Post*. December 1. www.washingtonpost.
com/opinions/global-opinions/swedens-anti-lockdown-experiment-flopped-
now-it-faces-a-wave-of-pandemic-pain/2020/12/01/9e90ee28-3344-11eb-8d38-
6aea1adb3839_story.html, accessed April 28, 2020.

3 Loss and Longing for the Field During COVID-19 in Australia, and Finding It Again Because "*Ngukurr* Is Everywhere"

Kate Senior, Richard Chenhall, and Frances Edmonds

Introduction

Confined largely to our homes, our immediate focus has been on living, adapting, and learning to do our jobs remotely. For some of us, life has been confined to a five-kilometer radius of the house, so even getting to the supermarket has become an expedition. Boundaries are everywhere, and most tangibly for us authors, travel has been halted between many states in Australia. For New South Wales and Victoria (the most populous states in the country), travel is now restricted to all other states and the closures appear to be indefinite. For the first time in 20 years, Kate Senior has been unable to visit the Ngukurr community where she has long been conducting fieldwork, and more importantly, has three generations of friends and people whom she calls family. This loss of physical contact cannot be easily mediated through technology; even a simple telephone call is often impossible due to lack of access to phones and the remoteness of the region.

Kate's process of separation and grieving for the field, shared by many other anthropologists, has prompted discussions about separation from the field and the "end of fieldwork," and how that process is negotiated and understood. It also raises continuing issues about the "digital divide" between Indigenous and other Australians and the unequal access to communication and technology that could help to build "bridging" social capital, and to create new opportunities for employment, education, and resourcing for Indigenous Australians.

In this chapter, written in May 2021, we provide an autoethnographic description and analysis by Kate Senior and her colleagues Richard Chenhall and Fran Edmonds about isolation and longing for the field and how we have negotiated and mitigated these. We begin by describing the restrictions on people's movements in Australia as a response to COVID-19, and how specifically the closure of state borders has affected not only our ability to undertake fieldwork, but also to maintain contact with people within the field and even to plan for a period where such movement may again

DOI: 10.4324/9781003187462-5

be possible. A discussion of loss and grieving for fieldwork under these circumstances becomes a basis for exploring experiences of separation from the field and whether it is possible to *be* an anthropologist when the field itself becomes inaccessible. We conclude with a hope-inducing description of how we found "the field" again, right where we were.

Ngukurr

Ngukurr is a remote Indigenous community of around 1,000 people in Southeast Arnhem Land. It was formerly the Roper River Mission and was established in 1908 as the Christian Missionary Society responded to the devastation of the tribes in the region, due to the rapidly expanding cattle industry there. The Mission bought people from seven different language groups together; as a result, the predominant language in Ngukurr is Ngukurr Kriol, which arose out of a necessity to communicate with each other and the missionaries. This Mission was intended both to bring Christianity and "civilization" to the local Aboriginal population and to keep them safe from mass killings by white settlers. The Eastern and African Cold Storage Company had driven these people off their lands to set up cattle stations and export the meat around the world. The missionaries did protect them from death by starvation or massacre, but discouraged their languages and traditional ceremonies, which nevertheless they still perform. More recent missionary work has focused on the preservation of languages and recording Ngukurr Kriol as a written language; the Bible has been translated into Ngukurr Kriol.

Ngukurr is a place of stark contrasts for the people who live there. In terms of social determinants of health such as employment, education, access to quality housing and a good diet, there is a serious deficit when compared to non-Indigenous Australians (Chenhall and Senior 2017). However, Ngukurr residents are able to retain contact with and spend time on their ancestral lands surrounding the community (Senior et al. 2018). Traditional beliefs center on a world created by ancestral spirits whose paths define the region and people's relationships with land. The Dreamtime, a religious/cultural worldview that refers to an eternal present where ancestors inhabit the land, is not fixed—it is ongoing and its powers of regeneration are encouraged and celebrated through ceremonies (Senior et al. 2018). However, Ngukurr retains a strong Christian element, with attendance at both Church and Fellowship groups. Few people see traditional and Christian belief systems as mutually exclusive. There has also been considerable effort to revitalize some of the traditional languages in the region.

The Ngukurr economy is largely based on government welfare payments. A Community Development and Employment Program (CDEP, in which people's welfare payments are linked to participation in community projects) has recently been reinstated. A local shop provides most of the food in the community, which is often expensive due to high freight costs. Some people, particularly those with access to a vehicle, are able to supplement store-bought food with hunting and fishing. Turtle and wallabies are the most commonly hunted animals. Non-residents of Ngukurr, as is the case with Indigenous communities across the Northern Territory, require a permit to enter the community from the Indigenous Controlled Lands Councils. No permits were given from March 2020, and by the time of writing are only just becoming available. Ngukurr avoided COVID by effectively closing its community.

COVID-19 and Fieldwork

> It's a sunny late winter day and Daphne Daniels, an Indigenous woman from Ngukurr, and Kate Senior, a white woman from Newcastle, are sitting at the General Washington Pub in Stockton, New South Wales. Stockton, situated on a peninsula across the harbour from Newcastle, which feels about as remote from Ngukurr in the Northern Territory as could possibly be. As they sip their drinks, they notice the muted television behind the bar; it's showing the film Lil Bois, made in Ngukurr in 2019 and starring Daphne's nephew Dwyane. Daphne and Kate stare at the television and everyone else in the bar stares at them, but no one says a word. "Ngukurr is everywhere" says Daphne. "Why don't we tell these stories?" The feeling after this meeting was of excitement, a new direction for our research, but this feeling was quickly eclipsed by the world events that happened in January. This was the last time Kate saw Daphne before the lockdown of 2020.

By Easter 2020, Australia had been in lockdown for several weeks; yellow signs had been posted throughout our community telling us not to congregate; parks and play equipment were sealed off with orange tape; the beaches were closed; and a big flashing sign was erected at the entry to our peninsula community telling people not to travel. There were still shortages in our local shop in Stockton—an inner-city suburb of Newcastle, New South Wales—notably of flour and chocolate for the long Easter weekend. The initial panic had subsided, replaced by a vague unease about how long this would all last and for us, a sense of loneliness—a deep and abiding longing to be with, to see and touch, other people.

On Easter I (Kate) was very surprised to get a Zoom call from my friend and colleague Daphne (her real name) in the remote community of Ngukurr in the Northern Territory of Australia. The connection wasn't great, but at least I could see her. She was worried about us: "Did we have enough food? Were the children okay?" I called my family together and we spoke to Daphne's mother and her children and grandchildren. We talked about their own, much more serious lack of food in the community (the food delivery truck hadn't come) and the fishing trips that people were going on. I could hear the crows in the background, children yelling, people interrupting

Daphne to ask for smokes—familiar Ngukurr sounds. For that moment, I felt connected, amazed that technology could bridge the gaps of lockdown and distance.

But we didn't manage another such call. Daphne's computer broke and then she lost her phone. The separation caused by COVID-19 and the closure of both the Northern Territory borders and entry to remote Aboriginal communities continued. For the first time in 23 years, I could not go to Ngukurr—I wasn't allowed to travel 5 kilometers from my home, let alone 3000! This was more than the loss of opportunity to do my work— it was a physical yearning to be in a particular place with particular people. The enforced separation caused by COVID-19 has allowed Richard, Fran, and myself to reflect on the *embodiment* of fieldwork—which, pre-COVID, was taken for granted—and on the meanings of physical and emotional connection, as well as on the continuing frustrations of the digital divide between Indigenous and non-Indigenous Australians. But we have also come to see this period of separation as an opportunity to think about the meanings of the field and how to engage in ethnography in different ways.

Australia's Response to COVID-19

Australia's international borders were closed on March 20, 2020. By March 21, schools across the country were closed and the state borders were closed to all but essential travel. Restrictions were progressively lifted from mid-May. On July 7, 2020, Melbourne went into a second lockdown that lasted until September. Once again state borders to Victoria were closed, and all travelers across state borders were required to undertake mandatory hotel quarantine. Since that period, several smaller outbreaks have occurred, resulting in more localized lockdowns (including in Northern Sydney over Christmas 2020, and in South Australia, Brisbane, and most recently Perth). Many Aboriginal communities, including Ngukurr in southeast Arnhem Land, where we work, self-imposed further travel bans, which restricted people from leaving or entering the community. This, for example, was the advice published in the *Ngukurr Nyus*, the Ngukurr community newspaper:

> Leaders say: "Don't drive to Mataranka, Katherine, Darwin, Minyerri or Numbulwar. Don't go past Roper Bar. You can go shopping at Roper Bar, but don't go past there." This message for Ngukurr is very important. Pay attention to this message. This message isn't from Government, it's from our community leaders.
>
> (*Ngukurr Nyus*, April 1, 2020)

These formal restrictions were combined with considerable fear in rural and remote areas about the spread of disease from the cities, and sometimes overt hostility towards visitors.

By May 2021, Australia had not succeeded in rolling out the COVID-19 vaccine, and it was not expected that the population would have had their two doses until the end of 2021. The delays in delivering a vaccine in Australia leave open the possibility of more sudden lockdowns and mean that planning for any sort of travel is very uncertain. Furthermore, people from remote communities are anxious about traveling, because they think they might miss an opportunity to be vaccinated if they are away from home.

In terms of Richard and my (Kate's) work as teaching academics and as members of boards and committees, we adapted fast, quickly transforming our work into various forms of online delivery. In Fran's case, her work during COVID-19 lockdowns was frequently defined by finding ways to continue her long-term engagement with Aboriginal artists in southeast Australia, who are involved in exploring and reclaiming their ancestral collections held in collecting institutions, and who have recently begun working with the Ngukurr community. Most often, Fran's contact with artists was through text messages—a way of sharing images and stories that can be kept and archived; occasionally Zoom meetings were possible (see Edmonds et al. 2021). Although we were able to work longer days due to time saved from commuting and organizing face-to-face archival visits, doing fieldwork from the perspective of how we had always defined it—as extended participation in a community—seemed impossible.

Remoteness and Communication

I (Kate) have at least 15 different phone numbers for my Ngukurr colleague Daphne listed on my phone. I have taken to naming them by her first name and the date. A phone is often the only way that people in Ngukurr connect with those outside the community, as computers and iPads are too expensive and difficult to obtain. Simultaneously, the phone is a most fragile and transient piece of equipment. Phones get lost, stolen, borrowed and taken to other communities. A recent conversation exemplified this "phone phenomenon":

KATE: Hello
RESPONDEE: Who d'at?
KATE: It's Kate, where's Daphne?
RESPONDEE: (silence)
KATE: "Is this Daphne's phone? I'm looking for Daphne.
RESPONDEE: Na, this phone is in Borroloola" [250 kms away].

Phones are easily damaged and don't function well when they become full of dust. They are also expensive, and often local people cannot afford credit for their "pay as you go" phones. Furthermore, although the community of Ngukurr has good mobile phone coverage, this is not the case for the outstations—smaller satellite communities on people's ancestral lands. In

Nulawan, 22 kilometres away, a weak phone signal could be obtained by climbing a rusty ladder to the top of the water tanks. This was something the adolescents were adept at; thus it is hardly surprising that much of their Facebook content contained aerial vistas of the community.

Communication has always been difficult. Often, pre-COVID, I would plan a trip to Ngukurr, but not actually be sure if anyone was expecting me until I got to the community. My trips were always punctuated by anxiety: "Perhaps they are not answering because they don't want me to come"; "What if everyone has gone away?" But such anxieties were easily remedied by simply driving around until I found the person I was looking for. After a long period of separation, it becomes much more difficult to read the silences as simply caused by a lost phone or being out of range. Silences become ominous and terrifying. "Is this the end? Have I lost touch? Can I come back from this?"

I describe these communication difficulties to illustrate the deep "digital divide" between Indigenous and non-Indigenous Australia. Again, the "digital divide" refers to the unequal access to information and communications technology (ICT) between different groups. In Australia, Indigenous Australians have lower access to ICTs by around 43%, compared to 64% of non-Indigenous households that have sufficient 24/7 Internet access (see Hunter and Radoll 2020). Baum and colleagues (2014) have argued that people's lack of access to ICT contributes to cycles of disadvantage and has adverse impacts on health. In our fieldwork, this divide is ever apparent. In Aboriginal communities, computers and cellphones have short life spans due to both environmental harshness and to the pathways they take among multiple family members across different communities. When an individual loses Internet access in a remote community, then it is very difficult to remedy the problem, as there are few available and accessible support services and retail outlets.

Loss and Grieving

I (Kate) began fieldwork in Ngukurr at the end of 1998, as part of my PhD research, with Richard joining me from about 2003 on to collaborate on various projects. More recently, alongside Fran, we have been exploring archival material relating to Ngukurr, which is held in archival collections located elsewhere. Stories relating to the archival material resound in the community today. Yet unlike the information available in the archives and associated with the collections, Ngukurr residents have their own stories, many of which I have heard on and off over the years.

These stories were told to me initially during my first three years in the community, when I lived in a small, moveable house—a *donga*—which in this case consisted of a small former shipping container converted into a two-bedroom home right in the center of the town, where I could watch what was going on and make endless cups of tea for visitors. Since that time, I have been back to Ngukurr every year, sometimes with colleagues or students. In 2006, my first child was born and since then, my now three children and my husband Andrew have also been regular visitors to the community. I keep a permanent collection of camping equipment at a small outstation 22 kilometers outside the community; thus I always felt reassured that it would take very little preparation to go to Ngukurr when necessary, as almost everything I needed was already there. To store my equipment and to live in while there, I have been given a shed (a concrete slab with a tin roof and a set of buffalo horns perched on the top). Andrew and I have added functionality by constructing hooks and shelves from old pieces of iron. When we arrive, we hang our enamel mugs on wire hooks over the window. It doesn't take much to make it feel like home.

It's a place I know the feel of through my shoes, the sharp burnt stubble of grass, crumbly mud cracks and deep red dust punctuated with sheets of rusty corrugated iron and treacherous strands of barbed wire—I have walked so much of it in the daily rituals of gathering firewood and water. But it is also a place where we sit and talk, huddled around the fire in the morning, under giant mahogany trees during the day, and back around the fire as the evening and the mosquitos set in.

The routines here are as different as possible from those of my everyday life back home. Doing fieldwork is a freedom from home and work that feels good because it is actually sanctioned "work." But for me, doing fieldwork is also an obligation, because the people with whom I work are people I call "family" and who call me the same. I have a need to stay in touch and be involved, and an obligation to my own children, who consider Ngukurr to be a kind of home—a place filled with family members and friends.

In addition to missing my Indigenous family and friends, my grieving for the field during the restricted travel associated with COVID-19 (from March 2020 until January 2021 for entry into the Northern Territory, with restrictions still persisting as of the time of writing for entry into remote Indigenous communities) was about my loss of identity as an ethnographer. What was I, if I couldn't do my work? But work was only part of it; I also felt a deep longing to be in that particular place—to feel it, smell it, hear it, live it. My feelings of loss were intense, and were amplified by the fact that the gulf could not be effectively breached through communication technology.

The Archive as an Ethnographic Past

The lockdown period slowed everyday routines and allowed time to think. Daphne's words "Ngukurr is everywhere" were our impetus to think in a new way: What are the stories about Ngukurr? We were particularly looking for stories about people from Ngukurr who had influence in the wider Australian community. Where are these stories kept and how could we and the community re-engage with them? This was work we *could* do, even from a distance. We were inspired by Michael Jackson's (2007) *Excursions,* wherein he wrote that the skills you acquire as an anthropologist can be used in a variety of contexts, even if extended fieldwork is not possible. As we tell our first-year students, once you practice observation and start thinking anthropologically, it's very difficult to stop. You become alert to juxtapositions of sounds, colors, ideas, words, and images, the intersections of biography and memory, the process of making the strange familiar and the familiar strange. And you become open to new insights and surprises, and to considering the gaps between what is observed and experienced and what is written. These practices and insights make the everyday world filled with the potential for storying and interpretation.

In our case, the familiar, everyday world became the library and a collection of archives; we decided to encounter the archive that contained information about Ngukurr as a world in itself and to consider it ethnographically. During COVID-19, rather than personally visiting institutional collections/archives, our "archival ethnography" (see Decker and MacKinlay 2020) involved multiple emails to collecting institutions and online database searches to access collections holding Ngukurr material culture and other information. This information had been "locked up" for 100 years or more, and made even more difficult to access due to imposed COVID-19 "lock downs."

Working with and being led by the Ngukurr community to reclaim their stories from the archives is an enlivening process, one connected to the enduring nature of stories in Aboriginal communities throughout Australia. For thousands of years, stories have transmitted knowledge across generations and cultural groups. This knowledge is connected to the past, located in the present, and is also future-oriented (Balla 2016). Since colonization, Aboriginal stories have frequently been collected, controlled, and circulated through non-Indigenous institutions, including museums, libraries, and universities, often excluding Aboriginal perspectives (Thorpe 2017).

With fresh excitement, we designed a new project using a combination of ethnography, life history interviews, and archival research that seeks to tell the stories of how people from a small community continue to disproportionately influence Australian society through their initiatives, travels, and engagements. Aboriginal influence has always been present in Australian non-Indigenous culture, through music, art, movies, and the land (although these representations have often been co-opted in various ways through the discourses of settler colonialism [Senior et al. 2021]). Historical stories about individual achievements are centered around justice and land rights and on Aboriginal activists such as Charlie Perkins, Vincent Lingari, and Eddie Mabo—all three of whom made significant contributions to furthering Aboriginal rights. However, stories that did not make the national headlines are often much hider to find, buried in academic and local information sources.

This project requires a multi-disciplinary approach, so in addition to our ethnographic engagement, we have, over time, developed a team of Indigenous and non-Indigenous anthropologists, historians, and community leaders who worked with Ngukurr community members to understand the legacy of these stories and to find ways to both preserve and use them as catalysts for working with young people in the community as they think about their own futures. This has become a three-year Australian Research Council Indigenous Discovery Project (200100042), located at the University of Melbourne. Led by Wiradjuri creative writer and scholar Associate Professor Jeanine Leane, it explores storytelling as archive-making.

Ngukurr, situated in southeast Arnhem Land in the Northern Territory of Australia, is usually preceded by the descriptor "remote." It is true that Ngukurr is geographically remote from the perspective of many Australians, being a full day's drive from the capital city of Darwin and 350 km from the nearest sizable town of Katherine. But "remote" also implies cultural difference, isolation, and otherness (Hinkson and Smith 2005). These characterizations are reinforced by cultural materials, archives, and historical texts held by institutions outside of Ngukurr in Southern Australia and overseas. These objects and artifacts exclude the perspectives and stories of those to whom they relate. The dominant narrative about Ngukurr perpetuates a story about isolation that focuses on a settled place of location, rather than on a community as a base for extensive movement and transfusion of ideas. For example, an important transfusion of ideas came through the association of many Ngukurr people with the Australian Communist Party in the 1960s and 1970s, with a focus on equal pay for workers and obtaining rights to land. These particular stories were not isolated to the community or even to the Northern Territory, but became an important unifying theme across Australia and internationally (Boughton 2001).

Positive stories about Ngukurr (rightly) focus on the perpetuation of culture and language, the enduring kinship system, and the importance of people's connection to the land and to Dreamings. Other stories—the sorts of stories perpetuated in the mainstream media—tell of continuing disadvantage, poor health, and poor educational outcomes. Common to both discourses is the sense that they are bounded within a community, and that this community is distinctly different from other places in Australia.

Narratives about remote Indigenous communities are largely framed by modernist constructions of culture that "[begin] with the bracketing of all that is contemporary" (Sullivan 2005: 192). Such constructions obscure the histories of remote—and ancient—Aboriginal communities that tell of ways in which people have innovated and engaged with the broader Australian society. The term "intercultural" refers to an approach that considers Indigenous and non-Indigenous social forms as relational, as being part of a singular relational field (Hinkinson and Smith 2005:158). The intercultural history of Ngukurr and its inhabitants' contacts with the broader Australian society have not received attention in academic discourse, yet this is an important history that is both long and complex, and needs to be fully understood.

Some impactful stories are of national significance, such as the story of Dexter Daniel's trade unionism and his key role in the Wave Hill Walk-off in the 1970s. Daniels talked to the elders working in many of the cattle stations and supported them to go on strike for equal pay and land rights. He was engaged in speaking tours of major Australian cities and internationally, and an ASIO (Australian Security Intelligence Organisation) file on suspicion of communism for his efforts was created about him (Bern 1976; Kimber 2011).

Other actions of local people resonated strongly, such as the determination of many Ngukurr residents to go to Deakin University to obtain teaching qualifications in order to Aboriginalize this Ngukurr educational institution and to ensure that all staff are Aboriginal people (Senior 2003). Other narratives in Ngukurr describe people's working relationships with various research institutes that regularly employ local Aboriginal people as research assistants, but less frequently involve them in dissemination of research findings at national and international conferences. Some stories remain at the family level, and include the web of interconnections that people have built and maintained with families in locations across Australia.

Remembering Stories from the Past and the Present

A project of this kind that remembers people from the past might not have been previously possible, due to the general Aboriginal cultural restriction on speaking the names of people who have died. This restriction, however, has always been partial in Ngukurr; for example, the airport and the hospital are both named in honor of deceased residents. Recently, there has been a surge of interest in remembering people and their stories that has frequently been supported through the rapid uptake of social media by Aboriginal communities (Carlson and Frazer 2018). This uptake is encapsulated in the work of local artists, who have been recreating scenes from historical events, often posting the progress of their artmaking on social media. Local people have also engaged with photographs taken from 1935–1942 by Donald Thompson, taking pleasure in finding images of their relatives and sharing stories about them (see Thomson 2005).

Telling Stories from the Archives

For Aboriginal people, galleries, libraries, archives, and museums (the "GLAM" sector) have historically been contested sites because they position themselves as the "experts" on Indigenous culture and heritage, while asserting colonialist/Western ideas about a hierarchical taxonomy of "race" and culture (Peterson et al. 2008). More recently, there have been concerted efforts by Indigenous communities globally to intervene in their archives, moving towards self-determining and decolonizing approaches that support Indigenous knowledge systems, with the intention of gaining control of and providing appropriate access to Indigenous cultural heritage

(Janke 2019). For the Ngukurr community, there have been minimal opportunities to access their cultural heritage, located "elsewhere," as information relating to their collections is relatively inaccessible and removed from the lived realities of people in the community. Our project has the potential to promote many opportunities for different forms of renewed interest in stories/events from the past, while impacting contemporary culture-making through intergenerational knowledge exchange, as well as through accessing and reclaiming archival collections (see Kral 2020; Treloyn 2013).

Unexpected Stories from the Ngukurr Archive

Our holistic approach to the archive, and making sure that we allowed time for deep immersion and for following interesting stories as they emerged, provided opportunities for unexpected findings. In part, this deep immersion was forced upon us by COVID-19. No longer able to spend time in our field, we followed the discussion initiated by our friends in Ngukurr and the cultural artifacts we had seen before COVID-19. We sent materials to certain people in Ngukurr; they in turn went out into the community and asked their friends and families about the objects and stories we had found in the archives. Stories were expanded as people re-membered the past and started to plan to re-engage more closely with the issues raised and objects discovered. At the time of writing, we have been able to follow two specific stories that trace the interconnections and influences of people and things from Ngukurr across Australia.

In Melbourne, a visit to Museums Victoria before COVID-19 uncovered a set of flowers made from feathers. Our Ngukurr colleagues, one of whom was able to accompany us on our visit, did not know what they were, but we took photographs of them, which we sent back to the community. An elder upon seeing them knew exactly what they were; he remembered his mother making them under the guidance of one of the missionaries. With this information, we were able to trace the flowers back to an enduring tradition of feather flower-making in southeast Australia, linked to Arnhem Land, most probably to a non-Indigenous nurse, Ruth Hancock, who was located in the Ngukurr region in the 1930s. Ruth grew up with Aboriginal craftspeople in South Australia and may have learned the skill from them, later taking the feather flower technique to Ngukurr (Hughes 2005). From what our research has uncovered to date, we anticipate that the feather flower skills were most likely transmitted on to missionaries in Ngukurr, who supported feather flower making due to their desire to cultivate craftwork within the community as part of a profit-making enterprise (Edmonds 2020; Edmonds et al 2021).

In April 2021, when travel was again possible, Daphne Daniels and artist Karen Rogers visited the Museum again to see the flowers, and then visited the Koori Heritage Trust, which is an Aboriginal cultural center located in the middle of Melbourne dedicated to preserving and continuing the art and culture of Aboriginal people from southeast Australia (see Faulkhead and Berg 2010 for further information). This Trust has a collection of at least 800 feather flowers, made predominantly by Aboriginal women from southeast Australia dating from the early–mid twentieth century until now (see Figure 3.1). Daphne and Karen were then able to engage in a feather flower making workshop in Melbourne, with the Mutti Mutti/ Wemba Wemba/Boonwurrung/Yorta Yorta artist, Maree Clarke, a senior knowledge holder from southeast Australia, who has spent many years revivifying stories from museum collections around the world relating to the material culture of her ancestors (Thorner et al. 2018). Together the women (Karen, Daphne, and Maree) hope to work alongside others in the Ngukurr community to revive the tradition of feather flower making. Embedded in the fragile, softly colored petals of this craft is a story about the influence of the missions in Australia and about the interconnections of Indigenous peoples and craft traditions across thousands of kilometers and over time. It is also a story about a past that wasn't written down, but survives as an elder man's boyhood memory of his mother's craft work.

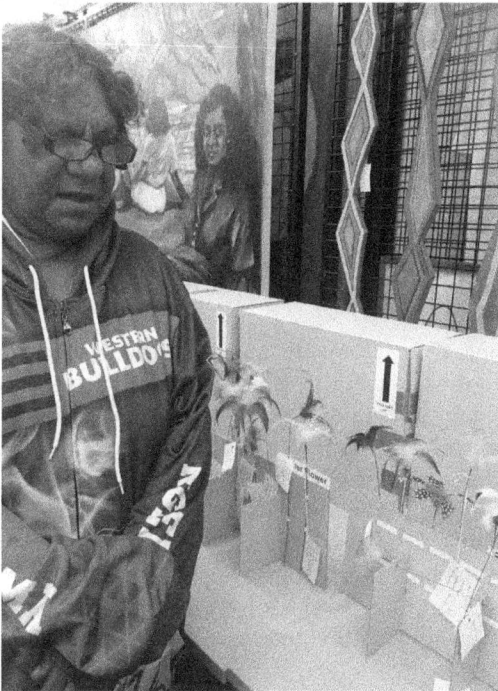

Figure 3.1 Karen Rogers exploring the Feather Flowers at the Koori Heritage Trust. Photograph by Kate Senior.

A very different type of story emerged in a small section of the University Library in Newcastle, New South Wales. The Cultural Collection there includes an archive of diaries and newspaper clippings collected by Merv and Janet Copley, members of the Australian Communist Party. This material recreates a rich description of what life was like in a regional Australian working-class town from the 1950s to the 1970s. Through these archives, it is possible to read the Copleys' emerging interest in the lives and situations of Indigenous peoples and their growing conviction of the importance of Aboriginal rights. They collected hundreds of newspaper clippings, which were eventually preserved in a file simply labeled "Aborigines 1960– 1970." As we immersed ourselves in the contents of these files, we found a personal connection, as the names Dexter and David Daniels leapt out at us—Daphne's great-uncle and her father. We knew that they were both activists, as we had already located Dexter's Australian Security Intelligence Organisation (ASIO) file. We hadn't known that there was a strong connection between Dexter Daniels and Newcastle. The Newcastle Unions raised money to support Dexter in his campaigns to address equal pay and land rights for Aboriginal people in northern Australia. Dexter marched in May Day rallies in Newcastle and is remembered by ex-members of the Australian Communist Party. Dexter's influence outside his own community is not well known in Ngukurr. As Karen said: "Nobody knows about what he did down here (in Newcastle)—it's important that people can know this story."

Karen and Daphne had the opportunity to work through the archive boxes (see Figure 3.2), and retrieved a great deal of information about their family members and their involvement in the struggle for equal rights for Aboriginal people. They were also able to talk to current Trades Union representatives in Newcastle to discuss ways to keep the story alive, so that people in Ngukurr and Australia could learn from it. Some ideas (which are still being worked out) include engaging Ngukurr artists to create a visual story of Dexter Daniels' struggles.

Karen and Daphne's trip to Melbourne and Newcastle from April 19–27, 2021 marked our first opportunity to re-engage in person with representatives from the Ngukurr community to explore the archive and its continuing meaning for the community. Yet travel between states in Australia is still fraught with uncertainty. On April 21, 2021, a man released from hotel quarantine traveled from Perth to Melbourne. On arrival, he found he was COVID-19 positive. All travelers at the QANTAS terminal at Melbourne airport between the hours of 6:30 and 7:30 pm were considered casual contacts and were required to self-isolate until they received a negative test result. Daphne and Karen caught a plane from Melbourne to Newcastle at 7:50 pm. Later that night, the window of exposure was reduced to 7–7:30 pm and Daphne and Karen were clear (so we thought) to travel home to Darwin. In this case, there was no consistent policy or

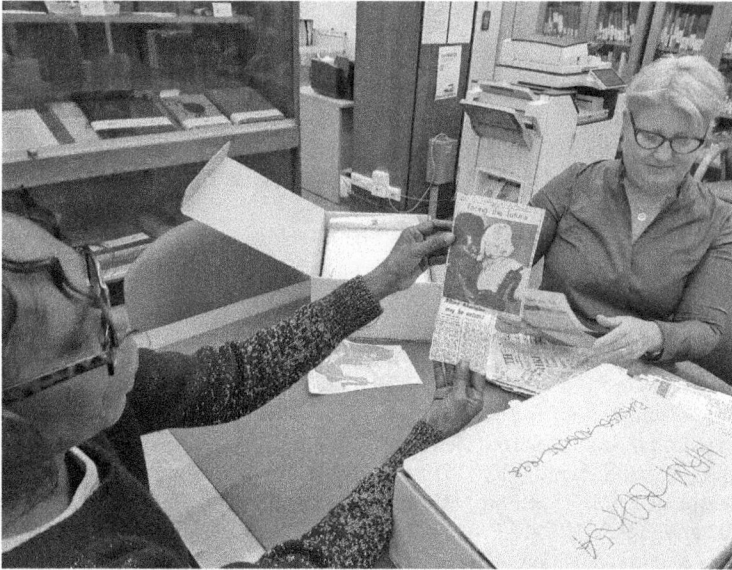

Figure 3.2 Daphne Daniels and Kate Senior exploring the Copley Archive. Photograph by Paige Wright, University of Newcastle Library. Used with permission.

evidence of communication between the states, and the Northern Territory still maintained the previous window of 6:30–7:30 as the exposure period. Daphne and Karen were detained at the airport and sent into compulsory self-isolation until they received a negative test result. This was an inglorious end to a highly successful trip and is a reminder of the continuing difficulties of maintaining links with communities across Australia.

Conclusion: Retelling the Stories

Drawing on our autoethnographic experiences of what could have been "the end of fieldwork" for us, we worked constantly to negotiate COVID-19 and to make sense of life under uncertain circumstances. Thus, rather than being the end of fieldwork, that period defined by COVID-19 marked a new beginning in our work with the Ngukurr community. The opportunities to engage with various archives, along with the time to follow leads and wormholes, opened up opportunities for us to discover new (to us) stories and to follow the interconnections between biography and history that we can now perceive, thanks to COVID. It is our hope that we will soon be able to return these stories to Ngukurr, and that the project of re-telling these stories, so that they can be re-encoded in societal memory, can begin.

References

Ardener, E. 2012. "Remote areas": Some theoretical considerations. *HAU: Journal of Ethnographic Theory*, 2(1): 519–588.

Balla, P. 2016. "Sovereignty: Inalienable and Intimate." *Sovereignty*. Australia: Australian Centre for Contemporary Art, pp. 11–16.

Baum, F., Newman, L., and Biedrzycki, K. 2014. Vicious cycles: Digital technologies and determinants of health in Australia. *Health Promotion International*, 29(2): 349–360.

Bern, J. 1976. Reaction to attrition: The Ngukurr strike of 1970. *Mankind*, 10(4): 213–220.

Boughton, B. 2001. "The Communist Party of Australia's Involvement in the Struggle for Aborginal and Torres Strait Islander People's Rights 1920–1970," in R Markey (ed.), *Labour and History: Historical Essays*. Wollongong: University of Wollongong Press, pp. 263–294.

Carlson, B., and Frazer, F. 2018. Yarning circles and social media activism. *Media International Australia*, 169(1): 43–53.

Chenhall, R., and Senior, K. 2017. Living the social determinants of health: Assemblages in a remote Aboriginal community. *Medical Anthropology Quarterly*, 32(2): 177–195.

Decker, S., and McKinlay, A. 2020. "Archival Ethnography," in R. Mir and A-L. Fayar (eds.), *The Routledge Companion to Anthropology and Business*. London: Routledge, pp. 14–31.

Edmonds, F. 2020. "Feather Flowers and Photographs." *Pursuit*. Melbourne: University of Melbourne pursuit.unimelb.edu.au/articles/feather-flowers-and-photographs

Edmonds, F., Clarke, M., Senior, K., and Daniels, D. 2021. "Feather Flowers, 'Home' and a Global Pandemic: Collaborative Storytelling and the Relationality of Things," in A. Harris, M.E. Luka, and A. Markham (eds.), *Massive/Micro Autoethnography: Creative Learning in COVID Times*. New York: Springer Publishing.

Faulkhead, S., and Berg, J. 2010. *Power and the Passion: Our Ancestors Return Home*. Melbourne: Koorie Heritage Trust Inc.

Hinkson, M., and Smith, B. 2005. Introduction: Conceptual moves towards an intercultural analysis. *Oceania*, 75(3): 157–166.

Hughes, K. 2005. "Same Bodies, Different Skin: Ruth Heathcock," in A. Cole, V. Haskins, and F. Paisley (eds.), *Uncommon Ground, White Women in Aboriginal History*. Canberra, Aboriginal Studies Press, pp. 83–107.

Hunter, B.H., and Radoll, P.J. 2020. Dynamics of digital diffusion and disadoption: A longitudinal analysis of Indigenous and other Australians. *Australasian Journal of Information Systems*, 24(1805): 1–21.

Jackson, M. 2007. *Excursions*. Durham, NC and London: Duke University Press.

Janke, T. 2019. *First Peoples: A Roadmap for Enhancing Indigenous Engagement in Museums and Galleries*. Canberra: Australian Museums and Galleries Associations Inc.

Kral, I. 2020. "Divided Digital Practices: A Story Australasian Indigenous Australia," in E. Morrell and J. Rowsell (eds.), *Stories from Inequity to Justice in Literacy: Confronting Digital Divides*. New York: Routledge, pp. 34–50.

Kimber, J. 2011. "'That's Not Right': Indigenous Politics, Dexter Daniels and 1968," in M. Nolan (ed.), *Labour History and Its People: The 12th Biennial National*

Labour History Conference, Australian National University 15–17 September 2011, Canberra: Australian Society for the Study of Labour History Canberra Region Branch, pp. 153–164.

Peterson, N., Allen, L., and Hamby, L. 2008. *The Makers and Making of Indigenous Australian Museum Collections*. Melbourne: Melbourne University Publishing.

Senior, K. 2003. *A Gudbala Laif? Health and Wellbeing in a Remote Aboriginal Community— What Are the Problems and Where Lies Responsibility?* Canberra: Australian National University PhD thesis.

Senior, K., Chenhall, R., Hall, J., and Daniels, D. 2018. Re-thinking the health benefits of outstations in remote Indigenous Australia. *Health and Place*, 52: 1–7.

Sullivan, P. 2005. Searching for the intercultural, searching for the culture. *Oceania*, 75(3): 183–194. doi.org/10.1002/j.1834-4461.2005.tb02879.x

Thomson, D. 2005. *Donald Thompson in Arnhem Land*, compiled by N. Peterson (ed.), Melbourne: Melbourne University Press.

Thorner, S., Edmonds, F., Clarke, M., and Balla, P. 2018. Maree's backyard: Intercultural collaborations for Indigenous sovereignty in Melbourne. *Oceania*, 88(3): 269–291.

Thorpe, K. 2017. *Aboriginal Community Archives, Research in the Archival Multiverse*. Melbourne: Melborne University Press.

Treloyn, S., Charles, R.G., and Nulgit, S. 2013. "Repatriation of Song Materials to Support Intergenerational Transmission of Knowledge about Language in the Kimberley Region of Northwest Australia", in M.J. Norris, E. Anonb and M-O. Junker (eds.), *Endangered Languages Beyond Boundaries: Proceedings of the 17th Foundation of Endangered Languages Conference*. Bath, UK: Foundation for Endangered Languages, pp. 18–24.

Part II

Conceptualizing and Negotiating the Pandemic Across Professions, Cultures, and Countries

4 "As Soon as People See You Cough, They Say You Have the Disease"

Negotiating COVID-Related Stigma and Health-Seeking Behaviors in Kenya

Violet Barasa

Introduction

Since the onset of the coronavirus pandemic in China in late 2019, the world has experienced unprecedented and far-reaching economic and social impacts. In low- and middle-income countries (LMICs), these impacts have been greater, due to pre-existing poverty and its accompanying conditions such as overcrowding, poor access to water and sanitation, and weak healthcare systems that become quickly overwhelmed by rising cases of infections (Farmer and Sen 2003; Leach and Dry 2010; Leach 2017; Ali and Ali 2020). However, as with other high-profile infections, response mechanisms overall tend to be rooted in purely biomedically driven measures such as lockdowns, quarantines, and testing and administering vaccines. Unfortunately, this often means that socio-economic dynamics such as stigma and its impacts on health inequalities receive little attention, despite their enormous burdens on people's lives. Stigma intersects with other forms of social inequalities to exacerbate the negative impacts of disease on vulnerable populations (Roelen et al. 2020).

In Kenya, for example, healthcare facilities throughout the country have reported a sharp fall in the number of patients attending hospitals and clinics for the treatment of non-COVID diseases since the outbreak hit in early March 2020 (Ayoyi 2020). This situation has mainly been blamed on the social stigma associated with coronavirus infection, which often leaves patients and their families more traumatized than the disease itself (ibid.; see also WHO 2020 on how stigma impacts health-seeking behaviors). Some media outlets have reported on doctors and nurses refusing to attend patients with high temperatures due to the association of fever with COVID-19 (KTN 2020), yet fever can also be a symptom of numerous other bacterial and viral infections (Feikin et al. 2011), and as John Crump (2014) rightly observed, fever is a leading reason for people to seek healthcare in the tropics.

DOI: 10.4324/9781003187462-7

For those living with chronic illness, COVID-related stigma has affected the ways in which they seek treatment. My own mother suffers from chronic comorbidities and the pandemic has fallen especially heavy on her. She was turned away numerous times from the health facility that she previously frequented as a high blood pressure (HBP) patient, either because the clinicians were afraid that her HBP reading was a symptom of COVID-19, or there were simply no healthcare personnel at the hospital—perhaps too afraid to come to work in case they caught the dreaded virus. Thus she had to manage her symptoms at home using over-the-counter-medications, which undoubtedly left her health in worse condition.

My mother's experiences with health services are not isolated. The stigma surrounding COVID-19 in Kenya, fueled by rumors and misinformation, has led to many people changing how they seek treatment for medical issues. Some Kenyans mused on social media about how little they had heard from family and friends reporting illness of any kind during the year 2020. Many suspected that ill people and their families chose to keep news of an illness private due to the risk of *any* kind of illness being associated with the coronavirus. As one person put it on their social media feed, "Nowadays in the Matatus [public transport minibuses in Kenya], if I have to cough, I hold my breath in for some time so that the cough does not come out, because as soon as people see you cough, they say you have the disease."

In this chapter, I first introduce the concept of stigma and situate it within health and illness research, exploring some key literature that highlights how stigma has shaped societies' responses to public health emergencies in times of epidemics and pandemics. I review the example of Ebola in West Africa to draw comparisons around how stigma shapes societal responses to these emergencies, including in the current pandemic. I then highlight some examples of the impact of stigma on mental health, drawing on the Great Influenza pandemic as it affected Europe and North America and the SARS epidemic as it affected Asia, and link these to the literature suggesting rising mental health issues in the present pandemic. I then present the case study of Kenya, looking at drivers of stigma and how it has shaped health-seeking behaviors in the context of COVID-19 containment measures. I conclude by providing some recommendations for beneficial policies and practices.

Methods and Materials

My data collection drew on personal accounts, including that of my mother and how her vulnerability, resulting from several medical complications, put her at heightened risk of facing stigma during the COVID-19 pandemic in Kenya. I also draw from first-hand accounts of two friends who posted on Facebook about being stigmatized after returning to Kenya from the United Kingdom and Dubai respectively, because these places were known to be experiencing high infection rates for COVID-19. My cyber-ethnographic sources came from multiple media reports about stigma within health facilities in Kenya that led to patients being neglected by healthcare providers due to fear of potential viral transmission. Further, I explored reports in the media on police brutality during the lockdowns and its highly negative impact on healthcare-seeking behaviors, particularly for at-risk populations. I also searched the Internet for articles and blog entries that highlighted the impact of stigma as experienced by individuals and/or their families.

My thematic analysis involved reviewing the various sources of material and noting converging and diverging themes, using an iterative process until the themes were firmly established. My findings point to two main drivers of stigma in the context of Kenya: inadequate access to healthcare for at-risk populations, and misinformation and lack of health literacy in the population, including among government officials and biomedical professionals.

Situating Stigma in Health and Illness

The concept of stigma is well established in the literature. Stigma represents what is viewed as a characteristic outside of the norm, and which attracts disapproval or discreditation of an individual or a group within a given sociocultural context (Goffman 1963; Link and Phelan 2001; Bos et al. 2013). Link and Phelan (2001) define "stigma" as the co-occurrence of four processes: (1) labeling human differences; (2) stereotyping such differences; (3) separating those labeled from "us"; and (4) status loss of and discrimination against those labeled. This discrimination can be direct, as in humiliation and name-calling, or it can be indirect and subtle—for example as experienced through exclusion, shunning, and avoidance of contact with the stigmatized person. Those at the receiving end of stigma often experience feelings of shame, self-devaluation, and a crisis of identity and belonging. As Pescosolido (2013) additionally showed, stigma can be a mark of disgrace that sets a person apart from others, with huge implications for the stigmatized individuals and/or groups. Stigma has long been associated with patterns of inequality and injustice. And as Mulea and colleagues (2009) have shown, stigma can have far-reaching consequences for those experiencing it. According to Matthew Claire (2018: 454), stigma may have evolutionary roots, serving "sociobiological functions by categorizing and excluding individuals who may threaten a community through the spread of disease or perceived social disorder." Although it is mostly individuals or smaller groups who suffer stigmatization, even whole countries can be stigmatized, as was shown for Sweden by Rachel Irwin in Chapter 2 of this volume.

In the context of health, studies have shown that stigma is indeed often experienced by those affected by disease, including patients and healthcare workers and their families and friends. In epidemic and pandemic situations, stigmatization leads to people being labeled, stereotyped and discriminated against due to their perceived association with the disease, which can include personal or work-related exposure, and/or vulnerability due to pre-existing illness, disability, or old age (WHO 2020b; Ramaci et al. 2020). The World Health Organization (WHO 2020b: 1) has recommended guidelines for addressing COVID-related stigma, as it acknowledges that: "Stigma can negatively affect those with the disease, as well as their caregivers, family, friends and communities. People who don't have the disease but share other characteristics with this group may also suffer from stigma."

Stigma greatly hampers efforts to contain disease outbreaks, as people experiencing symptoms may not attend health facilities due to fear of being stigmatized both inside and outside of these settings. Roulene and colleagues (2020) rightly argue that stigma puts up barriers to treatment-seeking and undermines adherence to treatment, which inevitably leads to negative health outcomes among those affected. Having accurate data on COVID-19 cases is essential for understanding the national and global burden of the disease and management practices and preventive efforts, yet stigma can cause people to hide illness symptoms and not disclose crucial information regarding their human contact history (ibid.), thereby exacerbating viral transmission. Stigma can also, as Peprah and Gyasi (2020) observed, become a motivator for people to delay healthcare seeking and can discourage the adoption of healthy behaviors.

During the Ebola epidemic in West Africa (2014–2016), patients, their families, and the healthcare workers who attended them experienced severe forms of stigma, including being shunned by friends and colleagues at workplaces, schools, and churches; being refused service at shops; and being excluded from social events (ERAP 2014; Karamouzian and Hategekimana 2014). Pepra and Gyasi (2020) have studied the socio-economic impacts of COVID-19. Their research shows that the pandemic and its concomitant contagions have resulted in prejudices and in community rejection and intense stigma against people of Asian backgrounds living in the USA and Europe because the virus originated in China. Across Sub Saharan Africa, evidence is emerging of pervasive social stigmatization of people who have recovered from COVID-19 and their families. Studies such as that of Adom and Mensah (2020) and Asare (2020) show that stigma and discriminatory behaviors are directed towards frontline healthcare workers (HCWs) and the most at-risk populations, including the elderly and chronically ill persons in Ghana. As Karamouzian and Hategekimana (2014) demonstrated, this trend is similar to the stigmatization of Ebola survivors in Nigeria, Sierra Leone, Guinea, and Liberia.

Stigma directed towards HCWs causes higher levels of stress and burnout, compromising their ability to care for patients. In Italy, for example, Ramaci and colleagues (2020) studied the impacts of stigma on HCWs at the height of a surge in COVID infections in the country in early 2020 and found that workers experienced stigma from family members and friends, who feared they were being put at risk of passing on infections to others. These authors argue that it is therefore essential to understand the effects of stigma, related to the intensity and frequency of exposure to the ongoing pandemic, job demands and self-esteem, and its impacts on HCWs' outcomes. In particular, it is essential to investigate whether these variables are potentially capable of producing changes to the quality of professional life.

(Ramaci et al. 2020: 2)

COVID-19-related stigma has generated barriers to contact tracing, prompt testing, and treatment in many countries, particularly in Sub Saharan Africa (Asare 2020; Ghana News Agency 2020), where people's levels of health literacy are low (see Chapter 6). This too can lead to underreporting of COVID-19 cases and contribute to fatalities (Pepra and Gyasi 2020).

Numerous media reports across the African continent document incidences where people suspected of having COVID-19 or those who have recovered from the disease have been ejected from their homes and shunned by the public, and one was publicly lynched. This horrific incident was perpetrated on a middle-aged man with a history of convulsions, who lived in the Kenya-Uganda border town of Malava; he was lynched by an angry mob after being accused of being a "super-spreader" of the virus, despite the victim not having been tested for COVID-19. In another instance, a young man who spent time in the hospital with COVID-19 symptoms reported being treated as an outcast by his neighbors after completing treatment and returning home. In an interview, the man described how "screaming ambulances sent to pick him up from home with medics dressed like astronauts did not help the situation," as this not only traumatized the children but also publicly advertised his COVID-positive status to the entire neighborhood (Waruru 2020: 1).

The WHO has acknowledged that stigma is a major problem that has been slowing efforts to contain the pandemic in Kenya and across Africa. WHO's COVID-Incident Manager for Africa, Ngoy Nsenga, remarked that "stigma in the community is a distracting factor hindering interventions to contain the spread. People might hide for fear or refuse seeking treatment even when they have coronavirus-like symptoms, endangering themselves and others" (WHO 2020b: 12).

Stigma and Mental Health Issues

Mounting evidence suggests a correlation between COVID-related stigma and a rise in mental health problems. The experiences of individuals discharged from quarantine and self-isolation across the world show that many of them suffer from some form of mental health issues resulting from a mix of emotions of anxiety and feelings of worthlessness due to not being able to participate in nor contribute to the running of the household, especially when isolating for long periods of time (WHO 2020a; Javed et al. 2020). Peprah and Gyasi (2020) also show that recovered patients find it difficult to integrate back into their communities, as they may still have to practice caution, particularly when around elderly relatives. Feelings of helplessness, anger, and sadness have also been reported among recovered COVID patients, sometimes resulting from broken relationships, as loved ones may harbor unfounded fears of contracting the disease from personal contact (ibid). According to Ramaci and colleagues (2020), stigma and discrimination may tend to persist in the long term, even after quarantines have ended and the epidemic has been contained. This persistence may result from an ongoing loss of status: once stigma is attached to a given person, it is challenging and complicated to undo; thus, even after the original reason for their stigmatization has disappeared (if it does), it may take quite a long time for their former social status to be restored (if it ever is) (Link and Phelan 2001).

Bao and colleagues (2020) have urged governments to prioritize mental healthcare in their strategies to combat COVID-19, as there is strong evidence to suggest that suicide rates often increase during pandemics. For example, Wasserman (1992) showed that deaths by suicide increased in the USA during the 1918–1919 Great Influenza pandemic. Cheung and colleagues (2008) also found that suicide rates increased in Hong Kong during the severe acute respiratory syndrome (SARS) epidemic.

While true figures on suicide rates during the current pandemic are yet to be established, some researchers are urging caution based on these experiences with previous pandemics. For example, in their article on "Suicide Risk and Prevention during the COVID-19 Pandemic," Gunell and colleagues (2020) highlight how stigmatized people with psychiatric disorders may witness worsening of symptoms due to loneliness, anxiety, depression, and post-traumatic stress disorder (PTSD), which can lead to suicide. Roelen and colleagues (2020) urge integration and consideration of the socio-cultural, economic, and political contexts in which transmissions occur to enhance understandings of the impacts of diseases on different people in different places. While some measures, such as forced quarantines and physical distancing, may be well-meaning, these can cause severe distress that may lead to heightened mental health problems, particularly in people who already experience these issues.

Drivers of COVID-19-Related Stigma in Kenya and Their Impacts

In this section, I review the official responses to COVID-19 by the Kenyan government, in order to explore how these responses may have exacerbated social stigma for patients and their families, including impacts on health-seeking behaviors for rural people suffering from comorbidities. I include a personal account from my mother to exemplify how her experiences reflect the broader impacts of COVID-19 on rural health-seeking behaviors in Kenya.

Access to Health Services for At-Risk Populations

There is plenty of evidence showing that public health emergencies and the strategies to contain them cause fear and anxiety among the population, especially among those at the greatest risk of contagion. Perhaps more importantly, such emergencies divert attention and resources away from other serious health issues such as chronic conditions, particularly in LMICs where these conditions are overrepresented (Correia 2020).

In Kenya, since March 13, 2020 when the first case of COVID-19 was reported there (Kagwe 2020), the government initiated measures to contain the spread of the virus. These measures included the cessation of movement, night curfews, requirements for citizens to stay at home, and a ban on all forms of gatherings. Law enforcement officers were deployed to ensure that the public adhered to these measures, and frequently, they beat people and arrested those found to be in violation of these regulations.

However, major risk factors for mortality from COVID-19, including comorbidities (diabetes, hypertension, respiratory diseases, cardiovascular disease, etc.), are common in Kenya, as is the case across LMICs, and these have put at-risk populations at even greater risk due to the government's containment measures (Ahmed et al. 2020). Ahmed and colleagues (2020) studied the impacts of lockdowns on access to healthcare in informal settlements in Africa and Asia; they found that access to all healthcare services decreased during COVID-19 lockdowns. They highlighted barriers to health-seeking as including increased costs of healthcare; reduced household income; increased challenges in physically reaching healthcare facilities; and people's fears of infection and stigmatization.

At the hospitals, a simple temperature check (see Figure 4.1) became a criterion for admitting patients into the dreaded COVID isolation wards.

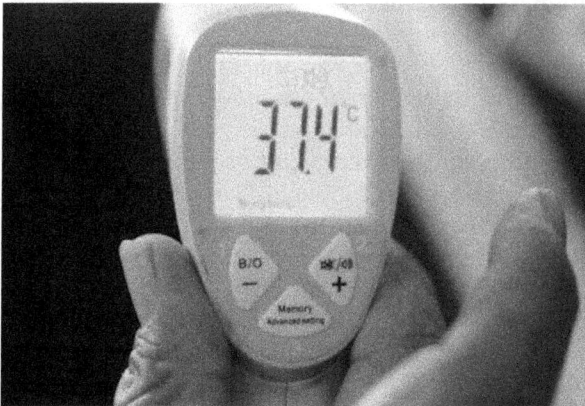

Figure 4.1 An Infrared Thermometer Showing the Presence of Fever. Public domain photo.

Nurses were said to have routinely sent anyone with a temperature above 37 degrees Celsius to these wards, even when there were no other accompanying symptoms associated with coronavirus infection. One woman told *The Standard Newspaper* of the moment her temperature check turned into a medical frenzy at a health facility that she attended for her regular ante-natal check-up. She recalled, "The nurse said my temperature was 37 degrees Celsius, so I must have it [the coronavirus]. So she sent me to this dark room where there were three other people. I was the only pregnant woman there. Nobody came to see us until I ran away after about an hour of waiting" (quoted in Awindi 2020: 22).

Obviously, a suspected fever alone cannot guarantee that someone will test positive for COVID-19. While the presence of fever is a major disease symptom (WHO 2020b), it is nonetheless a non-distinguishing syndrome, as it can also signal a variety of other diseases that share symptoms with COVID-19, such as tuberculosis, pneumonia, bronchitis, the common flu, and pulmonary embolism (ibid). In Kenya, patients who could be suffering from these other diseases have found themselves held in quarantine facilities, only for their test results to come back negative. This has adversely impacted their health-seeking behaviors and those of many others who hear their stories, with health facilities across the country recording a significant fall in the number of patients presenting with respiratory syndromes.

I now present as an example the case of my own mother, who suffers from a host of chronic illnesses and who, pre-COVID, frequently visited nearby medical facilities in her hometown; she recounted to me how COVID-related stigma has impacted her treatment-seeking habits:

Since the beginning of this illness in Kenya, it has been terrible for me because of my fever and breathing issues due to hypertension. I have been on medication for hypertension for a long time, and I always know that when my breathing becomes heavy, I go to the hypertension clinic in the hospital [there is a weekly clinic run at her local hospital where she gets her prescription for managing the condition]. But corona changed everything; now people say I breathe heavily because I have corona. When I go to the hospital, the doctor says he cannot see me because the nurse said my temperature is too high, that I need to be tested for corona. But for me, nothing has changed in my symptoms, they are the same as before corona. So I don't understand why they [doctors, nurses, community] associate them with corona.

During the first lockdown [April 2020], the hospital could not take me in on a number of occasions because the blood pressure clinic was shut due to a lack of doctors. As I had run out of my regular medication, I tried to purchase them in the pharmacy at the hospital but the supplies had been interrupted due to transport bans between Nairobi and Webuye [Webuye is her hometown], so I went without medicine for weeks. I became seriously ill and was rushed to the hospital one night, but when we reached the hospital, the doctor fled because I was breathing so heavily and my body was hot. I was abandoned in the examination room for 5 hours before a nurse came and told me that I needed to get a COVID test. By the time we left the hospital [without any COVID test, medical check-up, or prescription], it was already late into curfew hours, which meant that we could get into trouble with the police if found traveling. It was all too much, and at home, the neighbors started avoiding me because they thought I must have had COVID to have gone to hospital during curfew hours. I was very scared and anxious the whole time and simply prayed that the lockdown would be lifted soon.

I ask my mother what she thinks will happen after the pandemic is over, if ever, and she continues:

> I cannot look at the doctors the same way again, or the people who have said I have corona. I think it is unkind to label people like me, who are ill and already suffering. It is difficult, and the sooner this thing ends, the better for people like me to resume access to health services. I hope it ends soon, and that I will be alive long enough to prove that I did not have COVID.
>
> (Personal communication, April 2, 2021)

My mother's account is echoed in multiple other experiences of people with medical emergencies and chronic illnesses dealing with stigma in the face of COVID lockdowns in Kenya. National and international media have run numerous news articles describing how people with medical emergencies, including women in labor, died as a result of not being able to access appropriate healthcare due to physical distances and the blanket ban on travel during curfew hours. Although health facilities did remain open, fear of being stigmatized, coupled with a lack of staff and shortage of medicines at the facilities during lockdowns, deterred patients from visiting these facilities. For example, the Associated Press described how pregnant women were at risk of death during Kenya's COVID-19 curfew (Odula 2020). The *Guardian* newspaper highlighted the police brutality that characterized COVID-19 curfews, where, as previously mentioned, police officers beat up people found to be breaking curfew rules, regardless of their reasons, even when travel was to access emergency medical attention (Namu and Rilley 2020).

These scenes, which were common across the country, seriously undermined efforts to combat viral spread, as they inadvertently became super-spreader events in themselves, with no social distancing or mask wearing taking place, revealing an extreme lack of health literacy among Kenyan government officials, who completely failed to think through the implications of their well-intended prevention policies and what forms their implementation should take.

Misinformation and Misconceptions

Stigma often thrives on misinformation and misconceptions about the unknown, leading to the apportioning of blame for disease transmission. For example, Boyce and Cataldo (2019) found that in Pakistan, symptoms of dementia were misconceived as being a normal part of aging, or as even resulting from the sufferers' misdeeds. These misconceptions resulted in stigma for people with these symptoms. In parts of Africa, including in Tanzania, children born with albinism—a skin condition that inhibits the body's absorption of melanin—are ostracized and the condition is often blamed on witchcraft, sorcery, or ancestral curses. People living with albinism can therefore face life-threatening stigma. In their investigation of the drivers of Albino killings in Tanzania, Burke and colleagues (2014) found that cultural beliefs and myths attribute magical powers and sub-human characteristics to people with Albinism, who are killed to meet a market for body parts believed to bring wealth and fortune.

Misinformation and misconceptions about disease causation shape public opinion, which perpetuates stigma (Nyblade et al. 2019). Rumors and conspiracy theories relating to COVID-19 are already widespread (Ali 2020; Correia et al. 2020; WHO 2020b; see also Chapters 6, 16, and 18, this volume). Some prominent politicians in Africa, including the late president Magufuli of Tanzania, caused controversy by encouraging people to pray against the virus, which he dubbed as "satanic" and one that could only be cured by "divine intervention" (Bariyo and Parkinson 2020). In the US state of Florida, authorities arrested an evangelical preacher, Rodney Horward-Browne, for refusing to call off religious services in his church—a violation of the statewide ban on large gatherings (ibid). In Nigeria and Sudan, the BBC reported that politicians were wearing gadgets believed to kill the coronavirus by releasing some kind of bleaching agent (BBC News 2020).

In Kenya, and especially among young people, COVID-19 has become *the* talking point for social media feeds that are awash with misinformation. Numerous memes have been generated poking fun at how the public has reacted to the pandemic, with many posters musing on how they no longer hear much news about family and friends being ill, due to the fear that any illness would make them become perceived as COVID-19 carriers.

Severe forms of stigma were directed especially at people who had recovered or were recovering from COVID-19. Peter Karagu, a 37-year-old Kenyan banker who went public about contracting the coronavirus, talked about how people he knew began treating him differently once they learned that he had recovered from COVID-19. Although it had been months after his full recovery, Karagu recounted that a local pharmacist refused to serve him and hurriedly shut the doors on him before embarking on the process of fumigating the entire pharmacy. He described his experience to a global health monitoring watchdog, Health Policy Watch:

> The reaction surprised me, the pharmacy owner knew me, so he had heard that I had been diagnosed with the disease. What really shocked me more is the fact that he and his workers were not just ordinary Kenyans, but medical professionals who should have known better.
>
> (Quoted in Waruru 2020: 1)

Karagu's statement about how this pharmacist "should have known better" reflects the lack of health literacy in Kenya even among medical professionals—also exhibited in their blanket approach of treating everyone with a temperature as having COVID-19, as described above.

Stigma in Kenya is also directed at anyone with a recent travel history to countries known to have high infection rates. For example, in one Facebook feed that attracted thousands of comments, a 27-year-old woman who traveled back into the country from the UK in March 2020 was ostracized by her close family and friends, and even after completing a mandatory 2-week quarantine, her close friend refused to pick her up from the hotel room where she had been quarantining. Upon arriving home, her family kept her isolated in their maize storage room for an additional two weeks for fear of contracting a disease for which she had not been diagnosed (Aloyi, Blogpost, July 22, 2020). Another traveler who had been to Dubai in May 2020 was branded a "COVID super-spreader" and was publicly mocked when she left her home to buy groceries at the nearby market, after completing a 14-day mandatory quarantine period. By her own account, she never experienced any symptoms associated with COVID-19 (Facebook feed, October 2020).

In Kakamega County Hospital in Kenya, a young woman who was due to give birth became a victim of coronavirus-related stigma when she was referred to a county referral facility for an emergency cesarean in June 2020. But the woman was abandoned by the doctors upon arrival at the facility because she was "coughing too much"; she later died from birth complications. She was posthumously diagnosed with pulmonary embolism, and tests for COVID-19 showed negative results (Ayoyi 2020). The woman's grieving mother lamented the negligence of the doctors, insisting that:

> They could have saved her life...But the doctors fled. They ignored her because she was coughing too much and they did not want to catch it from her. I pleaded with them to save my daughter, but they said they had to wait for the COVID-19 team to assess her symptoms
>
> (2020: 1)

As these experiences show, stigma can have profound impacts on people and their families, including long-term mental health impacts and even death (Gunell et al. 2020). Research shows that that stigma tends to persist during and post-epidemic, and therefore not paying attention to it as part of disease containment strategies could have both immediate and long-term deleterious public health impacts (Pepra and Gyasi 2020). Kenya's Health Ministry admitted that stigma was hindering efforts to contain the disease as community transmissions accelerated, particularly in rural areas where people refuse to submit to testing, thereby derailing the country's targeted testing strategy (Kagwe 2020).

Conclusions and Recommendations: Implications for Policy and Practice

Stigma, fueled by misinformation and misconceptions, hampers public health responses to disease outbreaks (WHO 2020b). Stigma intersects with other structural issues such as poverty, lack of education and health literacy, illiteracy, and inequalities in ways that increase the risk of disease transmission to vulnerable populations (Peprah and Gyasi 2020). As the examples above demonstrate, stigma creates barriers to prompt medical attention and puts lives at significant risk because it can act as a negative motivator for people to hide illness symptoms, delay healthcare-seeking, or refuse to disclose important medical history. Thus, stigma negatively impacts case reporting, thereby concealing the true impacts of the pandemic. In Turkey, for example, Kisa and Kisa (2020) showed that stigma led to underreporting of COVID-19 cases, which affected the level of resource allocation for fighting the pandemic.

Kenya, with a total population of around 54 million people, as of May 2021 had officially reported around 164,000 cases, around 3,000 deaths, and around 113,000 recovered. Clearly, these numbers are questionable, for the reasons described above; Ali (nd) terms this "politicizing statistics." And as Ramaci and colleagues (2020) found, stigma directed towards healthcare workers and volunteers can lead to higher rates of stress and burnout, and thus can compromise the quality and standards of service provision in fighting the outbreak.

So how can policymakers and ordinary citizens help fight COVID-related stigma in a context such as Kenya? The WHO (2020b) proposes strategies that include countering misinformation with facts about COVID-19, particularly through social media. For example, prioritizing the collection, consolidation, and dissemination of accurate country- and community-specific data on who is vulnerable, where and when they can seek help, in simple, non-technical language, can help to relieve the anxieties that come with this virus, which is ill-understood by those with low health literacy, who likely constitute a significant percentage of the global population, as other chapters in this volume illustrate.

It is also important to amplify the voices of local survivors of COVID-19, as doing so can help people "normalize" the disease as an ordinary experience with ill health rather than as an extraordinary one, as most people do recover from the disease. "Hero" campaigns that honor caregivers of COVID patients, including family and friends as well as healthcare workers, could motivate people to look out for each other rather than stigmatizing those affected by the disease. Nyblade and colleagues (2019) also propose participatory learning approaches that involve healthcare workers working with patients and their families and engaging them in interventions such as counseling, and gathering and spreading factual information about the virus in locally understandable terms. There is also a need for structural changes to policies, including restructuring the healthcare system to include departments that are charged with deliberately addressing stigma, targeting groups likely to experience stigma, and generating and implementing interventions that inculcate empathy and humanize the stigmatized individual or group.

References

Adom, D., and Mensah, J.A. 2020. The psychological distress and mental health disorders from COVID-19 stigmatization in Ghana. *Social Sciences & Humanities Open* [preprint]. https://papers.ssrn.com/sol3/papers.cfm?abstract_id=3599756. Accessed May 10, 2021.

Ahmed, S.A.S., Ajisola, M., Azeem, K., Bakibinga, P., Chen, Y-F., Choudhury, N.N., et al. 2020. Impact of the societal response to COVID-19 on access to healthcare for non-COVID-19 health issues in slum communities of Bangladesh, Kenya, Nigeria and Pakistan: Results of pre-COVID and COVID-19 lockdown stakeholder engagements. *BMJ Global Health* 5(8): e003042.

Ali, I. 2020. Impacts of rumors and conspiracy theories surrounding COVID-19 on preparedness programs. *Disaster Medicine and Public Health Preparedness*, 1–6. https://doi.org/10.1017/dmp.2020.325

Ali, I. (nd). Politicizing statistics and statisticizing politics: Global and political stakeholders deal with COVID-19. *Medical Anthropology*, Under review.

Ali, I., and Ali, S. 2020. Why may COVID-19 overwhelm low-income countries like Pakistan? *Disaster Medicine and Public Health Preparedness*, 1–5. https://doi.org/10.1017/dmp.2020.329

Asare, N. 2020. Stigma as a social death for COVID-19 survivors in Ghana. www.researchgate.net/publication/341342665_Stigma_as_a_Social_Death_for_COVID-19_Survivors_in_Ghana. Accessed May 13, 2020.

Awindi, S. 2020. At the crossroads: How COVID changed my life. Kenya Television Network, July 29.

Ayoyi, A. 2020. Low infection numbers fail to capture the impacts and stigma of COVID-19. Blog, accessed online on May 6, 2021: https://blogs.lse.ac.uk/africaatlse/2020/07/22/low-infection-numbers-kenya-capture-impact-stigma-covid19/

BBC News Africa 2020. Covid-19 in Africa: Fighting fake news about Coronavirus. www.bbc.co.uk/news/resources/idt-e7e3acde-9cdf-4b53-b469-ef6e87a66411.

Bao, Y., Sun, Y., Meng, S., Shi, J., and Lu, L. 2020. -nCoV epidemic: Address mental health care to empower society. *Lancet* 395(10224): e37–e38.

Bariyo, N., and Parkinson, J. 2020. Tanzania's Leader Urges People to Worship in Throngs against Coronavirus, *Wall Street Journal*, April 8. Accessed online on

May 6, 2021 through: www.wsj.com/articles/tanzanias-leader-urges-people-to-worship-in-throngs-against-coronavirus-11586347200?mod=article_inline

Bos, A., Pryor, J.B., Reeder, G.D., and Stutterheim, S.E. 2013. Stigma: Advances in theory and research. *Basic and Applied Social Psychology* 35(1): 1–9.

Boyce, P., and Cataldo, F. 2019. "MSM-ing" as a networking concept. *Medicine Anthropology Theory* 6(4): 214–237. https://doi.org/10.17157/mat.6.4.707

Burke, J., Kaijage, J., and John-Langba, J. 2014. Media analysis of Albino killings in Tanzania: A social work and human rights perspective. *Ethics and Social Welfare* 8(2): 117–134, doi:10.1080/17496535.2014.895398

Cheung, Y., Chau, P., and Yip, P. 2008. A revisit on older adult suicides and severe acute respiratory syndrome (SARS) epidemic in Hong Kong. *International Journal of Geriatric Psychiatry* 23: 1231–1238.

Claire, M. (2018). Stigma. In Ryan, J.M. (ed.) 2018. *Core Concepts in Sociology*. New York: Wiley Blackwell, pp. 145–154. Available at stigma_finaldraft.pdf (harvard.edu).

Correia, T. 2020. SARS-CoV-2 pandemics: The lack of critical reflection addressing short- and long-term challenges. *The International Journal of Health Planning and Management* 35: 1–4. Accessed April 13, 2021. https://doi.org/10.1002/hpm.2977.

Crump, J. 2014. Time for a comprehensive approach to the syndrome of fever in the tropics. *Transactions of the Royal Society of Tropical Medicine and Hygiene*, 108(2): 61–62. https://doi.org/10.1093/trstmh/trt120

ERAP 2014. Ebola survivors: Using a stepwise re-integration process to establish social contracts between survivors and their home communities. *Intervention Concept Note*. Brighton: Institute of Development Studies.

Farmer, P., and Sen, A. 2003. On suffering and structural violence: Social and economic rights in the global era. In *Pathologies of Power*. Berkeley, CA: University of California Press, pp. 29–50.

Feikin, D., Olack, B., Bigogo, G., Audi, A., Cosmas, L., Aura, B., et al. 2011. The burden of common infectious syndromes at the clinic and household level from population-based surveillance in rural and urban Kenya. *PLoS ONE* 6: e16085.

Ghana News Agency 2020. Stop Stigmatizing COVID-19 Patients. *Communities-Upper West Minister*. https://newsghana.com.gh. Accessed April 14, 2021.

Goffman, E. 1963. *Stigma: Notes on the Management of Spoiled Identity*. New York: Simon and Schuster.

Gunnell, D., Appleby, L., Arensman, E., Hawton, K., John, A., Kapur, N., et al. 2020. Suicide risk and prevention during the COVID-19 pandemic. *Lancet Psychiatry* 7(6): 468–471.

Javed, B., Sarwer, A., Soto, E.B., and Mashwani, Z. 2020. The coronavirus (COVID-19) pandemic's impact on mental health. *The International Journal of Health Planning and Management*. https://doi.org/10.1002/hpm.3008.

Kagwe, M. 2020. First case of coronavirus disease confirmed in Kenya. Ministry of Health, Government of Kenya. Available at: www.health.go.ke/wp-content/uploads/2020/03/Statement-on-Confirmed-COVID-19-Case-13-March-2020-final.pdf. Accessed May 8, 2021.

Karamouzian, M., and Hategekimana, C. 2014. Ebola treatment and prevention are not the only battles: Understanding ebola-related fear and stigma. *The International Journal of Health Policy and Management* 4(1): 55–56.

Kisa S., and Kisa, A. 2020. Under-reporting of COVID-19 cases in Turkey. *The International Journal of Health Policy and Management* . https://doi-org.ezproxy.sussex.ac.uk/10.1002/hpm.3031. Accessed May 11, 2021.

Leach, M., Bett, B., Said, M., Bukachi, S., Sang, R., Anderson, N., et al. 2017. Local disease–ecosystem–livelihood dynamics: Reflections from comparative case studies in Africa. *Philosophical Transactions of Royal Society B* 372(1725): 1–18.

Leach, M., and Dry, S. 2010. *Epidemics*. London: Earthscan.

Link, B., and Phelan, J. 2001. Conceptualizing stigma. *Annual Review of Sociology* 27(1): 363–385.

Muela, R., Peeters Grietens, K., Toomer, E., and Hausmann-Muela, S. 2009. A word of caution against the stigma trend in neglected tropical disease research and control. *PLOS Neglected Tropical Diseases* 3(10): e445.

Namu, J., and Rilley, T. (2020). Nine weeks of bloodshed: How brutal policing of Kenya's Covid curfew left 15 dead. Guardian Newspaper, October 23, 2020. www.theguardian.com/global-development/2020/oct/23/brutal-policing-kenyas-covid-curfew-left-15-dead. Accessed May 3, 2021.

Nyblade, L., Stockton, M.A., Giger, K., Bond, V., Ekstrand, M.L., McLean, R., et al. (2019). Stigma in health facilities: Why it matters and how we can change it. *BMC Medicine* 17(25). https://doi.org/10.1186/s12916-019-1256-2.

Odula, T. 2020. Pregnant women at risk of death in Kenya's COVID-19 curfew. July 25, 2020. Associated press. https://apnews.com/article/virus-outbreak-ap-top-news-health-africa-international-news-2e1a7d8b8401e4c06df52085994cf4ba. Accessed May 6, 2021.

Peprah, P., and Gyasi, R.M. 2020. Stigma and COVID-19 crisis: A wake-up call. The *International Journal of Health Planning and Management* 36: 215–218. doi:10.1002/hpm.3065

Pescosolido, B.A. 2013. The public stigma of mental illness: What do we think; what do we know; what can we prove? *Journal of Health and Social Behaviour* 54: 1–21.

Ramaci, T., Barattucci, M., Leddda, C., and Rapisarda. 2020. Social Stigma during COVID-19 and its Impact on HCWs Outcomes. *Sustainability 2020* 12: 3834. doi:10.3390/su12093834

Roelen, K., Ackley, C., Boyce, P., Farina, N., and Ripoll, S. 2020. COVID-19 in LMICs: The need to place stigma front and centre to its response. *The European Journal of Development Research* 32: 1592–1612. https://doi.org/10.1057/s41287-020-00316-6

Waruru, M. 2020. Stigma blots Kenya's COVID-19 War—Some patients fearful of seeking treatment. *Health Policy Watch*. https://healthpolicy-watch.news/stigma-blots-kenyas-covid-19-war-as-country-abandons-contract-tracing/ Accessed May 10, 2021.

Wasserman, I.M. 1992 The impact of epidemic, war, prohibition and media on suicide: United States, 1910–1920. *Suicide Life Threat Behav* 22: 240–254.

WHO 2020a. Warning on lockdown mental health. *Euobserver*. https://euobserver-com.ezproxy.sussex.ac.uk/coronavirus/147903. Accessed May 3, 2020.

WHO 2020b. *Social Stigma Associated with COVID-19. A Guide to Preventing and Addressing Social Stigma*. Geneva: IFRC, UNICEF, WHO. www.who.int/docs/default-source/coronaviruse/covid19-stigma-guide.pdf.

5 How US Maternity Care Providers Conceptualize COVID-19 and Negotiate Practice Changes

The Tensions Between Organizational Protocols and Childbearers' Needs

Kim Gutschow and Robbie Davis-Floyd

Introduction: Changing Practices and Attitudes Towards COVID-19 among US Maternity Care Providers

This chapter illuminates shifting maternity care practices and protocols among community- and hospital-based providers across the US in response to the COVID-19 pandemic during 2020.[1] Following up on an earlier article (Davis-Floyd, Gutschow, and Schwartz 2020) that summarized how providers had shifted their practices and attitudes during the first few months of the COVID-19 pandemic in 2020, we expanded our questionnaire and the set of providers we contacted to discuss how protocols and attitudes had further changed in response to new evidence and experiences by late fall of 2020. Here, our focus is on the emergent ways in which a range of hospital-based and community-based maternity care providers—obstetricians, midwives, nurses, and doulas—responded and adapted to COVID-19.

Methods

Between August and October 2020, we conducted an email survey of maternity care providers to discover how their practices and attitudes towards COVID-19 had shifted in response to new evidence. We used snowball sampling to enable our respondents to forward our questionnaire to other providers. All of our respondents replied to our survey questions via email. All gave explicit written consent for their comments to be used, and most indicated that they wished to be identified, while a few preferred pseudonyms. Unless otherwise indicated, real names will be used for our respondents.

By November 2020, 28 providers had responded to our survey, one-third of whom were obstetricians (including a maternal-fetal medicine specialist), while the remainder were midwives (certified professional midwives—CPMs—and certified nurse midwives—CNMs), doulas, and a labor and

DOI: 10.4324/9781003187462-8

delivery nurse. Our respondents came from Texas, Arizona, Arkansas, Virginia, North Carolina, Florida, Illinois, Idaho, Oregon, Massachusetts, and California. Critically, CPMs, who only attend births at home and at free-standing birth clinics, are legal and licensed in 36 US states, with legislation long pending in the 14 holdout states, where their legalization is blocked primarily by state obstetric associations. In contrast, CNMs are legal, licensed, and professionally regulated in all states; they attend births mainly in hospitals, though some few of them attend "community births," meaning births at home or in freestanding birth centers. Rather than labeling these "out of hospital births" (OOH), we will define them in terms of what they are—births in communities—rather than what they are not.

We frame our provider responses within a summary of the most recent labor, delivery, and newborn care guidance in response to COVID-19 in the USA as of December 2020. Our literature review of this guidance drew on a repository on "COVID-19, Maternal and Child Health, and Nutrition" compiled monthly by the Johns Hopkins Center for Humanitarian Health, and keyword searches for critical terms.[2] Our chapter is organized around the salient themes that emerged from our literature and questionnaire data.

Findings: Negotiating Shifts in Attitudes and Practices

Shifts in Attitudes Towards COVID-19: From Fear to Action

Looking back with the hindsight of current knowledge, we cannot stress enough how disruptive and confusing the evidence around SARS-CoV-2 and COVID-19 was in the early months of 2020. The prior coronavirus epidemics of SARS and Middle East Respiratory Syndrome (MERS), and experiences with Ebola and Zika viruses, compounded the fear and trepidation about rates and routes of transmission of SARS-CoV-2 and its specific impacts on pregnant women. Rates of obstetric complications from COVID-19 were alarming (Boelig et al. 2020), and significant increases in maternal deaths, stillbirths, and rates of postnatal depression were reported (Ellington et al. 2020).

For a small number of pregnant women, the most serious complications of COVID-19 included severe pneumonia, cardiomyopathy, thrombosis, and multiorgan diseases that require intensive care and mechanical ventilation (Schwartz and Morotti 2020). A pooled meta-analysis of several early studies indicated the following rates of maternal and newborn complications for infected childbearers: 41% preterm delivery before 37 weeks; 15% preterm delivery before 34 weeks; 15% preeclampsia; 19% premature rupture of membranes (PROM); 91% cesarean delivery; 7% perinatal deaths; 43% fetal distress; and 9% of newborns admitted to a NICU (Di Mascio et al. 2020). While miscarriages and stillbirth were rare, women who were asymptomatic during labor and delivery fared much better, and some preterm births were provider induced (Boelig et al. 2020).

Providers had to respond to patient fears and misinformation, as well as to a fundamental lack of evidence regarding how SARS-C0V-2 would impact fetal, maternal, and newborn health and outcomes. Maternal-Fetal Medicine (MFM) specialist Charles Deena (a pseudonym) explained his Illinois hospital's initial struggles:

> As for safety protocols, a lot of this had to do with where COVID-positive people were allowed to labor (on L&D [labor and delivery ward]? In a separate unit?), how to deal with particular emergencies in a COVID+ patient (i.e. maternal code, need for intubation, need for emergency cesarean delivery or operative vaginal delivery), and contingency planning for patients who needed advanced life support.

Homebirth obstetrician Stuart Fischbein of Los Angeles summarized how the hospitals in his area used COVID-19 as a pretext to abandon their relatively recently introduced humanistic practices in ways that compromised maternal health and agency:

> The pandemic has exposed the medical model of maternity care and clarified how they really think. The Mother-Baby Friendly moniker that they were all so proud of labeling themselves went out the window immediately. Little or no concern for the psychological well-being of the mother is clear by their separation policies…The individualization of care and respect for autonomy in decision making should not go out the window because of fear.

Fischbein notes how quickly these humanistic *policies of connection* (Davis-Floyd 2018a) were reversed in favor of the traditional model of obstetrics and its *policies of separation*, which, decades ago in the USA, resulted in routinely separating laboring people from their partners and families and mothers from their newborns (Davis-Floyd 2003)—and then did so again after the pandemic struck.

Regarding childbearers' fears, Fishbein noted, "Main fear is not about health. It is about hospital restrictive policies and separation from their baby and support system." Doula Merino echoed:

> Not being able to have the support that they want because of hospital support person restrictions is the number one fear that I have heard the most. Another is the limited support options because of the fear, anxieties, risks of COVID-19 for themselves/infant(s).

L&D nurse Lauren Hicks from Texas explained how client fears were reduced by stringent hospital protocols around PPE and testing:

> The mothers I have worked with have expressed a generalized fear of contracting the virus in the hospital. For a lot of them, going to the

hospital is one of the first times they have left their homes outside of OB/ GYN [obstetrician/gynecologist] visits…The precautions taken by the facility seem to ease the fears pregnant mothers and their families have.

Many of our providers reported that the most significant changes in their protocols involved strict use of PPE, testing, hygiene, telehealth, and restrictions on support people and rooming in, which we discuss in turn below.

Negotiating Practice Shifts: Testing for COVID-19, Using PPE, and Incessant Sanitizing

Both hospital- and community-based providers suffered severe shortages of PPE in March and April 2020 (Davis-Floyd, Gutschow, and Schwartz 2020). Many of these initial shortages had resolved by the fall of 2020, although the spread of COVID-19 across the USA brought increased stress to hospitals and communities that had not experienced a first wave. L&D nurse Hicks explained how her hospital was ensuring a steady supply of PPE for all staff:

> The major changes in the practices and protocols at the hospital I work at are geared towards protecting patients and healthcare staff from each other… .Our facility has enough PPE but is taking precautions to not run out. Every nurse in the emergency room and labor and delivery unit has to wear an N95 at all times, goggles during patient interactions, and face shields during deliveries, because there is always a chance that a patient will come to the unit that needs emergent care and is COVID-19 positive. All other nurses wear surgical masks at all times. The only time masks can be removed is in the designated break room. The nurses that have to wear N95 masks wear their mask until a string breaks or it gets dirty, which normally take two days. Every six hours a PPE "czar" comes by the unit to see if any supplies are needed such as gloves, shoe covers, and sanitizing wipes. Face shields are assigned to staff members and are used until they break.

Doula Stevie Merino, who attends both home and hospital births, stated a common problem:

> It has been difficult for me to access sufficient PPE because I am not a medical provider. Many of the sites that I normally would purchase from are directing [PPE] understandably to medical providers/locations. Thankfully, many in my community have been great at supporting me with PPE … .I use continuous PPE gear when visiting homes or at births, even when clients and others have become more relaxed with it.

CNM Dinah Waranch reported that, although hospitalized birthgivers were required to wear masks throughout, in her home and birth center practice,

"During labor and birth the mother is *not* masked [due to the heavy breathing she needs to be making]. Midwives are masked. Support people [are] masked.... .Some [clients] roll their eyes at masks." Waranch illustrated:

> [My client] is unmasked and I make a gesture across my face for her to mask up as I am. [She] rolls her eyes, puts on a mask, and stomps into the room. "Masks are communist. They are un-American." Loudly through her mask, defiant. I am opinionated too. "Communism isn't so evil," I am smiling, teasing, but my dagger glints. Then reaching deeply for my mature, inner midwife, I say. "If you prefer not to wear a mask, let's sit outside in the park a few feet away from each other. I can do your intake history on my phone." How easy it was then to create a peace between us, to open to each other across the picnic table beside the pond; the story of her motherhood, unique but mutually understood. Our angers soften...

In addition to PPE, all providers reported a strong emphasis on hygiene and sanitation. Representing our other community midwife respondents, CPM Sarita Bennett said that she instituted "a short break between clients to allow time to wipe things down and ask that children not come along to prenatal visits because we can't wipe down toys every time." Also echoing other community-based midwife respondents, CPM Jessica Willoughby reported:

> Cleaning, everything, all the time, between every patient. It. Is. Exhausting. We also have a hand sanitizer and an alcohol wipe station at the front door...I always felt like the birth center was a sanctuary from the craziness that happens in the mainstream medical model. Now with COVID, I feel like our tranquil borders have been breached! I hate the super vigilance and paranoia I feel with the obsessive cleaning.

It took many months for universal testing for COVID-19 to become readily available both in hospitals and in communities, causing great hardships for providers and childbearers alike. The irregular access to testing and frequent delays in test results for much of 2020 across the USA represented a lost opportunity for US maternity care institutions. Regular access to testing with rapid results would have enabled providers and patients to limit inadvertent transmission, anxiety about attending clients who might be infected but were asymptomatic, as well as reduced fear among their clients about hospitals and clinics as sites of contagion. A systematic review and meta-analysis of 30 population-based studies conducted in September 2020 revealed that 95% of all obstetric patients were asymptomatic (Yanes-Lane et al. 2020). In the future, careful distinctions may be made between asymptomatic but infected individuals and the smaller number of infected persons with symptomatic COVID-19. This distinction mirrors the critical distinction between being HIV positive and having a diagnosis of AIDS.

Some of our community birth providers required their pregnant clients to be tested, while others did not. Community-based CPM Shea Childs in Arkansas notes that she would not test asymptomatic clients, but feels differently about symptomatic clients, "If they were symptomatic at 36 weeks or more, I may [test], but that has not come up." Community-based midwife Jessica Willoughby requires her staff but not her clients to get tested regularly: "We do not require COVID testing. I've never even sent a mom to get tested. If she's asymptomatic we just treat everything as normal. If she's sick we ask that she stay home, and we can do telehealth. I've never had a patient be sick in labor." Many community-based providers work with a clientele who are low risk for birth complications as well as COVID-19, and who follow social distancing and masking guidelines.

In contrast, our hospital-based providers were very serious about mandatory testing, reporting that all childbearers are routinely tested before admission to hospital for labor as well as for out-patient pregnancy consults. Yet there were difficulties, as CNM Jennifer Bagg of Florida explained: "We have started testing all pregnant patients for COVID weekly starting at 36w. We do the rapid antigen tests, but the whole process from start to finish takes over 30 minutes and severely negatively impacts our already very busy patient flow."

Telehealth/Telemedicine

Our providers indicated a rise in telehealth, especially for doulas who reported attending to their clients virtually, using devices positioned in the sight line of the laboring person. Given that providers in the room could shut off or move the device out of range without consent of the laboring person, and that the essence of doula care is physical touch and presence, many doulas and their clients were unsatisfied with virtual support. In contrast, many providers in both hospitals and communities were comfortable using telemedicine for prenatal care. While homebirth midwives stated mixed opinions about telehealth, hospital-based providers were more comfortable with this form of care. We will need longer-term and more systematic studies to determine whether the rise of telemedicine in maternity care continues after the pandemic passes.

Negotiating Restrictions on Labor Support: Impacts on Maternal Mental Health and Health Equity

By mid-March and into the summer of 2020, many hospitals across the USA negotiated COVID-19 by excluding labor support people—partners and doulas—due to fears of viral transmission (Davis-Floyd, Gutschow, and Schwartz 2020). In the USA, an Executive Order by New York State Governor Cuomo on March 28, 2020 explicitly allowed one support person to attend the person in labor in all New York hospitals, and other hospitals in other states later adopted this policy. By October 2020, most of our respondents reported that their hospital allowed at least one support person, and sometimes even for women who tested positive. CNM Diana Jolles from Arizona stated that her hospital began excluding all support people in April 2020, but reallowed them back in September 2020. Even freestanding birth centers were limiting support people, as confirmed by several of our provider respondents.

Doula Stevie Merino explained how confusing hospital policies were, as well as how the limitations on support people put her clients and doulas in difficult situations:

> Every hospital's policies are different, which has also been difficult to navigate and keep up with…There are a very few hospitals that see doulas as an essential part of the birth team, which has allowed me and partner/support person to be present in the room. In quite a few instances, I have been chosen over a partner to be present in labor. This was an intentional and very difficult decision on all parties.

By not considering doulas as "essential personnel," hospital protocols devalued their services and limited the ability of childbearers to advocate for themselves and their newborns (Castañeda and Searcy 2020). Even when hospitals allowed a single support person, the strict rules insisting that this support person was forbidden to leave the labor room further limited or prevented continuous support in labor, as many families could not afford for the partner to stay the entire time. This rule fell especially heavily on minoritized and low-income childbearers, who have been struck hardest by the virus (Obinna 2020; Norton et al. 2020). Further, it penalized women who already had small children at home with limited childcare, as their partners might have to choose between tending to their children or their birthing partner, who is already facing increased stress and isolation (Norton et al. 2020). Doula Merino noted, "Many are not having the experiences that they envisioned in terms of family, friend, community support due to social distancing recommendations. This isolation has had and will continue to have dramatic effects on new parents."

The restrictions denying labor support for childbearers who tested positive could indeed mean isolation and mental suffering, as MFM specialist Deena confirmed:

> COVID-19 positive pregnant people who labor in our hospital do so in a negative pressure room on a floor above labor and delivery, have one-to-one nursing, and only one provider (no residents) at the delivery. As for the experiences of people laboring alone…the stories I heard from my colleagues working on the COVID floor is that it was heartbreaking— extremely isolating and really difficult to help people through, especially

since we knew (and still know) so little about perinatal outcomes associated with the virus.

L&D nurse Hicks described the alienating scene that seropositive mothers faced in their negative pressure rooms:

> COVID-19 positive women…were not allowed to have a support person with them, and the newborn was immediately removed after delivery… Nurses are encouraged to cluster care while in the patient's room. When nurses are caring for COVID positive patients, a primary nurse is allowed to go into the room while another nurse acts as a runner to get any supplies or medications the primary nurse needs.

Yet via negotiations, some hospital protocols changed, as Hicks explained: "[Women testing] positive are still being treated differently, but our protocols have recently improved. Now, COVID-19 positive mothers can have one companion with them."

The denial of labor support is especially critical for women of color, who have been disproportionately affected by SARS-CoV-2, and who already face formidable disparities in maternity care and obstetric outcomes (Norton et al. 2020; Obinna 2020; Ellington et al. 2020). Well before COVID-19 struck, between 2014–2017, the pregnancy-related mortality for non-Hispanic Black women (41 deaths/100,000 live births) was three times that of non-Hispanic white women (13.4 deaths/100,000 live births) and quadruple that of Hispanic or Latina women (11.6 deaths/100,000 live births) (CDC 2020a). Evidence shows that the racial disparities in maternal outcomes are related to the chronic stress of structural racism and providers' implicit racial bias (Bridges 2011; Eichelberger et al. 2016; Davis 2019; Obinna 2020).

By defining doulas as visitors, not essential personnel, childbearers are being denied critical advocates during labor and the postpartum period when they are isolated due to COVID-19 restrictions. A Cochrane meta-analysis of deliveries in 17 countries found that women receiving continuous labor support from a doula had shorter labors, were *more likely* to have spontaneous vaginal delivery and report positive childbirth experience, and *less likely* to have a cesarean delivery, to use any form of intrapartum analgesia, to have a baby with low (<5) Apgar score, and to experience postpartum depression (Bohren et al. 2017). Yet a Canadian study (Fortier and Goodwin 2015) showed that doula presence was not viewed favorably by half of the obstetricians and one-fourth of nurses in the study. Given this level of hostility to doulas, we are not surprised that the COVID-19 pandemic provided quick justification to exclude them from labor and delivery rooms, with adverse consequences for women during labor and birth.

Negotiating Mother-Newborn Separation and Transmission of SARS-CoV-2

Most of our hospital-based providers reported that mothers testing positive for SARS-CoV2 were separated from their newborns at birth, not allowed skin-to-skin contact, and discouraged from breastfeeding, based on the assumed possibility of mother-to-newborn viral transmission. As MFM specialist Deena noted, "Some hospitals are sequestering newborns in the NICU [Neonatal Intensive Care Unit] if mothers are COVID-19 positive for up to five days, despite any evidence suggesting that this is beneficial."

Obstetrician Michael White confirmed that his hospital separated mothers who tested positive from their newborns, while L&D nurse Hicks explained that her hospital had separated seropositive mothers from newborns, yet there had been positive change: "Recently at my facility they have been allowed to breastfeed and have skin-to-skin contact with their newborns . . . I am so glad that now my facility is treating COVID-19 positive patients almost like any other patient." Obstetrician Walters noted that his unit never separated mothers and newborns, stating, "Babies need contact with their mom and they need breastmilk. We do allow breastfeeding and skin-to-skin, and advise hand washing and masks." We note with irony that unless mothers or newborns who tested positive were critically ill, they were usually sent home together within two days after birth even if they had been separated in the hospital. CNM Waranch responded to this paradox, stating: "No logic [to that], but then why expect logic from an illogical system?" Obstetrician Marco Giannotti added:

> When the pandemic first started, I was a big proponent of keeping positive moms with their babies and breastfeeding. (There just was not any data present indicating otherwise.) I received a lot of pushback from our Neonatologists and Pediatricians. Shortly afterwards, the American Academy of Pediatrics confirmed that asymptomatic COVID positive moms should not be separated from their baby, and that breastfeeding should continue as normal.

CNM Kylea Liese noted that her hospital separated mothers and newborns in contradiction to AAP policy:

> The rationale per peds [pediatrics] is "hospital policy" though they have acknowledged their own professional organization no longer supports this policy...the World Health Organization (WHO), Centers for Disease Control (CDC) and American Academy of Pediatrics (AAP) all recommend that mothers and babies stay together and breastfeed (if desired).

When the AAP (2020) issued its first neonatal guidance on April 2, it recommended separating newborns from mothers and discouraging skin-to-skin contact and breastfeeding. By August 2020, evidence had accumulated that the risk of vertical transmission even for mothers testing positive for SARS-CoV-2 was rare, and that most infected newborns recovered quickly without hospitalization. Nevertheless, the effects of the earlier guidance separating newborns from mothers proved difficult to undo for some time. For example, a CDC survey of 1,344 hospitals in the USA between July and August 2020 (Perrine et al. 2020) confirmed that for mothers with suspected or confirmed COVID-19, in a significant number of hospitals, rooming-in, skin-to-skin care, and breastfeeding were either discouraged or prohibited. All of these policies were in contradiction to WHO, ACOG, and AAP guidance by the time, which now encouraged rooming-in, skin-to-skin contact, and breastfeeding for all mothers, even those testing positive for SARS-CoV-2, unless they were too ill to do so (Perinne et al. 2020).

By August 2020, the CDC (2020b) had updated its recommendations, stating that mothers with suspected or confirmed SARS-CoV-2 infection should discuss risks and benefits of rooming in with their providers, and that healthcare providers must respect maternal autonomy in the medical decision-making process. As rationale for encouraging rooming-in even for mothers with COVID-19, the CDC noted that:

> Early and close contact between the mother and neonate has many well-established benefits. The ideal setting for care of a healthy, term newborn while in the hospital is in the mother's room, commonly called "rooming in." Current evidence suggests the risk of a neonate acquiring SARS-CoV-2 from its mother is low. Further, data suggests that there is no difference in risk of SARS-CoV-2 infection to the neonate whether a neonate is cared for in a separate room or remains in the mother's room.
>
> (CDC 2020b)

By February 2021, the AAP (2021) had further revised guidance concerning mothers who test positive for SARS-CoV-2 with updated recommendations that encouraged rooming-in, immediate skin-skin contact, and breastfeeding. These recommendations clearly stated that the risk of vertical transmission from mother to newborn was highest for mothers who gave birth within 14 days of the onset of COVID-19 symptoms. This newer guidance was based on a nationwide Perinatal COVID-19 Registry that included over 10,000 newborns (AAP 2021). A CDC surveillance report including 923 infants born to mothers with COVID-19 reported that 2.6% of the newborns tested positive for SARS-CoV-2, but among the subset of those newborns whose mothers first reported COVID-19 symptoms in the past 14 days, 4.3% tested positive for the virus (AAP 2021).

This newer evidence suggested that the timings of the onset of infection and the display of COVID-19 symptoms are important in evaluating the risk that mothers testing positive for the virus pose to newborns. The guidance also noted that symptomatic maternal infection at time of delivery was associated with increased risk of preterm birth and perinatal morbidity, but did not quantify those risks. Finally, newborn death directly attributable to perinatal infection with SARS-CoV-2 was "extremely rare" (AAP 2021). Mother-to-baby transmission can occur in three ways: intrauterine or placental transmission, intrapartum transmission, or postpartum transmission. An analysis of newborns whose mothers tested positive for SARS-CoV-2 revealed a very low perinatal transmission rate to newborns (Schwartz et al. 2020; Schwartz, Baldewijns, and Benachi 2020; Schwartz and De Luca 2021).

By June 2021, AAP guidance emphasized that delayed cord-clamping,[3] breastfeeding, and immediate skin-to-skin contact should be continued as per usual practices, adding that infected mothers and visiting family members should wear a mask, and providers should wear full PPE while providing hands-on care to newborns. Breastfeeding was encouraged because viable infectious virus had not been detected in breastmilk, and mothers were urged to don masks and practice hand hygiene before breastfeeding. The CDC (2020b) guidance explicitly stated that while mothers with COVID-19 may choose to separate from their newborns,

> if after discharge they will not be able to maintain separation from their neonate, it is unclear whether temporary separation while in the hospital would ultimately prevent SARS-CoV-2 transmission to the neonate, given the potential for exposure from the mother after discharge.

All newborns should be tested before discharge, and infants who test positive for SARS-CoV-2 but have no signs of COVID-19 were to be discharged as usual and followed up by phone or telemedicine.

Newborns admitted to the NICU should optimally be admitted to single rooms or with at least 6 feet between isolettes, while providers should wear full PPE before providing hands-on care. NICUs should limit mothers and partners with confirmed COVID-19 until 10 days have passed from onset of symptoms, and yet because recovery can still include positive nucleic acid tests, NICUs should not require infected parents to produce a negative PCR test before entry to the NICU (AAP 2021). It is significant that this guidance attempts to distinguish between active COVID-19 cases and non-infectious individuals who test positive for fragments of the SARS-CoV-2 virus. In short, as we pointed out in our earlier article (Gutschow and Davis-Floyd 2021b), this guidance provides an important distinction between having the virus and having the disease.

One possible theory for why hospitals moved so quickly to isolate newborns from mothers is that this affirmed the *principle of separation* (Davis-Floyd 2018a) that can be found in many obstetric practices, some of which are based on little or no evidence (see Miller et al. 2016). Davis-Floyd

(2003, 2018c) has analyzed obstetric interventions that interfere with normal birth physiology as rituals that enact core technocratic values and generate a sense of control for providers, sometimes with little or no benefit for mothers or newborns (see also Gutschow, Davis-Floyd, and Daviss 2021). The emphasis on separation and control represents a major step back from recent humanistic changes in hospital birth across the globe, including access to labor support partners and doulas, immediate mother-newborn skin-to-skin contact, and rooming-in of mothers and newborns.

Community Birth during COVID-19

Some of our respondents reported an increased demand for community births in their areas. Yet for other providers and their clients, the rise of interest in community births did not always translate to a successful homebirth for a variety of reasons, as doula Stevie Merino explained:

> Many potential clients and current clients have reached out via email, social media, phone, and my website to ask for advice on how to find OOH [out-of-hospital] options...Unfortunately, however, many are unable to because of how far along they are in their pregnancy, insurance, cost of OOH options, high risk status, living situations, etc. I try to support however I can but also am realistic about people's access and the fact that less than 2% of people in the US still give birth in homes.

CPM Shea Childs from Arkansas described how she adapted to the growing demand for homebirth in her area by asking more pointed questions about families' motivations for wanting homebirth. For example, homebirth midwife Marimikel Potter CPM of Texas described her reasons for rejecting some would-be clients:

> When COVID-19 first got started, I got a bunch of calls from women wanting a homebirth just because they were afraid of hospital infection. I rejected all of them because it was clear to me that they weren't actually committed to homebirth, and that rarely works out well.

CPM Sarita Bennett agreed, stating:

> We didn't accept those last-minute transfers at the beginning of the pandemic because the reasons for transferring didn't give us confidence that the families were committed to our model of care and out of hospital birth. I've had several midwife friends regret that they accepted those transfers because they wound up with labor dystocias [slowed labor] and transports [to a hospital] way too often.

Here Bennett speaks to the facts that if a birthing woman truly feels safer in the hospital, then that is where she should be, and that an ideological commitment to homebirth is generally key to a successful outcome at home.

CPM Vicki Penwell, who runs a midwifery school in Boise, Idaho, saw a notable increase in demand for community births: "All the midwives all over the country that I have been speaking with recently are somehow managing to cope with client volumes of around 8 births per month—twice their normal load. They are really rising to the challenge!" Yet this increased demand can add significant risks to homebirth midwives as births begin to cluster and practitioner stress and exhaustion set in. This could become a quality of care and safety issue if the demand remains high for too long; it clearly indicates the need for more community-based midwives in the USA.

The Home/Hospital Divide in US Maternity Care

Many of our obstetrician respondents remained prejudiced against homebirths, as doula Merino described:

> Many of my clients or potential clients who have discussed [community birth] with their [obstetricians] have been told outright that it is still safer to birth in hospitals and it is actually "dangerous" to birth at home. This is quite ridiculous obviously and frankly a shame that even in the face of a pandemic that some hospital-based providers still do not see OOH providers as capable or see birth beyond a medical experience.

In response to our survey question on whether they might support homebirths during the pandemic, our obstetrician respondents largely responded by emphatically stating "NO."

Yet MFM specialist Deena had a very different view:

> I do support OOH among people who have a trained CPM/CNM... In the midst of the pandemic, I think a well-counseled person—understanding the risks and benefits of homebirth—with a good care team and easy ability to access higher order care would be great as a homebirth!

Deena's optimism was not shared by our other obstetrician respondents, whose negative opinions about homebirth indicate that there is a long way to go in educating obstetricians about the substantial evidence that exists showing excellent outcomes for planned, CPM-attended community births in the USA (Johnson and Daviss 2005; Stapleton, Osborne, and Illuzzi 2013; Cheyney et al. 2014).

Conclusion: Negotiating Integrated and Sustainable Maternity Care in the USA

Our provider responses show that in this highly disruptive pandemic time, US maternity care providers identified and negotiated ways in which their practices and maternity care needed to be shifted—and then shifted again in response to changing evidence. Initial, reflex reversions to past practices of separation have been giving way over time to a consumer-demanded return to more recently adopted humanistic practices of connection.

The COVID-19 crisis is an opportunity for identifying directions for future improvements in maternity care. The crisis highlights the fractures and dysfunctions within maternity care systems; it can also enable the birth and development of more sustainable, flexible, and stronger systems of care in which women experience more agency and better outcomes, while providers suffer less burnout and conflict (Gutschow and Davis-Floyd 2021a). We urge providers and policy makers to use this time of disruption to work towards leaner, more cost-effective, and *decentralized* maternity care systems that integrate midwives with obstetricians and community birth providers with hospitals, while working to dismantle the systemic racism and provider bias that prevent high-quality care for all (Gutschow, Davis-Floyd, and Daviss 2021; Daviss and Davis-Floyd 2021).

It is our hope that maternity care systems in the USA will become more integrated, and will recognize hospital- and community-based midwives and doulas as full participants in the care of mothers and newborns. In equalizing access to doulas, homebirth, and freestanding birth centers through coordinated insurance schemes and subsidies, we might also begin to improve health equity outcomes for minoritized populations in the USA and to de-racialize care more broadly (Profit et al. 2020). And we believe it critical that doulas be accepted as *essential* care providers, given the longstanding evidence that continuous doula support in labor reduces interventions and improves maternal and neonatal outcomes. We also believe that US community midwives can seize this pandemic moment to raise national awareness of their value, while obstetricians can become more aware and accepting of the high value and cost-savings of midwifery care and community births. In an analysis comparing the costs of in- vs out-of-hospital births, which also provides ample evidence of the safety of CPM-attended community births, Anderson, Daviss, and Johnson (2021) have shown that, if only 10% more US births took place at home or in freestanding birth centers, the cost-savings would amount to *$11 billion*, along with improved birth outcomes—or $321 million per percentage raise.

We emphasize the importance of teaching and transmitting midwifery skills and of the midwifery model of care (Davis-Floyd 2018b), which is woman-centered, facilitates normal physiologic birth, and is based on the *principle of connection*. As we have shown, this midwifery model can be applied in both home and hospital settings, in both disruptive and more stable times, in decentralized or shifting locations of disaster care (see Davis-Floyd et al. 2021), as well as in routine, institutionalized care (Gutschow, Davis-Floyd, and Daviss 2021). As CPM and DO Sarita Bennett put it, "I believe that the lesson we should be learning is that large volume, facility birth is not sustainable and that small, community-based midwifery centers are the answer for the vast majority of pregnant people" (Gutschow and Davis-Floyd 2021b). Bennet's words illustrate what we mean by a "decentralized" system of care.

We trust that the US maternity care system will continue to restore humanistic strides made in enhancing maternal and newborn health and well-being. We hope that providers will work more collaboratively, with obstetricians recognizing midwives as colleagues rather than subordinates and doulas as essential, rather than non-essential, personnel. We hope that community midwives in the USA can achieve autonomous practice without restrictive state regulations, and thereby be empowered to practice and promote the midwifery model of care. In this way, they can continue to flexibly adapt to the next disruption or crises that our society may face as *recognized frontline providers*—most especially when hospitals are overwhelmed. Finally, we hope that providers across the USA will seize the transformational moment of COVID-19 to transform the US maternity care system to be more sustainable, egalitarian, and resilient in the face of future pandemics and disasters.

Acknowledgments

We sincerely thank all the busy providers who responded to our email questionnaire and the IRB director at Williams College for providing expedited review.

Notes

1 This chapter is abridged, excerpted, and adapted from "The Impacts of COVID-19 on US Maternity Care Practitioners: A Follow-Up Study," by Kim Gutschow and Robbie Davis-Floyd, *Frontiers in Sociology*, May 27, 2021. doi: https://doi.org/10.3389/fsoc.2021.655401, with the kind permission of *Frontiers in Sociology*.
2 This literature repository can be found at: http://hopkinshumanitarianhealth.org/empower/advocacy/covid-19/covid-19-children-and-nutrition/).
3 Delayed cord clamping is beneficial to the newborn: as long as the umbilical cord is pulsing, the baby is receiving oxygenated blood that can ease the newborn's transition to breathing.

References

American Academy of Pediatrics (AAP). 2021. Frequently Asked Questions: Management of Infants Born to Mothers with Suspected or Confirmed COVID-19. See https://services.aap.org/en/pages/2019-novel-coronavirus-covid-19-infections/clinical-guidance/faqs-management-of-infants-born-to-covid-19-mothers/ Accessed June 10, 2021.

American Academy of Pediatrics (AAP). 2020. AAP Updates Guidance on Newborns whose Mothers Have Suspected or Confirmed COVID-19. www.aappublications. org/news/2020/05/21/covid19newborn052120 . Accessed June 10, 2021.

Boelig, R.C., Manuck, T., Oliver, E.A., Di Mascio, D., Saccone, G., Bellussi, F., et al. 2020. Labor and delivery guidance for COVID-19. *American Journal of Obstetrics and Gynecology MFM* 2(2), Supplement 100110. https://doi.org/ 10.1016/j.ajogmf.2020.100110

Bohren, M.A., Hofmeyr, G.J., Sakala, C., Fukuzawa, R.K., and Cuthbert, A. 2017. Continuous support for women during childbirth. *The Cochrane Database of Systematic Reviews* 7(7), CD003766. https://doi.org/10.1002/14651858. CD003766.pub6

Bridges, K. 2011. *Reproducing Race: An Ethnography of Pregnancy as a Site of Racialization.* Berkeley, CA: University of California Press.

Centers for Disease Control and Prevention (CDC). 2020a. Pregnancy Mortality Surveillance Program: Pregnancy-Related Deaths by Race/Ethnicity. www.cdc. gov/reproductivehealth/maternal-mortality/pregnancy-mortality-surveillance-system.htm. Accessed January 10, 2021.

Centers for Disease Control and Prevention (CDC). 2020b. Evaluation and Management Considerations for Neonates at Risk for COVID-19. August 3. www.cdc.gov/coronavirus/2019-ncov/hcp/caring-for-newborns.html

Cheyney, M., Bovbjerg, M., Everson, C., Gordon, W., Hannibal, D., and Vedam, S. 2014. Outcomes of Care for 16,924 Planned Homebirths in the United States: The Midwives Alliance of North America Statistics Project, 2004 to 2009. *Journal of Midwifery and Women's Health* 59(1): 17–27. doi:10.1111/ jmwh.12172.

Davis, D. 2019. *Reproductive Injustice: Racism, Pregnancy, and Premature Birth.* New York: New York University Press.

Davis-Floyd, R. 2003 [1992]. *Birth as an American Rite of Passage,* 2nd ed. Berkeley, CA: University of California Press.

Davis-Floyd, R. 2018a. "The Technocratic, Humanistic, and Holistic Paradigms of Birth and Health Care." In R. Davis-Floyd (ed.), *Ways of Knowing about Birth: Mothers, Midwives, Medicine, and Birth Activism.* Long Grove, IL: Waveland Press, 3–44.

Davis-Floyd, R. 2018b. "The Midwifery Model of Care: Anthropological Perspectives." In R. Davis-Floyd (ed.), *Ways of Knowing about Birth: Mothers, Midwives, Medicine, and Birth Activism.* Long Grove, IL: Waveland Press, 323–338.

Davis-Floyd, R. 2018c. "The Rituals of Hospital Birth: Enacting and Transmitting the Technocratic Model." In R. Davis-Floyd (ed.), *Ways of Knowing about Birth: Mothers, Midwives, Medicine, and Birth Activism.* Long Grove, IL: Waveland Press, 45–70.

Davis-Floyd, R., Gutschow K., and Schwartz, D.A. 2020. Pregnancy, birth, and the COVID-19 pandemic in the United States. *Medical Anthropology* 39(5): 413–427. https://doi.org/10.1080/01459740.2020.1761804

Davis-Floyd, R., Lim, R., Penwell V., and Ivry, T. 2021. "Effective Maternity Disaster Care: Low Tech, Skilled Touch." In K. Gutschow, R. Davis-Floyd, and B.A. Daviss, *Sustainable Birth in Disruptive Times,* 261–277. New York: Springer Nature.

Daviss, B.A., Anderson, D.A., and Johnson, K.C. 2021. Pivoting to childbirth at home or in freestanding birth centers in the US during COVID-19: Safety, economics and logistics. *Frontiers in Sociology* 6: 618210. doi:10.3389/fsoc.2021.618210

Daviss, B.A. and Davis-Floyd, R., eds. 2021. *Birthing Models on the Human Rights Frontier: Speaking Truth to Power*. Abingdon, UK: Routledge.

Di Mascio, D., Khalil, A., Saccone, G., Rizzo, G., Buca, D., Liberati, M., et al. 2020. Outcome of coronavirus spectrum infections (SARS, MERS, COVID-19) during pregnancy: A systematic review and meta-analaysis. *American Journal of Obstetrics and Gynecology Maternal Fetal Medicine* 2(2) Supplement 100107, May 1, 2020. https://doi.org/10.1016/j.ajogmf.2020.100107

Eichelberger, K.Y., Doll, K., Ekpo, G.E., and Zerden, M. 2016. Black Lives Matter: Claiming a space for evidence-based outrage in Obstetrics and Gynecology. *American Journal of Public Health* 106(10): 1771–1772. doi:10.2105/AJPH.2016.303313.

Ellington, S., Strid, P., Tong, V.T., Woodworth, K., Galang, R.R., Zambrano, L., et al. 2020. Characteristics of women of reproductive age with laboratory-confirmed SARS-CoV-2 infection by pregnancy status—United States, January 22–June 7, 2020. *MMWR Morbidity and Mortality Weekly* (MMWR) 69: 769–775. http://dx.doi.org/10.15585/mmwr.mm6925a1

Fortier, J.H., and Godwin, M. 2015. Doula support compared with standard care: Meta-analysis of the effects on the rate of medical interventions during labour for low-risk women delivering at term. *Canadian Family Physician* 61(June): e284–292.

Gutschow, K., and Davis-Floyd, R. 2021a. Introduction. In K. Gutschow, R. Davis-Floyd, and B.A. Daviss (eds.), *Sustainable Birth in Disruptive Times*. New York: Springer Nature, 1–28.

Gutschow, K., and Davis-Floyd, R. 2021b. The impacts of COVID-19 on US Maternity Care Practitioners: A follow-up study. *Frontiers in Sociology*. https://doi.org/10.3389/fsoc.2021.655401

Gutschow K., Davis-Floyd-R., and Daviss, B.A., eds. 2021. *Sustainable Birth in Disruptive Times*. New York: Springer Nature.

Johnson, K.C., and Daviss, B.A. 2005. Outcomes of planned homebirths with Certified Professional Midwives: Large prospective study in North America. *British Medical Journal* 330(7505): 1416.

Miller, S.E., Abalos, E., Chamillard, M., Ciapponi, A., Colaci, D., Comandé, D., et al. 2016. Beyond too little, too late and too much, too soon: A pathway towards evidence-based, respectful maternity care worldwide. *Lancet* 388: 2176–2192. https://doi.org/10.1016/S0140-6736(16)31472-6

Norton, A., Wilson, T., Geller, G., and Gross, M.S. 2020. Impact of hospital visitor restrictions on racial disparities in Obstetrics. *Health Equity* 4(1): 505–508. https://doi.org/10.1089/heq.2020.0073

Obinna, D.N. 2020. Essential and undervalued: Health disparities of African American women in the COVID-19 era. *Ethnicity & Health*. doi:10.1080/13557858.2020.1843604

Perinne, C.G., Chiang, K.V., Anstey E.H., Grossniklaus, D.A., Boundy, E.O., Sauber-Schatz, E.K., et al. 2020. Implementation of hospital practices supportive of breastfeeding in the context of COVID-19—United States, July 15–August 20, 2020. *Morbidity and Mortality Weekly Report* (MMWR) 69(47): 1767–1770. doi:10.15585/mmwr.mm6947a3

Profit, J., Edmonds, B.T., Shah, N., and Cheyney, M. 2020. The COVID-19 pandemic as a catalyst for more integrated maternity care. *American Journal of Public Health* 110(11): 1663–1665. https://doi.org/10.2105/AJPH.2020.305935

Schwartz, D.A., Baldewijns, M., Benachi, A., Bugatti, M., Collins, R.R.J., De Luca, D., et al. 2020. Chronic Histiocytic Intervillositis with Trophoblast Necrosis are Risk Factors Associated with Placental Infection from Coronavirus Disease 2019 (COVID-19) and Intrauterine Maternal-Fetal Severe Acute Respiratory Syndrome Coronavirus 2 (SARS-CoV-2) Transmission in Liveborn and Stillborn Infants. *Archives of Pathology & Laboratory Medicine*. https://doi.org/10.5858/arpa.2020-0771-SA

Schwartz, D.A., and De Luca, D. 2021. The public health and clinical importance of accurate neonatal testing for COVID-19. *Pediatrics* 147(2): e2020036871. https://doi.org/10.1542/peds.2020-036871

Schwartz, D.A., and Graham, A.L. 2020. Potential maternal and infant outcomes from Coronavirus 2019-nCoV (SARS-CoV-2) infecting pregnant women: Lessons from SARS, MERS, and other human coronavirus infections. *Viruses* 12(2): 194. https://doi.org/10.3390/v12020194

Schwartz, D.A., Morotti, D., Beigi, B., Moshfegh, F., Zafaranloo, N., and Patanè, L. 2020. Confirming vertical fetal infection with coronavirus disease 2019: Neonatal and pathology criteria for early onset and transplacental transmission of severe acute respiratory syndrome Coronavirus 2 from infected pregnant mothers. *Archives of Pathology & Laboratory Medicine* 144(12): 1451–1456. doi:10.5858/arpa.2020-0442-SA.

Searcy, J.J., and Castañeda, A.N. 2020. COVID-19 and the birth of the Virtual Doula. *Medical Anthropology Quarterly* 19, June. http://medanthroquarterly.org/2020/06/19/covid-19-and-the-birth-of-the-virtual-doula/.

Stapleton, S.R., Osborne, C., and Illuzzi, J. 2013. Outcomes of care in birth centers: Demonstration of a durable model. *Journal of Midwifery & Women's Health* 58(1): 3–14.

Yanes, M., Winters, N., Fregonese, F., Bastos, M., Perlman-Arrow, S., Campbell, J.R., et al. 2020. Proportion of asymptomatic infection among COVID-19 positive persons and their transmission potential: A systematic review and meta-analysis. *PLoS ONE* 15(11): e0241536. https://doi.org/10.1371/journal.pone.0241536

6 Health Literacy and Information Fatigue

Understanding People's Beliefs and Behaviors as They Negotiate COVID-19 in Germany

Mayarí Hengstermann

Introduction

By the end of January 2021, almost 60,000 people had died in Germany in connection with a coronavirus infection. With 4,379 infections per 100,000 inhabitants, the highest number of infections in relation to the number of inhabitants was found in Saxony, followed by Berlin, with 3,241 cases per day.[1] Although the pathogen responsible for Severe Acute Respiratory Syndrome Coronavirus 2 (SARS-CoV-2) was rapidly identified, one of its particularities was that at the time, many factors remained unknown, especially with regard to effectively preventing contagion. The first few months of the pandemic resulted in extreme uncertainty and fear, which prompted people to strictly follow the measures recommended. Additionally, the level of trust in scientists, governments, and health institutions was key to maintaining the expected behaviors to prevent the virus from spreading. However, people's initial trust was later transformed into skepticism or incomprehension due to persistent uncertainty, opening a wide window to allow doubt and disinformation to spread and to permeate people's beliefs and behaviors. Worldwide, no other disease since the Great Influenza pandemic of 1918–1920 has been such a collective concern; that pandemic has highlighted the power of the consequences of COVID-19 (C-19) (Bavel et al. 2020). Personal and social responses to C-19 can therefore be better understood and explored if the relevance of health literacy (HL) is acknowledged, and vice versa (ibid.; Lunn et al. 2020).

The coronavirus pandemic has taken multiple directions and has been sharpened by the many existential questions and emotional circumstances posed by any major infectious disease. Some of these issues are fundamental and concerned with individual and collective practices, perceptions, desires, hopes, and fears (Kramer et al. 2014). Examining behavioral responses to the preventive measures against C-19 spread shows that these are strongly linked to individual biases and cultural norms that prompt and justify specific

DOI: 10.4324/9781003187462-9

practices that encompass complex dynamics. Because of this complexity and variability, public health recommendations are not necessarily followed and information that is supposed to be normative can backfire. Thus, health promotion strategies are more successful when messages are clear, effective, and relevant, including perspectives from the target group. My goals for this project were to explore the subjective experiences of German individuals and how they make sense of the new reality created by the pandemic.

Methodology

For this ethnographic research project, I utilized a phenomenological and health literacy approach. I conducted interviews between November and December 2020 in Berlin, Germany. Interpretative Phenomenological Analysis assisted an in-depth exploration of ten narratives from people aged 35 to 55 years, of different genders, beliefs, and occupations, as will be shown throughout. I recruited participants via personal relationships and through snowball sampling. I did not intend this ethnographic research to be exhaustive, as I also autoethnographically draw on my personal experience as a German citizen dealing with the same issues as my interlocutors. For the interviews, I utilized a series of five short open-ended questions to help start and lead the dialogue, placing particular emphasis on understanding people's comprehensions of and responses to the C-19 official health campaigns.

Reflecting on Biomedical Concepts and Frameworks: The Politics Surrounding COVID-19 in Germany

On January 28, 2020, the Bavarian Ministry of Health reported the first COVID-19 case in Germany. The patient, in the Upper Bavarian district of Starnberg, was medically monitored, housed in isolation and later reported to be in good clinical condition. This case in Germany turned out to be the first known case of human-to-human transmission outside of Asia: a 33-year-old man who was infected by a colleague who had traveled from China.

Two months later, in March 2020, lockdown measures were imposed to prevent contagion from spreading in the country. Restaurants, bars, cinemas, museums, concert halls, gyms, swimming pools, non-essential shops, schools, universities, and workplaces were shut down, and a ban was placed on groups of more than two people meeting in public. While some people were experiencing anxiety and uncertainty, others thought that the preventions were an overreaction—an opinion shared by many, not only in Germany but also in many other countries.

During the first wave's peak, Germany was recording more than 6,000 new cases daily. With new infection rates significantly reduced from the highs at the beginning of April 2020 and a death toll significantly lower than those of its neighbors, in early May 2020, Germany became the first major European Union (EU) country to begin easing restrictions such as travel bans and lockdown, while leaving many preventive measures in place. These measures' effects were manifested in changing personal and social practices, and in new ways of redefining private and social interactions, matters of work, leisure, religious practices, personal and social rituals, intimacy, and relationships.

Protests directed against the governmental measures started to occur in Germany in early April 2020, on the basis that such guidelines contradicted the rights of personal freedom; the protestors even criticized scientists for at times apparently contradictory findings. From being afraid of viral infection, some people switched to being angry about having to use face masks, distressed over not being able to socialize or continue with their routines, and distraught due to the consequences of these prohibitions. Thousands of people from different political views across Germany gathered under the umbrella of "Resistance 2020," with right-wing extremists and left-wing alternatives becoming the main opponents of the measures, insisting that the pandemic was created to establish a "corona dictatorship" and using expressions such as "fake news."

According to this group, the preventive measures were against people's dignity (protective mask requirement), rights and freedom (curfews, travel bans, prohibition of exercise in gyms, restrictions on gatherings), and prosperity (mass unemployment, inflation). In addition to these beliefs, this group believes that C-19 is simply another flu virus. Its members wore caps made of aluminum foil at large protests they held in Berlin during the summer of 2020 without wearing masks—and also without respecting the social distancing measures—as statements of their views. These aluminum hats constitute a reappropriation of the expression "tin foil hat," often used by the media to express their criticisms of how the government and the mainstream media deal with the pandemic. "Tin foil hat" is associated with conspiracy theories and paranoia. This expression has been largely spread in popular culture (music, movies, books) since the beginning of the twentieth century. Its main feature is the belief that the tin foil hat gives protection against strong electromagnetic radiation and prevents "mind control." German Neo-Nazis, for example, have been arguing that the measurements to contain the virus, including vaccines, are vehicles used by the German government to control and destroy the "white population"; they believe that the government wants to implant a chip into white people's bodies and kill them. Conspiracy theories have helped to exacerbate the problems of mistrust and weariness, arguing that the virus was purposefully produced in China by Bill Gates and other powerful actors to create chaos in order to rule the world.

On August 29, 2020 in Berlin, 38,000 people gathered to protest the COVID-19 safety measures, including vaccination; they included an eclectic mix of right-wing extremists, anti-vaccine activists, New Age followers, and conspiracy theorists, who spread misinformation and infused civil disobedience. During this gathering, far-right extremists attempted to storm Germany's parliament building before the police were able to disperse this crowd and arrest some of them. The interior minister declared "zero tolerance" for such behavior, resulting in the introduction of a fine for failing to wear a face mask, a ban on major public events, and later on the re-introduction of shutting down businesses, which is still in place at this time of writing (May 2021). These government actions have served as a platform for the far-right Alternative for Germany party (AfD) to use the coronavirus preventive measures to infuse resentment and split the polls. However, opinion polls still show vast support for the prevention measures.

Such behaviors can be attributed to factors such as feelings of confusion, anger, resentment, and fear, and to a lack of health literacy. When critical decisions need to be made, but we lack the appropriate knowledge, then we normally trust specialists. Health literacy works under the assumption that a population should be—or should be facilitated to be—able to understand the severity of a disease as well as how to navigate health-related information. C-19 involves and requires a variety of closely linked informed approaches, particularly by virologists, infectologists, epidemiologists, medical specialists, and institutions that engage with the disease, including the government, creating an overwhelming "infodemic" and underpinning ideas and behaviors that can be a source of conflict between perceptions of risk and measures taken—or not taken—to avoid that risk.

Whether Germans were for or against the government's preventive measures, knowledge of the presence of the virus became ubiquitous in people's lives. Over time, the information provided by scientific authorities moved from uncertain and unclear findings and explanations to relatively clear research outcomes within the academic realm, yet which still seemed abstract to the population. Alongside this information disconnect, a rich new etymology emerged, permeating and materializing new experiences. Whereas words such as "contagion," "virus," "prevention," and "isolation" were already understood, new terms such as "social distancing," "super-spreader," "self-quarantine," and more specialized terminology like "incubation period," "R-number," "incidence," "asymptomatic carriers," "viral shedding," and "herd immunity" appeared. The rapid and increasing information overwhelm—the infodemic—therefore started to become problematic. While this type of scholastic jargon is key to understanding the virus and its effects for those who can understand such terminology, an endeavor to develop a common and easier lexicon that would allow a better understanding of prevention, care and treatment for the general public would have been beneficial but was not always forthcoming. *Wirrologen*, a neologism linking the German term for virologist and "warren" (confusion), is an example of people's reactions to this terminology. This linguistic issue is essential to understanding peoples' perceptions of an abstract risk vs a real danger (Ali and Davis-Floyd 2020). Two of my interlocutors stated:

> We are now overflowed with information. I know it's not always right, but accessing the information on social media is much easier than reading something written by experts. They keep repeating the same things but you never get what's their point.
>
> (Markus, age 44, carpenter)

> If you hear the news today, the things they say will be different in a week, so why bother?
>
> (Nora, age 37, architect)

Fact-checking is therefore not straightforward but needs the guidance of various experts to explain the facts on the basis of which the decisions are made and what are the alternatives, especially when these differ among (federal) governments. For example, lack of full explanation of all reasons for and aspects of a preventive measure was perceived by my interlocutors as unreliable information, creating anxiety and uncertainty. Although viruses exist outside of politics, people's perceptions of them and actions around them can easily become politicized. Many German individuals and groups expressed their political resistance to preventive measures in terms of ideologies leading to behavioral contestations. Consequently, a few months after the pandemic started, people became less willing to obey the guidelines and began to engage in risky behaviors.

The Importance of Health Literacy and the Prevention Paradox

Since the 1970s, the term *health literacy* (HL) has been used mainly in the context of school education concerning appropriate behaviors to maintain or restore an individual's health, as well as in connection with adult education and empowerment as an important part of community development (Sørensen 2012). Within the medical care system, HL refers to an individual-focused approach to improving patient knowledge and the ability of individuals to act accordingly. For instance, population-wide strategies to curb C-19 have been key, yet these successful prevention programs have trivialized the severity of the disease by slowing its spread, thereby making it appear less dangerous, resulting in a *prevention paradox*.

In health promotion, HL describes practical knowledge and skills for dealing with health and disease, within one's own body and within the living conditions that shape health or illness (Sørensen 2012). These skills are primarily imparted or passed on throughout childhood, during formal education, and via societal practices. HL is thus an integral part of social-based resources, the acquisition and use of which is strongly influenced by people's backgrounds.

In addition to everyday practical experiences, HL also includes specialized knowledge, such as about individual and collective health risks or about measures to improve health-relevant living conditions (Wallerstein 2006). These shape the possibilities and motivations of individuals to develop health knowledge from their respective living environments and to use it in different fields of action (e.g., family, work, daily life, healthcare systems) for health maintenance and promotion. HL is thus primarily understood as a resource that can help individuals gain more control over their health and health-influencing factors. Ideally, both individual health gains and improvements in the general conditions for health can be achieved by increasing HL (Lee et al. 2004). For health promotion, this connection between individual skills and structural conditions is an important starting point for a critical application of the concept. Measures to promote HL are to be embedded in the context of the lifeworlds and the relevance system of the target group. This includes promoting HL from a user-oriented perspective and linking the interventions to the needs, ideas, and lifestyles of the target group—which in the case of COVID-19 is the entire population of Germany (Berkman et al.2010).

The Impacts of Health Literacy and of Its Lack

Health literacy is an essential personal competence, crucial for clinicians, healthcare systems, and lay people. Yet it is difficult to operationalize in best practices. The significance of HL competence becomes evident when new healthcare strategies are introduced into public settings. This significance can be observed in the rollout of the C-19 preventive measures. Following measures such as hygiene procedures, social/physical distancing, isolation, use of masks, and quarantine indicates public compliance, achieving significance and positive impacts for these public health measures. However, among the general public, these strategies often seem abstract and irrelevant to or interfering with their daily lives; thus, many resist or refuse to implement them. Additionally, with the start of mass inoculation in 2021, doubts and fears about the vaccine's safety, even among healthcare workers, have been present. A survey taken during April and June 2020 showed early on that the willingness of Germans to get vaccinated against COVID had declined, from 70% to 61%.[2] The main concern has been how rapidly the vaccines were developed, prompting apprehension. Side-effects of some of the vaccines, news about deaths apparently related to the vaccines, and a lack of information about how these vaccines work were the main reasons for this apprehension. This, along with the slow pace of vaccination programs, has contributed to the fact that only around 4.3 million people had received two vaccines by the beginning of April 2021; both doses appeared necessary to provide full protection, but much later it became clear that a third "booster" dose was also needed[3]. Such vaccine refusal stems from the concerns noted above and also from distrust of pharmaceutical companies and the government, conspiracy theories, and lack of clarifications of the efficacy of the vaccines.

One of my study participants works in a psychiatry unit, and another takes care of disabled people; the rest of these interlocutors work outside of the healthcare realm. Yet all participants regard themselves as either relatively knowledgeable or as experts concerning their understanding of science in general. Nevertheless, during our interviews, each referred to whether or not to implement the preventive measures as a personal decision, rather than as the result of respect for the scientific evidence. For example, why some are against being vaccinated involved *perceptions* instead of scientific understandings. Moreover, opinions shared on social media or by peers were taken more seriously than scientific evidence:

> First they said that we need to follow the measures because a vaccine would take time. I heard it takes more than 10 years to create a vaccine, so why should I trust one that has been developed in just a few months? I don't know, I won't trust any vaccine that has been developed so fast, there is not enough data to be sure it is 100% safe.
>
> (Martin, age 41, nurse)

> What does it mean that a vaccine is only 70% effective? If it's not 100% effective, why should I risk being vaccinated?
>
> (Michelle, age 52, unemployed)

Concerns around the safety and side-effects of vaccines have not been addressed in terms of health promotion. Nor have pharmaceutical companies, experts, or the government delivered suitable explanations to the general public regarding the fact that every decision to slow down or stop viral spreading is based on research results. The general appeal continued to be primarily based on calling upon "people's trust and cooperation"; this appeal is disconnected from people's individual understandings and needs for clear explanations.

Health Campaigns

Since the pandemic started, official health campaigns have been overshadowed by the immense amounts of false or misinformation regarding the coronavirus. Consequently, the World Health Organization (WHO) started a global campaign, "Stop the Spread," to encourage people to "check information with trusted sources such as WHO and national health authorities."[4] In Berlin, the Senate took a different approach, initiating a campaign in which people who were non-compliant with the preventive mask-wearing measure—known as "anti-maskers"—were blamed for negligence. Since Berliners are known for having a grouchy attitude as a way

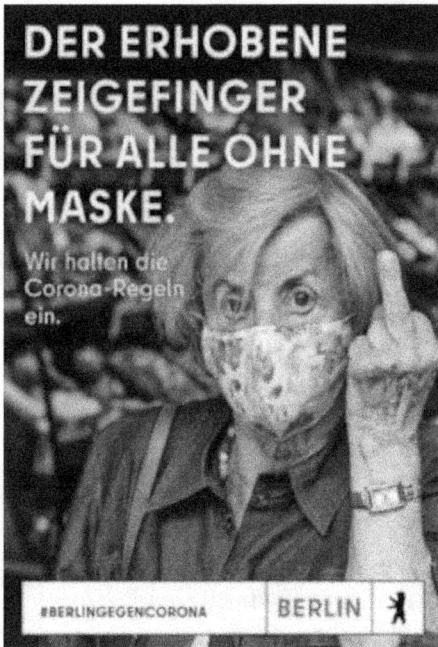

Figure 6.1 The Campaign Poster. The literal translation of the heading is "The middle finger for everyone without a mask. We adhere to the corona rules." Public domain.

of "being funny," this health campaign opted for an illustrative approach in which an old woman shows her middle finger to people who do not wear a mask (see Figure 6.1).

This public health response was not only non-educational, but also mask wearing was confusingly presented as being an optional, personal choice. In addition, this poster could easily be misinterpreted as saying "Screw people who don't wear a mask" instead of "Screw COVID-19." This misinterpretation is visible in this comment by one of my interlocutors: "Yeah, I have seen that [campaign] and I feel the same, I say, 'Fuck them all to make me wear a mask as if I were a dog wearing a muzzle'" (Stephan, age 43, postal service worker).

This campaign, which many experienced as offensive, was later changed. Along with this form of "raising awareness," the *Ordnungsamt* (Office of Order)—a squadron responsible for maintaining public safety and order, normally well-known for issuing parking fines—was the first to be in charge of enforcing mask-wearing and social distancing. These two institutional methods of "educating the public" were not responsive to people's questions, such as: "What does it mean when someone can be pre-symptomatic?" "Why do I need a mask if I'm outside?" "If I got the virus, am I now immune?" "If I get the vaccine, can I still spread the virus?" and so on. Thus, a lack of health literacy in terms of basic understandings of viruses, spread, and contagion—which should have been provided by clear public health responses to such questions—have resulted in poor choices around how to behave or to follow instructions.

The absence of appropriate information has caused many people to decide to just carry on with their daily lives and only follow the measures if reprimanded for not doing so. Containment of the virus has therefore been particularly challenging, and the rapid viral spread across the country can be seen as being primarily caused by personal attitudes towards the measures resulting from lack of HL and of governmental clarity. Examples of obfuscating messages spread by the government and health authorities include:

- Meetings in groups no larger than four...with some exceptions;
- Wear the mask before entering the restaurant and then take it off once seated;
- A negative test result doesn't mean you don't have the virus;
- Only FFP2 masks can protect you but you can wear a self-made one;
- We don't know if a vaccine can protect you from a reinfection, vs
- Vaccinated people should regain all their rights.

Given these extremely mixed messages, it comes as no surprise that participants were reluctant to follow preventive measures due to distrust and misunderstandings; they perceived official information as unreliable, contradictory, and authoritarian in its intent. Thus, it is clear that measures to promote HL should be embedded in the context of daily life and the relevance system of the target group. This includes promoting HL from a user-oriented perspective, linking the interventions to the needs, comprehensions, and lifestyles of the target group—which, again, in this case would be the German population as a whole, in all its diversity.

I now turn to a closer examination of some of two of the most important preventive measures in terms of health literacy: handwashing and mask-wearing as they played out in Germany during COVID-19.

Health Literacy as Related to Handwashing and to the Prevention Paradox

"We thought by 2020 we'd have flying cars but no, here we are teaching people to wash their hands." This supposedly funny remark was posted in Memes on Instagram®, Facebook® and other social media for several weeks as the preventive measures were put in place. The simplistic idea that we had regressed to our childhood years to learn how to wash our hands properly was preposterous for many. "Washing hands for at least 20 seconds" has long been one of the WHO's guidelines to save people from infections, as hands are the main pathways of germ transmission. However, in lower-resource countries, many people still lack or have inappropriate access to water, soaps and drains to wash their hands. And many in all countries wash their hands insufficiently: they don't wash them for long enough, nor at the right times, and they may not use soap, thinking that water will suffice. Since pathogens are not visible, it can be hard to believe that they are present and can cause deadly diseases. *Intellectual awareness often does not translate to actual practice.*

Washing hands correctly and using masks were the first key procedures to the "AHA formula" of Germany's guidelines, introduced by the Ministry of Health. With winter approaching and the second wave beginning, this changed to "AHAL" to allow schools to reopen. (AHAL stands for *Abstand halten* (keep your distance); *Hygiene-Maßnahmen beachten* (observe general hygiene rules); *Alltagsmaske tragen* (wear your mask every day); *Lüftung* (ventilation)). That these practices have been marked as key gives a brief insight into how health literacy needs to be discussed and implemented in more detail, engaging with practices of "functional knowledge"—meaning health literate knowledge of understanding the need for and implementing behaviors specific to preventing diseases. For example, even when people do wear masks, we can still observe inappropriate behaviors, such as the myriad ways of mask wearing that avoid appropriate mouth and nose coverage.

One difficulty is that these guidelines are perceived as curtailing and controlling, since the interlinkage between national healthcare recommendations and policies and the ideas of the private sphere are crosscutting and undercutting personal and social frameworks through the expansion of public health responses to C-19. The individual fears of the transgressive power of government policies, even when these benefit people's health, are equally embedded in the lack of understanding of *how* such measures impact people's health. The Robert Koch Institute—the German government's central institution for the identification, surveillance and prevention of infectious diseases—and German universities have always been regarded as the main contributors to research. Some of these are coextensive with governmental institutions, and such partnerships are often instrumental in bridging the gap between research outcomes and policies. However, in the process of providing information to the civil sector as a result of this association, the "facts" occasionally become ambivalent, confusing, and challenging for lay people to understand, as demonstrated above. Academic scientific research is based on trial and error, in which hypotheses can be proposed and tested, sometimes confirmed and sometimes refuted; this ongoing process makes it possible to gain further knowledge. But when this process is shared outside the world of academia, perceptions and people's reactions point to emerging complications. This results in another difficulty, which is that although simple messages provided to the public are more beneficial than complex ones—which would depend on high degrees of HL to understand—their simplicity paradoxically disguises their underlying complexities and may lead to contestations of and a concomitant decrease in their importance—in what I referred to above as the "prevention paradox."

Health Literacy and Mask Wearing

Starting on April 6, 2020, the use of masks became compulsory in the neighboring country of Austria, initiating the first discussions of adopting the same regulation in Germany, which in turn initiated a mask-wearing policy by the end of that month. Masks then had to be worn everywhere, all the time (with fines being issued for failure to wear a mask as a form of discipline), except in homes and in open places where physical distancing could be maintained. Yet the type of mask that should be used was continually debated. And to what extent a protective mask, regardless of whether it was medical or self-sewn, actually offered protection against transmission was controversial. The Robert Koch Institute therefore carefully formulated the recommendation on its website: "It can be assumed that makeshift masks can also reduce the risk of infecting others because they can reduce the spread of the droplets produced by coughing, sneezing or speaking."

The "It can be assumed" part of this recommendation diminishes its strength right at the start. Nevertheless, the message sent did indicate that wearing a mask could help to reduce infection rates—yet mixed messages concerning which masks are more appropriate have been continual. Additionally, the information provided was primarily focused on the reasons why people who belonged to a high-risk group needed to be a priority. According to the recommendations of the Robert Koch Institute, wearing so-called "non-medical" everyday masks could reduce the risk of infection for the person wearing them, but more importantly, these masks protect others if the wearer is a carrier of C-19. Yet our experience in Germany was that people who do not perceive themselves as being vulnerable or are not having contact with people at risk simply did not wear a mask (Wise et al. 2020; Tunçgenç 2021). The recommendations revolving around ambiguous linkages were often perceived as inconsistent, incrementing people's feelings of distress and/or information fatigue. Conspiracy theorists were using this vagueness as evidence that the pandemic was just a hoax. Thus, as the number of infections increased, problematic behaviors became increasingly visible:

> Wearing a mask offers more problems than solutions. I can't properly breathe and I can't see peoples' expressions. I feel disconnected. Surely, it can't be healthy to wear a mask for so long, lacking oxygen, anyway, so, I don't wear it. I carry a mask with me and put it on to enter a place if they ask me to, but then I leave it on my chin. People can't make me do something I don't want to. I don't want to do something that harms me more than doing good. I think people from East Berlin are even more

reluctant to follow those dictatorial measures. I can understand why some call it a "corona dictatorship."

(Matthias, age 39, health worker)

You wear a mask inside the bus or train but you have people sitting by your side and they are not wearing their mask properly—it's all nonsense.

(Steffi, age 55, teacher)

My research highlighted a variety of other factors as to why some people do wear masks when they are not being observed, even at a collective level, such as perceptions of self-vulnerability or of risk, along with emotions that these two factors trigger—both important factors to approach in any health campaign:

When I'm with one of the people I take care of, I ask him if it's okay if I don't wear a mask. They can be without one if they choose to. Using a mask makes people feel detached and what we need is the opposite to be in balance. Social connection is healing, not wearing a mask. There have been people ill with more threatening illnesses and they get cured if they are with people who love them. Viruses are everywhere, so why should this one be different?

(Matthias, age 39, health worker)

I do now use the mask because it would be expensive if they caught me without one, for example at the train, but you can't really breathe with it. You can't tell me that wearing a mask is healthy. So, if I take the train to somewhere and there are not people around, then I just take it off or I start drinking water or eating something so people can't tell me to put it on.

(Taby, age 38, NGO coordinator)

Taby elaborates:

I believe that a good diet is more important than wearing a mask to protect ourselves. One person from our group says that we actually need to get in contact with more people in order to protect ourselves, live more in tune with nature—only like that can we teach our body to protect itself. [In following preventive measures], we're doing something that is against nature.

Taby's statement is revelatory of the opinions and ideology of many others in Germany, who believe that if they lead healthy lives, their immune systems will protect them from COVID infection, or from becoming seriously ill should they get infected.

In terms of HL, the regular use of masks is key to controlling and preventing an increase in contagions. However, C-19 health promotion in Germany has been individual-centric, with a strong emphasis on "individual responsibility," thereby neglecting a systematic and more compelling campaign in health education. The development and applicability of HL in this case totally depends on the respective counterpart: the willingness and ability of people to contribute to their health competence. Yet, with the increasing importance of the measures introduced, HL's development should gain pertinence as an explicit target or outcome variable as a criterion of evidence-based health promotion (Brigs 2020; Lunn et al. 2020). Nevertheless, in late summer 2020, many individuals and groups became increasingly less aware of all the measures approved by public health institutions. The AHAL formula sufficed to underline what proved to me to be an emerging problem concerning health behaviors, as indicated in the quotations above and in the following section.

Understanding C-19 within a Phenomenological Approach

Institutionally speaking, C-19-driven measures are increasingly carried out via political establishments. As the pandemic's impacts became visible, political and academic institutions became active "partners" in the C-19 negotiations and operations. One of the results of this partnership, as also shown above, has been that information has not always been clearly communicated, causing problems and challenges:

> Not being able to go wherever you want, not being able to visit your parents or grandparents if they don't live with you, people on the street telling you off if you come too close or you're not wearing a mask, people tracing you down with those lists,[5] that all stuff is Stasi[6] performance.

> (Michelle, 52, unemployed)

In addition, as noted above, my participants found it difficult to trust and navigate C-19 information from official media outlets. Fact-checking was considered overwhelming or inadequate, and a lack of the necessary health literacy to deal with academic information also contributes to reduced competence when dealing with this type of data. We know from previous research that a "one-size-fits-all" approach to persuasion and behavioral change is likely to be limited in efficacy (Singer and Baer 2018). Clear communication from health authorities and scientific experts is essential, including paraphrasing and clarifying information according to different target groups. This pandemic has revealed how public reliance for information about C-19 on social networking and non-academic media constitutes a model of knowledge exchange that threatens and diminishes acceptance of officially established preventive measures (see Kramer 2014; Briggs and

Hallin 2016). Because HL arises in a multitude of different contexts (family, peers, workplaces, associations, etc.), intersectoral interventions—programs or activities affecting health outcomes undertaken by sectors external to the official health sector—to promote HL are important to improve understanding and the corresponding ability to act appropriately.

In this era of the Internet and social media, there are many alternative "realities" delivering innumerable versions of facts competing for "the truth." Information and language are important elements that provide structure to people's everyday lives. This way of looking at C-19 responses enables rich insight into the sense-making practices concerning health literacy processes, since it recognizes the existence of an individual lens through which perceptions and knowledge are created and filtered. Phenomenological theorists argue that certain essential features of the lifeworld include a person's sense of selfhood, embodiment, temporality, spatiality, sociality, discourse and mood-as-atmosphere (Ashworth 2003). These interconnected "fractions" operate as lenses through which we assess information; thus, health campaigns should consider these socially-shared dimensions (Dahlberg et al. 2008). The successes of fake information, rumors, and conspiracy theories partially stem from the fact that their messages are personal as well as societal, while scientific facts are abstract and cannot easily be understood and applied, and require very high levels of health literacy—not held by the general population—to understand. As Taby representatively described:

> I can't do all this for too long. I'm sure there are more people like me that think that we should just get infected and have this behind us to keep working, to keep living. This is just another flu virus. A few friends are getting depressed. I'm sure the majority of people are suffering from other things and not from corona.

The social and psychological determinants of health and personal wellbeing are important aspects that enable the understandings of people's ideas of personal exposure, risk and consequences, which have not been part of the German preventive measures campaign.

Conclusions: Health Literacy, Information Fatigue, and the Prevention Paradox

Health literacy follows a long path and relies on understanding information and "facts" that are often incomplete and contradictory, and which require constant verification, since the very nature of science is that it lives in a continuous state of development. C-19 is an excellent example of how HL plays a significant role in the use of available data to acquire information and justify specific behaviors. It also has the particularity of constantly providing new evidence, which can be beneficial and/or can generate fear, anxiety, distress, and information fatigue, reducing people's abilities to focus on what is important.

This ethnographic research reveals that many Germans considered the information concerning C-19 too technical, unreliable, contradictory, inconclusive, or insufficient—the prevention paradox. These contradictions resulted in measures being perceived as deceiving, increasing uncertainty about health protection actions, and resulting in a direct negative impact on responses to the preventive health measures, which in turn is now having a direct negative impacts on the inclination to get vaccinated. Important messages were lost in a politicized campaign, decreasing credibility and public trust. The obvious solution is for the authorities—the government and the scientists—to agree on messages before they are published and to make sure that they are clear, well-explained, responsive to people's primary questions and concerns, and directly relevant to people's everyday lifeworlds and within their health literacy levels. In addition, I suggest that the government and educational institutions should work to increase the health literacy of the population to better prepare them for improving health in times of normality and for possible future epidemics or pandemics.

Notes

1 www.rki.de/DE/Content/InfAZ/N/Neuartiges_Coronavirus/Fallzahlen.html
2 www.dw.com/en/coronavirus-vaccine-germany/a-54146673.
3 www.rki.de/DE/Content/Infekt/Impfen/ImpfungenAZ/COVID-19/COVID-19.html
4 www.who.int/news-room/feature-stories/detail/countering-misinformation-about-covid-19
5 Referring to the policy of keeping visitor attendance records for innkeepers, which was mandatory at the beginning of the reopening of restaurants and cafes in June 2020. People needed to leave personal information such as name, address, and telephone number to be contacted—i.e. tracked—in case an outbreak was reported at that place. In addition, information on the time and duration of attendance, table and seat numbers of the guests was also recorded.
6 The Ministry for State Security, the official security service of the German Democratic Republic, created in 1950 with the aim of spying on the population, primarily through a large network of citizens who worked as informants, who reported anyone who was in opposition to the political measures of the time.

References

Ali, I., and R. Davis-Floyd. 2020. The interplay of words and politics during COVID-19: Contextualizing the universal pandemic vocabulary. *Practicing Anthropology* 42(4): 20–24. https://doi.org/10.17730/0888-4552.42.4.20

Ashworth, P. 2003. An approach to phenomenological psychology: The contingencies of the lifeworld. *Journal of Phenomenological Psychology* 34: 145–156.

Bavel, J.J.V., K. Baicker, P.S. Boggio, V. Capraro, A. Cichocka, M. Cikara, et al. 2020. Using social and behavioural science to support COVID-19 pandemic response. *Nature Human Behaviour* 4: 460–471.

Berkman, N.D., T.C. Davis, and D.L. McCormack. 2010. Health literacy: What is it? *Journal of Health Communication* 15(2): 9–19.

Briggs, C.L. 2020. Beyond the linguistic/medical anthropology divide: Retooling anthropology to face COVID-19. *Medical Anthropology* 39(7): 563–572.

Briggs, C.L., and D.C. Hallin. 2016. "Making Health Public: How News Coverage Is Remaking Media." *Medicine, and Contemporary Life.* London: Routledge.

Dahlberg, K., H. Dahlberg, and M. Nystrom. 2008. *Reflective Lifeworld Research.* 2nd Edition. Lund, Sweden: Student literature.

Kramer, A.D.I., J.E. Guillory, and J.T. Hancock. 2014. Experimental evidence of massive-scale emotional contagion through social networks. *Proceedings of the National Academy of Science of the United States of America* 111(24): 8878–8790.

Lee, S.Y., A.M. Arozullah, and Y.I. Cho. 2004. Health literacy, social support, and health: A research agenda. *Social Science Medicine* 58(7): 1309–21.

Lunn, P., et al. 2020. Using behavioural science to help fight the coronavirus. *ESRI Working Paper* No. 656. March 2020. [Working Paper]

Sørensen, K., S. Van den Broucke, J. Fullam, G. Doyle, J. Pelikan, Z. Slonska, et al. 2012. (HLS-EU) Consortium Health Literacy Project European. Health literacy and public health: a systematic review and integration of definitions and models. *BMC Public Health* Jan 25: 12–80.

Singer, M., and H. Baer. 2018. "Critical Medical Anthropology." In Ray H. Elling (ed.), *Critical Approaches in the Health Social Sciences Series.* London: CRC Press.

Tunçgenç, B., M. El Zein, J. Sulik, M. Newson, Y. Zhao, G. Dezecache, et al. 2021. Social influence matters: We follow pandemic guidelines most when our close circle does. *British Journal of Psychology.* https://doi.org/10.1111/bjop.12491

Wallerstein, N. 2006. *What is the Evidence on Effectiveness of Empowerment To Improve Health? Health Evidence Network Report.* Copenhagen, Denmark: World Health Organization Regional Office for Europe.

Wise, T., T.D. Zbozinek, G. Michelini, C.C. Hagan, and D. Mobbs. 2020. Changes in risk perception and self-reported protective behaviour during the first week of the COVID-19 pandemic in the United States. *Royal Society Open Science.* September 16; 7(9): 200742. doi: 10.1098/rsos.200742. PMID: 33047037; PMCID: PMC7540790.

7 "Flexible Lockdown" in Switzerland
Individual Responsibility and the Daily Navigation of Risk and Protection

Nolwenn Bühler, Melody Pralong,
Célia Burnand, Cloé Rawlinson,
Semira Gonseth Nusslé, Valérie D'Acremont,
Murielle Bochud, and Patrick Bodenmann

Introduction: The Swiss Response to COVID-19

What characterizes the responses of Switzerland to the COVID-19 (C-19) pandemic and how does it shape individuals' daily life navigation of risk and protection? To shed light on the variety of responses to C-19, this chapter focuses on this small, multilingual, mountainous country of 8.5 million inhabitants. Located in central Europe, it is also one of the wealthiest countries in the world, renowned for its cutting-edge biotech sector and the excellence of its hospitals. Comprising 26 states (*Cantons*), Switzerland's healthcare system works on a federalist basis in which each Canton is in charge of managing the health of its population.

At the end of February 2020, as attention was riveted on the dramatic situation in Italy, the first cases of C-19 were identified on Swiss ground, suddenly reminding the population that the country was not immune to the coronavirus. By the beginning of March, cases were more than doubling every day. On March 16, 2020, a state of emergency was declared and the Swiss federal authorities closed schools and non-essential shops, and banned all gatherings in public spaces of more than five people. However, unlike in most neighboring European countries (with the exception of Sweden; see Chapter 2), there was no complete lockdown. The health and political authorities called on the population to behave in responsible and civic ways and to adopt *gestes-barrière* ("barrier gestures") to protect the healthcare system, those medically considered as being at risk, and healthcare workers.

This form of lockdown, with no sanctioning nor formal obligation to stay home, which we refer to as *flexible lockdown*, represents a Swiss specificity, in contrast to other forms of lockdown in France, Italy, Germany, and the UK (Desson et al. 2020; Hirsch 2020), and to Sweden, which never implemented any form of lockdown (see Chapter 2). Flexible lockdown was based primarily on the principle of *individual responsibility*, which lies at the core of Swiss values, along with a *culture of consensus*. Health

DOI: 10.4324/9781003187462-10

authorities adopted individual responsibility in their public communications and favored transparency, acknowledging the multiple uncertainties and appealing to individuals' common sense, as did medical experts. How is this principle of individual responsibility enacted and experienced in the daily lives of Swiss people navigating between viral exposure to C-19 and protective measures? In this chapter, we question the "moral economy" (Fassin 2005) of responsibility at stake in the Swiss context during the C-19 pandemic, and present the first results of the medical anthropology project described below.

Methods and Materials

This chapter presents the preliminary results of a medical anthropology study called SociocoViD, which was developed as part of an epidemiological project on transmission and immunity to SARS-CoV-2 in the Canton de Vaud, Switzerland. SociocoViD is funded by the Swiss National Science Foundation (NRP 78 Covid-19, SNSF). This qualitative project aims to complement the epidemiological quantitative methods used in the project called SerocoViD by shedding light on how living conditions impact viral exposure, the adoption of protective practices, and the emergence of additional vulnerabilities[1] that might increase health inequities related to gender, ethnicity, and socioeconomic status.

We collected data through qualitative semi-directed interviews (videoconference or in-person) and observations of participants' living environments whenever possible. Three groups of the population, also participating in the epidemiological arm of the study, were included: (1) Index cases (the first to be tested positive with C-19) and members of a representative sample of the general population who were randomly selected (20 interviews); (2) Asylum seekers (9 interviews at the time of drafting the chapter); and (3) Employees of essential services (three interviews at the time of drafting the chapter). Data collection is ongoing and, in this chapter, we draw only on interviews and observations with the first group. We complement our empirical analysis with media and official sources, available online. Approval from the Ethical Commission of the Canton de Vaud was granted in May 2020 and then amended in December 2020 to include the second two groups of the population described above. All translations of the quotations below are by the authors.

Containing COVID-19 via Individual Responsibility

Gestes-barrière as Core Protection Measures

A wind of panic blew throughout Switzerland in March 2020 when the first cases of C-19 were diagnosed there. Facing a dramatically uncertain future, and due to fear of shortages, people rushed to purchase in large amounts household goods such as non-perishable food items and hygiene products, especially for handwashing. Located next to Italy, the Canton of Tessin was the first to report a diagnosed case of C-19 and to face the gravity of the pandemic. While dramatic images of overwhelmed Italian care units made the news, the federal health authorities did not choose to implement containment measures similar to those of Italy, instead calling its population to individual responsibility by urging symptomatic people to self-isolate and to wash their hands frequently (Dussault 2020). Although other countries mandated mask wearing, it was not part of the early preventive measures implemented in Switzerland, except for sick people and healthcare professionals. The fact that there was a shortage of masks in Switzerland at that time probably contributed to this policy choice. The federal health authorities justified not requiring mask wearing for the general population with the fear of generating a sense of false security, due to the lack at that time of proven efficacy of protective masks. It was only in early July 2020, that, observing an upsurge in cases, some Cantons made mask wearing obligatory in stores (RTSinfo 2020a); the Federal Council also mandated this measure on public transportation.

Social distancing and *gestes-barrière* represent core measures that have been upheld during the pandemic in Switzerland. These *gestes-barrière* consisted of hygiene and distancing measures, such as sneezing in the elbow, washing hands regularly, stopping handshaking, and maintaining a two-meter distance between individuals. *Gestes-barrière* refer to what are elsewhere called "preventive measures," yet the French-speaking countries' use of the term "barrier gestures" conveys a specific meaning—it implies a physical protection between viral exposure and the self, illustrating how the virus is perceived as a threat against which protection is required. In France for example, the metaphor of war, used by the President when announcing the first lockdown, reveals how *gestes-barrière* are conceived as defensive walls erected against a viral enemy. In contrast, in the French-speaking part of Switzerland, the use of the term *gestes-barrière*[2] refers more to their paradoxical social dimension, as the "obstacles [necessary] to enter in contact, the gestures that distance one from drawing near" (ZHAW 2020).[3] They can be understood as flexible, situational, and relational boundaries aimed at reducing viral circulation. Both material and symbolic, they are made and negotiated in daily practices. They separate the inside of bodies from a potentially infectious outside, the safe spaces and relations from the risky ones; they allow people to situate and define themselves, but may also generate other kinds of risky exposures, as we will demonstrate below. Respecting *gestes-barrière* was done in the name of solidarity, with healthcare workers, especially those practicing in intensive care units, spotlighted as heroes on the frontline.

Throughout the C-19 pandemic, *gestes-barrière* have remained core measures of containment resting essentially on individual responsibility. Despite their apparent simplicity and obviousness, these low-tech measures are complex to navigate in daily life, leaving individuals to choose when and how to adopt them. They also reveal the deep entanglement of the biological and the social at work to try to contain viral transmission. The use of the term "social distancing," simultaneously indexing spatial, physical distance, and social relationships, shows well how the two levels cannot be disentangled. The entanglement between the viral and the social is negotiated by individuals in their daily lives, as we demonstrate below.

The Implementation of "Flexible Lockdown"

Witnessing a significant increase in the number of cases—+500 per day—on March 16, the Swiss Federal Council declared an "extraordinary situation"—an action justified by the law on epidemics (Art. 7, *Loi sur les épidémies* 2010), enabling the federal authorities to take control over the Canton authorities, and to become the legitimate political decision-makers able to impose measures at the national level (RTSinfo 2020b). In one of the many press conferences that have punctuated the pandemic in Switzerland, the Minister in charge of the health system, Alain Berset, justified this measure by stating the need for uniformity across Cantons, with the purpose of increasing the population's understanding of the pandemic. The measures announced on this day aimed to facilitate the avoidance of social contacts by closing public spaces such as restaurants, bars, schools, and stores, with the exception of essential services. Persons at risk due to other illnesses or age were asked to stay home, while the rest of the population was asked to avoid superfluous contacts, leaving the definition of "superfluous" to individual responsibility. It was "highly recommended," but non-mandatory, to stay at home, with the exceptions of grocery shopping, bringing help to others, work, and medical appointments. Fines were imposed for not following some of the recommendations, such as avoiding outdoor gatherings of more than five people (RTSinfo 2020c). However, their application was left to the Cantons and the local police authorities. In the case of essential services, companies were to accommodate workplaces according to certain security criteria, and in cases where this was not possible, to authorize working from home.

These initial measures were characteristic of what we designate "a flexible regime of pandemic management," including flexible lockdown. These measures were constantly readjusted over time according to epidemiological statistics on viral transmission rates, the capacities of intensive care units, and the numbers of available medical materials—masks, medical ventilators, C-19 tests, and now vaccines. Acknowledging from the very beginning the complexity of the situation, the health authorities adopted a communication style of transparency, recognizing scientific uncertainties, and favoring flexibility as the only viable way of navigating risk—a middle ground between caution and strictness. By comparing the pandemic to a "marathon," these authorities asked the Swiss people to take responsibility, be patient, act on common sense, and respect the preventive measures in the name of solidarity with others. Calls for individual responsibility were heightened in importance when the flexible lockdown was released in May 2020, yet took a slightly different form as the importance of supporting the economy slowly overtook the fear of viral transmission (RTSinfo 2020d).

The trust and flexibility that health authorities manifested towards the population through the valorization of individual responsibility placed the weight of the moral responsibility to navigate between risk and protection on individuals. The normative character of the flexible regime appeared, for example, when groups of the population were specifically pointed to and blamed for their "irresponsible" behaviors. For instance, situations in which young people reunited in higher numbers than authorized and threw wild parties made breaking news, but no retribution was addressed to employees going to their offices when working from home was supposedly mandatory. Moreover, this flexibility and the importance of individual responsibility increased differentials between groups of the population, as not all were in the same conditions for navigating risk and protection.

Solidarity and Individual Responsibility as Core Swiss Values: *Unus pro omnibus, omnes pro uno*

In Switzerland, the valorization of individual responsibility is embedded in a moral economy of solidarity, which is at the core of public health values and of epidemiological reasoning, but also has neoliberalist origins. Over past decades, the public health sector, and more generally public services, have slowly been dismantled and privatized in Switzerland. Investments in prevention and health promotion are insignificant in comparison to investments in high-tech biomedical sectors. Investments in healthcare tend to rely on individualistic measures based on individual choices around healthy or unhealthy behavior, regardless of the structural inequities that lead to ill health (Berg, Harting, and Stronks 2021) and cause unequal access to care. However, when C-19 spread in the Swiss population, threatening the health sector as much as the economic sector, calls for solidarity took central stage, reviving the Swiss motto from the Latin: *Unus pro omnibus, omnes pro uno* ("One for all, all for one") (see Hebeisen 2020). Expressions of solidarity were visible on social networks such as Facebook, or through the applause for the healthcare workers that came from balconies every evening at 9pm during the first lockdown. This notion of solidarity rested on individual responsibility, which was invoked and even defended as a Swiss political core value.

An example comes from a letter written by the local politician Hodgers (2020) to a French senator who had criticized Switzerland for its "laxity" and absence of strict measures. Recalling the importance of civic attitudes, a culture of consensus, trust in the authorities, and the political weight granted to citizens in the democratic culture characterizing this federalist country (where the population is asked to vote several times a year and individuals can bring forward issues for vote by referendum), Hodgers defended Switzerland's choice by stating:

> that the only way of slowing down viral progression is the population's understanding of the health rules. [We insist] that the adherence of the population is a tool much more efficient than police forces who have other priorities to deal with [...] and that nothing justifies generalized controls.

The valorization of individual responsibility is a way of recognizing people's agency and intelligence; it is embedded in the context of solidarity to justify the protection measures adopted, but also carries a hint of neoliberalism. From the very beginning of the pandemic, the economic sector feared the consequences of prioritizing health by implementing strict protection measures. By asking the federal council to change its pandemic management paradigm, considered to rely on "strict and sometimes arbitrary interdictions"—such as the closure of restaurants and non-essential stores in early 2021—the federation of Swiss businesses (Economiesuisse 2021) defended individual responsibility as the only way out of the crisis. These closures slowed business activities; thus the economic sector representatives insisted even more on the value of individual responsibility to counter them and, in so doing, to boost the economy.

To question the implications of this moral economy of solidarity among individuals themselves, we draw on Fassin's work on "moral economies." Fassin (2005: 1257) states: "the moral economy [is] the production, distribution, circulation, and use of moral sentiments, emotions and values, and norms and obligations in social space." In what follows, we focus on daily lives as relevant sites for understanding the moral implications of navigating risk and protection through the negotiation of *gestes-barrière*.

By analyzing the pandemic experiences of 20 persons living in the Canton de Vaud, who are part of: (1) index cases (again, the first cases to be diagnosed during the first wave) registered by the health authorities; and (2) members of the general population who were randomly selected in the epidemiological part of the project described in the Methods section (Serocovid, Unisanté), we aim to explore how individual responsibility is internalized and translated into a moral responsibility embedded in logics of blame and guilt. Focusing on reconfigurations of living conditions during the pandemic and on logistical, practical, and symbolic negotiations of risk and protection measures, we shed light on the ambivalence of the flexibility and responsibility left to individuals, illustrating the constant work of negotiation of risk and protection in relation to others. The concept of "care" is useful here to capture this practical and moral activity of risk navigation. Laugier (2016: 208) defines "care" as "a practical response to specific needs (...), an activity necessary to maintaining persons and connections, work carried out both in the private and the public spheres, and sensitivity to what matters." Care activities are most often invisible to the wider society and are carried out without monetary exchange and in the name of love, as feminist studies have shown (Delphy 1997; Falquet et al. 2010). In the following section, we show that individual responsibility to navigate risk and protection involves a continuous work of care of one's and others' health, embedded in everyday contexts, activities, and relationships.

Protecting Others before Protecting Oneself

"I think that it is people's duty. We have a son with a chronic disease. He can catch everything with his inefficient immune system [...] We are selfish, but respectful. We wanted to go on holiday and as we are immune now, we know that we will not infect anyone, but we renounced, we won't go because the authorities recommended not to. A rule is a rule, that's the way it is," said an interlocutor in her 50s, whose entire family contracted the virus at the very beginning of the pandemic. This quote illustrates individual responsibility to adhere to health authorities' recommendations, regardless of one's own desires. We can also observe that the flexibility left to individuals takes the form of moral and practical negotiations and arrangements, such as deciding to strictly adhere to recommendations after carefully weighing the risks and potential consequences of not adhering strictly.

In such personal experiences, the importance of protecting others from the virus before protecting oneself prevails. This practical and moral work of caring for others by mitigating their risks is well shown in the case of our interlocutor Sarah, a 26-year-old middle-class woman who contracted the virus during the first week of the semi-lockdown in March 2020. She was living with her boyfriend in the home of her sister, who had just had a baby. The four of them were sharing the two-bedroom apartment with Sarah's mother, who was visiting from France to support Sarah's sister in the care of her granddaughter. When Sarah received a call from the medical office of the contact tracing center of the Canton de Vaud informing her that she had tested positive for C-19, a solution needed to be found to protect the whole family. At first, they decided to keep sharing the apartment, with Sarah's sister and her newborn baby sleeping in one bedroom and Sarah's mother in the living room; Sarah and her boyfriend were supposed to stay in the second bedroom. Sarah's boyfriend was also experiencing C-19 symptoms, requiring him to go into quarantine for ten days. Having already spent three of those days in the apartment, they realized that the apartment was not the best place to protect the family as a whole, and so they spent that time in their van in a forest instead. In so doing, Sarah and her boyfriend achieved two goals: they protected Sarah's family from the risk of viral exposure and from the risk of experiencing anxiety and fear—a practical response, in Laugier's (2016) words, to the moral and logistical dilemma of how to protect others from viral contamination in a small apartment.

Vulnerable others who need to be protected can also entail household members considered at risk due to a pre-existing medical condition. This is the case with Robin, a 17-year-old man who lives with his parents and his brother in a house outside the main city of the Canton. Regarding his lockdown experiences, he started by explaining that his father was at greater risk of developing severe symptoms from C-19 due to a pre-existing medical condition, and because of this, Robin spent the first weeks of the pandemic "locked in the house." *Space availability is key when negotiating risk and protection.* While Sarah and her boyfriend had to leave a too-small apartment for their even smaller van, for Robin and his well-off family, space availability was not a problem. This period went by very fast for Robin because he could easily live in his "huge bedroom" by himself, share the very nice garden with his family, and grab his bike to go out for exercise and enjoy the particularly beautiful spring weather that Switzerland was experiencing in March 2020. Access to space is a key indicator of socio-economic status, and Robin's case illustrates inequity by showing that the wealthy have far more options for negotiating prevention measures than those of lower socioeconomic status.

The enactment of and navigation between risk and protective practices thus appear as shaped by moral responsibilities and moral sentiments. As in Sarah's and Robin's cases, we observe that people adopt *gestes-barrière* in their everyday lives primarily from fear of contaminating others, especially when those significant others are at high risk for C-19. We observe an internalization of the moral responsibility to protect others—to "care" for them, which leads them to accept the isolation and exclusion of self-quarantine when they consider that to be necessary. In Switzerland's flexible regime of pandemic containment, people navigate protective practices based on their practical and moral engagements with others and on the available physical space they have at their disposal, itself unequally accessed depending on socio-economic status and cities/countryside regions (Marti and Ferro-Luzzi 2021; Sallier 2021). However, this flexibility can also generate anxiety and guilt, as protecting and carrying the risk for others can transform into a burden—as the experiences of Claire and Mylène described below will illustrate.

What Are "Superfluous Contacts"? The Difficult Task of Maintaining Both Distance and Relationships

Both Sarah and Robin were able to find solutions to maintaining safe spaces and protecting their families and relationships, yet protective measures can be more difficult to adopt in certain contexts—especially for people involved in the "economy of care" (Mahon and Robinson 2011), which relates not only to healthcare activities, but more broadly to all services to people, such as teaching and other so-called "essential" activities. While schools closed and went online during the first flexible lockdown, primary and secondary schools have remained open since, classes being closed only under specific decisions of health authorities when more than two persons in the school were infected. In May 2020, when schools reopened, hygiene and distancing measures had to be implemented by the teachers themselves, who were in charge of making sure the children respected these measures. Claire, a primary school teacher, explained to us that keeping safe distances with the children within her classroom was an impossible and therefore quite absurd rule. According to her:

> It was a joke. We had to keep the two-meter distance with our students [ironic laughter]…There was a story that if they got too close, we had to put on a mask or something…or with the desks… it's a joke, they are so small. I go close to play with them. One of our colleagues was explaining to me that there was a student who was crying, she said, "I looked at her, I couldn't stay two meters away, I took her in my arms." (…) So we always had the feeling that we were doing something wrong, especially in one of the schools where they were very strict, very procedural, and [sighs] I was always afraid of…being wrong. I was always afraid that the principal would arrive and surprise me when I was not two meters away from my students. (…) And then we were told that the children did not transmit the virus, so I held on to that [laughter]. And then I took some of them in my arms…I couldn't stay away from my students, so very quickly I said to myself, "Well—come what may!" I was more afraid of bringing the virus here [to her home]—of confining the whole family.

For people who had to keep working in close contact with others during the pandemic, the private and public spheres became closely connected, both socially and biologically. In Claire's and her colleague's experience, the physical distance that they were required to keep from their pupils, as well as their new role as "hygiene police," prevented them from doing their care work with their students. In this context, her non-respecting of distancing protected the relationships Claire had built with her pupils at the expense of the possibility of viral risk. However, this non-compliance generated in Claire guilt, anxiety, and the fear of doing something wrong, revealing an internalization of blame and guilt over not following preventive measures that are logistically impossible to fully respect in her school. As with our other interlocutors, Claire's narrative is pervaded less by fear of the disease and more by the risk of becoming an agent of contamination who might lead to the need to impose lockdown measures on her family. Claire's experience underlines that the distinction between "superfluous" contacts and "necessary" contacts is complex and blurry. This distinction builds on scientific knowledge about the virus and the disease it causes, and on people's perceptions of risks and the relationships they feel the need to maintain and protect, both in the public and the private spheres. These domains blur into each other in everyday life, as all our interlocutors have demonstrated.

Mylène also experienced guilt and acted to protect herself from anticipated blame during the spring of 2020. Mylène is a young woman who works as a nurse in a regional medical center and who was in regular contact with C-19 patients, particularly during the first flexible lockdown. Even though she contracted C-19 at the very beginning of the pandemic, recovered, and no longer tested positive, she worried that she could still transmit the virus to other people:

> When I was working in units where there were C-19 patients, I didn't see my family. I usually waited a week before seeing anyone. I saw my colleagues and then I went straight home, knowing that a patient had coughed on me. I didn't want to be a vector. So I isolated myself, but it wasn't required by my hospital. It was difficult for me to carry this guilt of bringing something into [other people's] homes. So I limited a lot of social contacts during the first semi-lockdown—my sister too, although I generally see her every week. (…) It was hard at first. (…) My sister and her husband were really isolated. My sister does home schooling with her children, so she really didn't see anybody. Her husband was working from home…So I worried about being a vector of transmission within their home. (…) If something would have happened, it would have come from me…because I was the one who was working with other people.

Because Mylène was the only contact that her sister's family had during the first flexible lockdown, she felt extremely responsible for potentially bringing the virus to their home, which, according to her, had no other risk of contamination. However, because her relationship with her sister and her family is not a "superfluous" one, she created her own contextualized preventive measure by isolating herself for at least a week after being in contact with C-19 patients to allow her to see her sister a few days later without taking too many risks. Both an internalized guilt and her own form of relational vulnerability—the need to see her family—shaped Mylène's actions during the pandemic. The fact that she isolated herself before seeing her family can be understood as "the protection of forms of life" (Laugier 2016: 208) where *what matters* is protected, in this case protecting and maintaining a safe relationship with her family, both at the relational and the viral level.

Conclusion: A Flexible Solidarity?

Flexible lockdown in Switzerland is embedded in a moral economy based on individual responsibility. The degree of freedom provided to individuals can be read as a way of valuing agency and empowering people, yet it has also left them to handle the mental and logistical load that this entails. By the end of 2020 in Switzerland, guilt, anxiety, mental health issues, and other psychosocial impacts of protective measures had emerged as public issues, notably among children and youth, and had increased the diagnoses of mental health issues in clinical settings. For example, these issues were specifically debated in the news after child and adolescent psychiatrists alerted the media that consultations had increased by 40% in several Swiss hospitals in November 2020 (RTSinfo 2020e). This example of the dramatic consequences of the pandemic for mental health illustrates well the government priority given to viral risk, leaving other risks (social, economic, psychological, etc.) broadly considered to be of lower priority. This focus on viral risk, combined with the flexible lockdown policy in Switzerland, led to the individualization and internalization of the moral duty to protect oneself, others, and the healthcare system. Such protection requires, at both individual and collective levels, *to care*, in the sense of constantly paying attention to others to navigate and negotiate protective practices in a context where uncertainties prevail.

With the limited hindsight that we have today, we can say that playing the solidarity and individual responsibility cards has worked relatively well, as Swiss authorities are now (May 2021) gradually relaxing their recommendations for taking protective measures. Official statistics currently state that since February 24, 2020, Switzerland has witnessed 10,187 deaths out of 682,160 diagnosed cases. Peaks in new cases were reached in November and December 2020 before a new flexible lockdown was implemented to counter the pandemic's second wave. By this time of writing (mid-May 2021), only 206 new cases per 100,000 inhabitants have been detected and only 5 people per 100,000 are presently hospitalized (Confédération Suisse 2021).

Political and health authorities are again asking the population to show solidarity, this time by getting vaccinated. The goals are to protect the most vulnerable in biological terms, and also to achieve "herd immunity." However, we in Switzerland are starting to witness cracks in the edifice of our social solidarity, as a part of the population seems reluctant to get vaccinated (Pandelé 2021). While the low-tech *gestes-barrière* are negotiated in daily life through a moral economy of individual responsibility, popular involvement in and adherence to the solidarity principle seem to be different this time. Protecting others from viral exposure reveals low-tech logics of care for the vulnerabilities of others that tend to be embedded in the gift/counter-gift dynamics of relationships, as in "I protect you and you protect me." With the high-tech C-19 vaccination, solidarity becomes a more abstract element, as people are now asked to take what they perceive as personal risks to protect others. The gift/counter-gift dynamics seem to become unbalanced, as the logics of vaccination require a greater commitment from individuals and raise fears about possibilities such as vaccine side-effects, as well as data protection, digital tracking, and controlling access to public spaces and events via a "vaccine passport."

Moreover, the double facet of individual responsibility in its neoliberal version resurfaces, as employees working in companies providing services to individuals have been asked to get vaccinated outside of their regular working hours (RTSinfo 2021), while at the same time the economic sector promotes vaccination as the only way out of the crisis. This reveals the mutability of the Swiss value on solidarity. This value is promoted when it serves the economic sector and does not prevent the workforce from continuing to work, but tends to fade away when companies are the ones that could actualize that value for their employees in return. Thus the responsibility for protection remains an individual burden that some large companies are unwilling to alleviate. However, some companies have started to provide opportunities for their employees to get vaccinated during working hours. Favoring community-based public health initiatives, as the Canton de Vaud has started to do (Barras 2021), is crucial to keeping the value on social solidarity, which was so much put to the fore during this pandemic, from becoming an empty shell. We argue that the flexibility we can observe in the Swiss management of the pandemic rests on a flexible understanding of solidarity, which enables the conciliation of health and economic interests in situated ways. We see this value as distinct from the moral responsibility to protect others from the risk of viral exposure that we could observe at the individual level, which is internalized, and can be experienced as stressful, but also reveals logics of care for other's vulnerabilities.

Our data and analyses provide insight into how people have experienced the flexible lockdown in Switzerland and have morally and logistically navigated between risk and protection. We write this chapter within the context of the ongoing collection and analysis of data within our larger project as described above. We are interviewing middle-class people of all ages and genders from similar socioeconomic and ethnic backgrounds, and are currently expanding our project by conducting ethnographic interviews with asylum seekers and essential services employees. These interviews will complement and put into perspective the preliminary observations we report on herein.

Among these latest interviews, we have observed many of the same issues described above by our interlocutors for the first phase of this project. These include the importance of the living environment, especially the availability of space, and of daily socialities—familial, friendly, professional—in which dynamics of care are embedded. Our analysis confirms the importance of living conditions in understanding the navigation of risk and responsibility, and allows us to grasp how the moral responsibility to protect others might rely more heavily on certain people than others. Living conditions, including housing, access to space, and involvement in care work, whether in the domestic or the professional spheres, emerge as crucial factors that we will explore further as our study progresses, especially to understand how gendered, racialized, and classed is the moral responsibility of caring for others by preventing risk of viral exposure. Finally, we argue that the moral economy at stake in the flexible management of the pandemic in Switzerland, reveals a mutable notion of solidarity. This mutable solidarity might be experienced as a real caring attention to others' risks in personal daily lives, but is also a way of reconciling the interests of the economy with those of the health authorities in ways that rest on the shoulders of individuals who internalize the moral burden of protection under fears of blame and guilt, often more than they internalize fears of the virus itself.

Notes

1 Drawing on Katz et al.'s (2020) critique of the vague use of the term "vulnerable," we want to make clear that we understand vulnerabilities as relational and situated, and not as inherent to people themselves.
2 The term *gestes-barrière* was selected as the second most important word of 2020 for the French-speaking part of Switzerland, after *Coronagraben* (Corona Trench), used in the German-speaking part. The latter term indexes the significant differences in the approaches of the French- and German-speaking parts of Switzerland to the pandemic, at both the epidemiological and the policy levels in regard to protection measures, about which these two parts of the country often disagreed. The differential uses of these two terms demonstrates that the pandemic is experienced very differently depending on the social and cultural context in which one lives (ZHAW 2020).
3 In the German-speaking part of Switzerland, people speak more of *Hygiene- und-Verhaltensregeln*—hygiene and behavior rules.

References

Art. 7, Loi sur les épidémies. 2010. RS 818.101—Loi Fédérale Du 28 Septembre 2012 Sur La Lutte Contre Les Maladies Transmissibles de l'homme (Loi Sur Les Épidémies, LEp). Retrieved May 5, 2021 (www.fedlex.admin.ch/eli/cc/2015/297/fr#art_7).

Barras, F. 2021. Lutte contre le Covid—Pour l'économie, la vaccination en entreprise reste un accélérateur nécessaire. *24 heures*, May 12.

Berg, J., J. Harting, and K. Stronks. 2021. Individualisation in public health: Reflections from life narratives in a disadvantaged neighbourhood. *Critical Public Health* 31(1): 101–112. doi: 10.1080/09581596.2019.1680803

Confédération Suisse. 2021. COVID- 19 Suisse | Coronavirus | Dashboard'| Coronavirus | Dashboard. Retrieved May 18, 2021 (www.covid19.admin.ch/fr/overview).

Delphy, C. 1997. *L'Ennemi principal, tome 1: L'Économie politique du patriarcat*. Paris: Editions Syllepse.

Desson, Z., L. Lambertz, J. Willem Peters, M. Falkenbach, and L. Kauer. 2020. Europe's Covid-19 outliers: German, Austrian and Swiss policy responses during the early stages of the 2020 pandemic. *Health Policy and Technology* 9(4): 405–18. doi: 10.1016/j.hlpt.2020.09.003.

Dussault, A-M. 2020. Covid-19: Le Tessin appelle "au sens de responsabilité individuelle." *Le Temps*, February 25.

Economiesuisse. 2021. Déconfinement: Retour à La Responsabilité Individuelle! |
Economiesuisse. Retrieved May 3, 2021 (www.economiesuisse.ch/fr/articles/
deconfinement-retour-la-responsabilite-individuelle).

Falquet, J., H. Hirata, D. Kergoat, B. Labari, F. Sow, and N. Le Feuvre, eds. 2010.
Le sexe de la mondialisation: Genre, classe, race et nouvelle division du travail.
Paris: Presses de Sciences Po.

Fassin, D. 2005. Compassion and repression: The moral economy of immigration
policies in France. *Cultural Anthropology* 20(3): 362–387. doi: 10.1525/
can.2005.20.3.362

Hebeisen, E. 2020. Unus pro omnibus, omnes pro uno: éclairage du Musée national
suisse. *SWI swissinfo.ch.* Retrieved May 5, 2021 (www.swissinfo.ch/fre/culture/
blog-du-mus%C3%A9e-national-suisse_unus-pro-omnibus--omnes-pro-uno/
45761996).

Hirsch, C. 2020. Europe's coronavirus lockdown measures compared. *Politico.*
Retrieved May 5, 2021 (www.politico.eu/article/europes-coronavirus-lockdown-
measures-compared/).

Hodgers, A. 2020. La réponse d'Antonio Hodgers au sénateur qui accuse la Suisse
de menacer la santé des Français. *Heidi News.* Retrieved May 5, 2021 (/sante/
la-reponse-d-antonio-hodgers-au-senateur-qui-accuse-la-suisse-de-menacer-la-
sante-des-francais).

Katz, A.S., B-J. Hardy, M. Firestone, A. Lofters, and M.E. Morton-Ninomiya. 2020.
Vagueness, power and public health: Use of "vulnerable" in public health literature.
Critical Public Health 30(5): 601–611. doi: 10.1080/09581596.2019.1656800

Laugier, S. 2016. Politics of vulnerability and responsibility for ordinary others.
Critical Horizons 17(2): 207–223. doi: 10.1080/14409917.2016.1153891

Mahon, R., and F. Robinson. 2011. *Feminist Ethics and Social Policy: Towards a
New Global Political Economy of Care.* Vancouver, BC: UBC Press.

Marti, J., and G. Ferro-Luzzi. 2021. Revue Médicale Suisse—la revue médicale
francophone de référence pour la formation continue des médecins. *Revmed.
ch* (724).

Pandelé, Y. 2021. L'acceptation Des Vaccins Covid-19 Gagne Peu à Peu Du Terrain
En Suisse - Heidi.News. Retrieved May 9, 2021 (www.heidi.news/sante/
l-acceptation-des-vaccins-covid-19-gagne-peu-a-peu-du-terrain-en-suisse).

RTSinfo. 2020a. 19h30 – Vaud et le Jura rendent le port du masque obligatoire
dans les commerces. *rts.ch.* Retrieved May 14, 2021 (www.rts.ch/info/regions/
jura/11447540-vaud-et-le-jura-rendent-le-port-du-masque-obligatoire-dans-les-
commerces.html).

RTSinfo. 2020b. La Suisse en état de "situation extraordinaire" jusqu'au 19 avril.
rts.ch. Last accessed December 13, 2021 (www.rts.ch/info/suisse/11166687-la-
suisse-en-etat-de-situation-extraordinaire-jusquau-19-avril.html).

RTSinfo. 2020c. 19h30 – Des amendes de plusieurs centaines de francs pour des
rassemblements interdits. *rts.ch.* Last accessed December 13, 2021 (www.rts.ch/
info/suisse/11232178-des-amendes-de-plusieurs-centaines-de-francs-pour-des-
rassemblements-interdits.html).

RTSinfo. 2020d. On ne pourra pas tout contrôler, mais on compte sur la
responsabilité individuelle. *rts.ch.* Last accessed December 13, 2021 (www.rts.
ch/info/suisse/11311491-on-ne-pourra-pas-tout-controler-mais-on-compte-sur-
la-responsabilite-individuelle.html).

RTS. 2020e. Avec le Covid-19, les consultations en pédopsychiatrie bondissent de 40%. Retrieved May 9, 2021 (www.rts.ch/info/suisse/11746796-avec-le-covid19-les-consultations-en-pedopsychiatrie-bondissent-de-40.html).

RTSinfo. 2021. 19h30—Les Grands Employeurs n'offrent Pas de Pause Vaccin Payée. Last accessed December 13, 2021 (www.rts.ch/play/tv/19h30/video/les-grands-employeurs-suisses-noffrent-pas-de-pause-vaccin-payee-?urn=urn:rts:video:12185947).

Sallier, P-A. 2021. Bilan du dernier "semi-confinement"—Les villes bien plus touchées par la crise du Covid. *24 heures*, March 12.

ZHAW. 2020. Voici les mots de l'année 2020 en Suisse. *ZHAW Linguistique appliquée*. Retrieved May 30, 2021 (www.zhaw.ch/fr/linguistique/mot-suisse-de-lannee/communique-de-presse/).

8 Practicing Resilience while Negotiating the Pandemic

The Experiences of People with Rare Diseases in Poland

Katarzyna E. Król and Małgorzata Rajtar

Introduction

The World Health Organization (WHO 2020) and the American Centers for Disease Control and Prevention (CDC 2020), among others, have emphasized that people with "underlying medical conditions," including children with genetic and metabolic conditions, are at increased risk for severe illness from COVID-19 (C-19). Following health policy recommendations and a rapidly growing scholarly literature on the impact of the C-19 pandemic, webinars organized for people with rare inherited metabolic diseases (IMDs), including children, consistently characterized them as being "at risk" or "at higher risk" due to their chronic and/or long-term conditions. Already in March 2020, early on in the pandemic, British medical experts presented an Inherited Metabolic Disease & Coronavirus (COVID-19) Webinar that offered guidelines on "shielding and protecting people defined on medical grounds as extremely vulnerable from COVID-19" (Metabolic Support UK 2020). According to this webinar, "people with rare diseases and inborn errors of metabolism that significantly increase the risk of infections" are considered "extremely vulnerable." Along with people who have underlying respiratory problems and patients with bone marrow or organ transplants, patients who may suffer from metabolic decompensation were designated as "high risk" for contracting C-19 and for suffering greatly from it. In Poland, the National Consultant in Pediatric Metabolism issued recommendations on the management of IMD patients, warning that "in the case of COVID-19 infection, patients with inborn errors of metabolism (…) remain in a high-risk group of developing severe metabolic decompensation" (Sykut-Cegielska 2020). She also recommended the "unconditional isolation" of both patients and their families as the best preventive method (Sykut-Cegielska 2020). These recommendations have been forwarded by a large Polish patient organization for people with PKU (phenylketonuria) and other IMDs as well as by a few support groups on Facebook.

Since the outbreak of the C-19 pandemic, several surveys have been conducted with rare disease patients. These surveys consistently show the

DOI: 10.4324/9781003187462-11

detrimental effects of the pandemic on this patient community. For instance, according to the EURORDIS–Rare Diseases Europe (2020), a nonprofit alliance of over 930 rare disease patient organizations from 73 countries that had carried out a multi-country survey among people living with a rare disease in Europe, 84% out of almost 7000 respondents "experienced disruption of care." This disruption included, among other issues, the inability "to access diagnostic tests," "to receive therapies such as chemotherapies or infusions," and to have "their surgery or transplant postponed or canceled" (EURORDIS 2020). Data on the impact of the C-19 pandemic on patients with IMDs are "very scarce" (Elmonem et al. 2020: 286). A few surveys were conducted among patients with IMDs (e.g., Oge-Enver et al. 2021 for Turkey), patient organizations and healthcare providers in Europe (Lampe et al. 2020),[1] and in 16 specialized medical centers that treat patients with IMDs in Europe, Asia, and Africa (Elmonem et al. 2020). Like the EURORDIS survey, these surveys also focus on the management and treatment of people with IMDs during the pandemic. Specifically, the survey results underline changes in therapy regimens: most visits were canceled or postponed, and most treatments, such as rehabilitation, were reduced or suspended altogether. Additionally, about a quarter of IMD patients had trouble accessing medicines (Lampe et al. 2020). The C-19 pandemic has also severely exacerbated "the potential risk of missed or delayed diagnoses" (Elmonem et al. 2020: 288). Characteristic of the bleak conclusions drawn from these surveys, Lampe and colleagues state that "the continuing disruption of the proper follow-up of IMD patients might compromise their clinical condition and aggravate the course of the metabolic disease, from a medical, psychological, and also social point of view" (2020: 13).

Biomedical and social science scholarship foregrounds the concerns of rare metabolic disease patients about contracting the coronavirus and the impact of the C-19 pandemic on their access to treatment and care (Rajtar 2020b; see also Manderson and Wahlberg 2020 for the impact of C-19 on people with long-term medical conditions). As Christine Lampe and colleagues (2020: 2) aptly put it, "in ordinary situations, IMDs are neglected conditions, with limited resources and attention dedicated to these rare diseases. The COVID-19 pandemic has reduced attention even further." Nonetheless, we argue that this focus should be balanced by acknowledging and highlighting resilience practices that constitute day-to-day life with a rare metabolic disease.

A Short Note on Rare Diseases and Methods

There is no universal definition of a "rare disease" (von der Lippe et al. 2017). In the United States, for instance, rare diseases and disorders "are those which affect small patient populations, typically populations smaller than 200,000 individuals" (Rare Diseases Act 2002). For the European Union (EU), a disease is considered rare if it affects no more than 5 in 10,000 persons (Council of the EU 2009). There are about 8000 rare diseases; almost 50% of these affect children (Plan 2021: 4, 6). About 6–8% of the population in the EU is affected by a rare disease (Council of the EU 2009); the number of people living with rare conditions in Poland is estimated at 2–3 million (Plan 2021: 5).

Rare inherited metabolic diseases (IMDs) are a large and diverse group of individually rare single-gene disorders that "involve defects in metabolic pathways"; they are usually diagnosed early in life (Siddiq et al. 2016: 2; Pugliese et al. 2020). These are chronic, disabling, and potentially lethal medical conditions. Currently, 29 IMDs are diagnosed through newborn screening in Poland. Newborn screening "facilitates early detection, treatment and care" (WHO 2010: 3; but cf. Timmermans and Buchbinder 2013). In Poland (population 38.5 million), over 300 newborns with IMDs are diagnosed each year (Ołtarzewski 2018). Clinical presentations and management strategies of different IMDs are diverse. Nonetheless, they all require challenging diagnostic procedures that involve specialized laboratories; both acute and long-term treatment and patient monitoring require a multidisciplinary collaborative medical team (Elmonem et al. 2020). Furthermore, patients (often children) have to adhere to a highly specialized dietary regimen throughout their lives (see Pugliese et al. 2020; Siddiq et al. 2016).

In this chapter, we utilize data obtained from ethnographic research conducted among people with IMDs, specifically fatty-acid oxidation disorders (FAODs), organic acidemia disorders (OADs), and maple syrup urine disease (MSUD), their families, health professionals, and patient advocacy groups, as well as from our analysis of social media and webinars tailored to this group of patients and/or their caregivers in Poland, before and during the pandemic.[2] People with FAODs, MSUD, and OADs, among others, are prone to episodes biomedically known as "metabolic decompensation" (or "crisis") that may be triggered by fever, cold, infection, and stress, to name only a few. They may include poor feeding or loss of appetite, lethargy, and vomiting, and often require hospitalization. Emergency management of metabolic crises in children are an important issue in the lives of patients and their families (e.g., Siddiq et al. 2016).

Emphasizing IMD patients' "pre-existing vulnerability" (Adams 2020) resulting from "multiorgan impairments caused by their chronic condition" (Lampe et al. 2020: 8), biomedical scholars have observed that "children and adults with an IEM are particularly at higher risk of morbidity and mortality when infected with SARS-CoV-2 due to their chronic preexisting conditions and potentially vulnerable immune system" (Elmonem et al. 2020: 286; see also Metabolic Support UK 2020).

Vulnerability and Resilience

In public health discourses, people with rare diseases are regularly portrayed as a vulnerable population (Rajtar 2020a). During the COVID-19 pandemic, some of them, including IMD patients, have even been labeled as "extremely vulnerable" (Metabolic Support UK 2020). The surveys mentioned in the introduction to this chapter usually point to the need for "support and protect[tion of] fragile persons during crisis" (Lampe et al. 2020) and emphasize "the need to move towards more resilient and shock resistant healthcare systems that do not exacerbate the vulnerabilities of people living with a rare disease" and aim to protect them (EURORDIS 2020). In public health, biomedicine, bioethics, and social sciences scholarship, "vulnerability" is often understood in negative terms: helplessness, weakness, neediness, and powerlessness (e.g., Coyle and Atkinson 2019; Honkasalo 2018; Katz et al. 2020; Mackenzie 2013; Trundle et al. 2019). Vulnerable individuals and groups are understood as being at risk of or susceptible to harm as well as having "a limited capacity or resilience to absorb, adapt to or recover from that harm" (Coyle and Atkinson 2019: 278). "Structural" (Quesada et al. 2011), "inherent" (Mackenzie 2013), and "embodied" (Willen 2012 in Trundle et al. 2019: 199) vulnerabilities become a "target for specific interventions" (Mackenzie 2013: 38) that are often paternalistic and are "closely aligned to technologies of social control" (Honkasalo 2018: 5).

Resilience has "emerged as a counter-narrative to discourses of vulnerability and social suffering" in social sciences and public health (Panter-Brick 2014: 439). Catherine Panter-Brick emphasizes that "resilience-based approaches (…) offer models of research and practice predicated on strengths rather than on vulnerabilities, capabilities rather than deficits, resources rather than exposures, transformation rather than stasis" (2014: 438). In her research with families raising medically vulnerable children, Cheryl Mattingly argues that resilience "can supplement an overly narrow focus on obstacles, barriers, risks, and social inequalities (…) by offering complementary attention on the circumstances and activities that permit people to thrive, despite formidable barriers" (2016: 41–42). She also highlights that "well-being," "thriving," or "resilience" is not "a stable achievement or state of being," but rather "an ongoing practice" (2016: 39); it is, as she puts it, a "phenomenon embedded in the complexities and shifting character of people's lives and social circumstances" (Mattingly 2016: 47).

In the following, we will address two preventative measures against C-19 infection: handwashing and "social distancing," or rather "self-isolation" and "shielding." Drawing from Mattingly's insights on the complementarity of vulnerability and resilience (2016; see also Oudshoorn 2020) and especially on Catherine Trundle and colleagues' (2019) idea of "vulnerable articulations," we argue that people with IMDs and their families engage in daily practices of "hygienic vigilance." As they acknowledge uncertainty and vulnerability as a part of life, persons with rare metabolic disorders strengthen their resilience by "focus[ing] on building *resources* instead of dismantling dangers" (Palmboom and Willems 2014: 281, emphasis in original). Hygienic vigilance—a set of "positive vulnerabilities"

(Trundle et al. 2019)—has become an invaluable resource during the ongoing C-19 pandemic.

Practicing "Hygienic Vigilance"

Survey research carried out among the IMD community during the C-19 pandemic focused on the management and treatment of IMD patients. Nevertheless, researchers also indicated that, as such, C-19 is one of many other diseases and infections that may cause metabolic decompensation in IMD patients. For instance, Lampe and colleagues noted that

> in general, IMD patients receive detailed information from specialists *to avoid any metabolic decompensation due to other diseases or infections.* For COVID-19, *it was not necessary* to provide additional indications aside from the general information given at the local or national level.
> (2020: 9, emphasis added)

While analyzing the results of a survey conducted among Turkish IMD patients and their families, Ece Oge-Enver and colleagues (2021: 106) also emphasized that being "at risk of life-threatening acute decompensation even after regular infections," these patients "are used to following measurements for reducing risks of an infection on a routine basis." Unlike other survey-based publications, this article focuses on handwashing. Stating that most families with children who have rare metabolic disorders "wash their hands more than 10 times a day," the authors argue that "this high rate may have been found due to the trainings that all of the patients receive in our clinic after diagnosis about food and medicine preparation and hygiene rules" (Oge-Enver et al. 2021: 106). From this perspective, the C-19 pandemic has not introduced new hygienic rules and/or practices, such as frequent handwashing; rather it has simply built upon existing ones.

Our research has also confirmed that doctors and dietitians emphasized special diets and hygiene as crucial for the survival of newly diagnosed newborns and children with rare metabolic diseases well before the outbreak of the C-19 pandemic. For instance, in 2017, Rajtar interviewed Marta and Jan, the parents of an elementary school pupil, Kasia. Born before the introduction of newborn screening for IMDs in Poland (2013), Kasia was diagnosed with LCHADD after already experiencing a series of medical crises. The doctor who delivered the diagnosis told Marta and Jan that LCHADD is a life-threatening disease and that they must fulfill their physician's recommendations to the letter:

MAŁGORZATA: What were you told to do?
MARTA: Well, diet...
JAN: Diet and hygiene. Most of all [we are to] wash our hands so we won't expose the kid to any... so she won't get sick. No [exposure to] bacteria.

Aware of the life-threatening consequences of metabolic decompensation, Marta and Jan take their doctor's precautions very seriously, as does their daughter. According to her parents, Kasia does not catch cold as often as her school peers. She "monitors herself" (*pilnuje siebie*) and she can't be around anyone who sneezes or coughs at school:

MARTA: Well, she knows she has to wash her hands.
JAN: Her hands, her hands… Marta: During every break.
JAN: During every break [and] when she goes to the bathroom, she has to wash her hands. Marta: She has to wash her hands before eating a sandwich. She knows that too. And she knows that she is not to approach [anyone who is sick].
MALGORZATA: She knows how it works.
MARTA: Yes, she knows how it works. You have to keep saying this right from the beginning.
JAN: We keep telling her that.
MARTA: When someone sneezes or coughs, it's better for you not to huddle. Go somewhere else (…) So, she rarely gets sick. I would even say that she gets sick less than healthy children do.

Kasia's parents are far from unique when it comes to their insistence on avoiding illness at all costs. Explaining why she sent her son with VLCAD deficiency to private rather than state kindergarten, Iwona told one of the researchers in the project:

> I didn't send him to a state kindergarten because I was worried about illness. There are more than 200 children in our district. When an illness (*choroba*) strikes, it will hit all children more than once. Here [at the private kindergarten], the ladies knew that and told me in advance about the virus there. Then I didn't send Wojtek to school; he stayed at home. He went back [to the kindergarten] after they called me saying "Well, it's over. He can come back."

Like many IMD patients and their families, Kasia, Wojtek, and their caregivers engage in what we call "hygienic vigilance." Hygiene, as the late Valerie Curtis (2007: 660) defined it, is "the set of behaviours that animals, including humans, use to avoid infection." Even before the C-19 pandemic, handwashing as well as self-isolation and shielding (see below) (Metabolic Support UK n.d.) stood at the core of hygienic vigilance, which people with rare metabolic disorders and their families practiced daily. As even a common illness may lead to metabolic crisis and possibly have life-threatening consequences for Kasia, her metabolic disease makes her "inherently" vulnerable (Mackenzie 2013). To redress her vulnerability and prevent any exposure to illness, Kasia and her parents remain cautious: they stay away from possible sources of transmission. Such habituated behavior has prepared them well for the C-19 pandemic.

Similar to Iwona, who refrained from sending Wojtek to kindergarten during "regular" flu outbreaks, other parents of IMD children followed such precautions during the C-19 pandemic. Thus, many parents decided to practice shielding for at least two more weeks after the official re-opening of nurseries and kindergartens in May 2020. Zofia, the mother of a LCHADD child, raised the question about sending children back to kindergarten on an online support group for IMD people:

ZOFIA: Hi! Have you sent your kids back to kindergarten/nursery after the re-opening? Or are you holding back (*wstrzymujecie się*)?
EWA: Michał has attended kindergarten since the 1st of July.
OLGA: I'm keeping Zuzia [at home] as long as possible.
ANNA: Julia has been in kindergarten since June, around two weeks after they re-opened.
MICHAŁ: Tomek went back to kindergarten in June; so far so good.

On March 14, 2020, in a futile, albeit globally utilized move to contain the spread of the novel coronavirus by imposing "a crude and extreme version of lockdown" (Caduff 2020: 469), the Polish Ministry of Health (2020) declared a state of epidemic that resulted in the closing of borders and severe restriction of movement. Although the restrictions were eventually lifted in June (Ministry of the Interior and Administration 2020), like their European counterparts, the Polish government strongly encouraged citizens to enjoy their summer holidays while traveling within the country. This "unprecedented" response to the pandemic "has pushed the world into a space of fragility and uncertainty" (Caduff 2020: 476). Moreover, the experience of being immobilized and/or country-bound was novel to most of the population; however, this was not the case for IMD persons and their families. Even before the C-19 pandemic, children with IMDs seldom participated in school trips that lasted more than a day and/or traveled a great deal with their families in general. Reflecting on the travel restrictions that her family is subjected to due to Wojtek's condition, Iwona said:

People tend to ask me, why don't you go abroad? I don't go [abroad], because I'm already afraid to travel within Poland, so going abroad is out of the question. (…) Yes, we don't travel far. We only travel within Poland. I check the destination in advance, so I know how to get to the hospital if necessary. I sleep well when I know where the hospital is and where I can turn to. I check it beforehand, otherwise I don't go.

Over a year into the C-19 pandemic, "social distancing" and "self-isolation" have become familiar rules to live by, thus reshaping our understandings of space, human, and non-human relations. In the case of some IMD patients, social distancing interpreted as simply "staying at home" (Metabolic Support UK n.d.) is not enough. Rather, shielding is called for. "Shielding" is "a measure to protect people who are clinically extremely vulnerable by minimizing all interaction between those who are extremely vulnerable and others" (Metabolic Support UK n.d.). By recommending "not leaving your home at all and minimizing all non-essential contact with other members of your household" (Metabolic Support UK n.d.), shielding may be interpreted as an extreme form of hygienic vigilance. In March 2020, the National Consultant in Pediatric Metabolism in Poland recommended "unconditional isolation" and emphasized that for IMD patients and their families "to stay at home in the circle of your closest family members who do not have contact with others outside [the family] is currently the best solution" (Sykut-Cegielska 2020). These recommendations triggered conversations among concerned parents in online support groups. For instance, Joanna, the mother of a boy with MCAD, shared their experience of self-isolation and shielding: "It's scary. Our son has asthma [on top of MCAD], so we are completely isolated at home. My husband is the sole 'link' with the outside world."

Since IMD patients and their caregivers had practiced episodic self-isolation and shielding before, this practical knowledge facilitated adhering to lockdown rules during the C-19 pandemic. This resonates with Ritti Soncco's (2020) observations of another group of the chronically ill. In her research with Lyme disease patients in Scotland, Soncco noted that the governmentally imposed new "social patterns...are very familiar" to her interlocutors. Patients with a compromised immune system had preexisting skills of self-surveillance and self-isolation. Thus, unlike the rest of the population that had to come to terms with "strange and frightening 'states of pandemic,'" people with chronic conditions perceived them as "continued 'states of normality'" (Soncco 2020).

Webinars organized for Polish IMD patients during the C-19 pandemic echoed the European survey results that we discussed at the beginning of this section (Lampe et al. 2020: 9) by emphasizing the need for continuation of treatment management and hygienic vigilance. Although these meetings' agendas featured presentations discussing best practices during the pandemic, doctors underlined that the risk of contracting C-19 infection is similar to that of any other disease or illness; hence, the same rules of general vigilance apply. The webinar attendees (who included both of us), were instructed that the main risk factor related to C-19 infection is a persistent fever, which can lead to metabolic decompensation. Yet, fever can be caused by numerous factors, such as stress or even the standard stages of bodily development—for instance, growing teeth. Thus, during a March 2021 webinar on low-protein diets for IMD patients, a doctor wanted to "impress upon" (*uczulić*) and "encourage parents to remain vigilant" (*zachować czujność*) and closely observe their children for any symptoms of possible decompensation in the exact same way as before. During a July webinar devoted to the special treatment of IMD patients during the C-19 outbreak, a doctor named a few important practices that should be carried out, such as constant communication with other parents of IMD patients, cooperation with patient advocacy groups, and regular dietary check-ups. These guidelines did not significantly differ from the pre-COVID-19 recommendations; in fact, adherence to special diets remains the most important issue in the management and treatment of IMDs. As a "highly medically supervised population" (Lampe et al. 2020: 13), IMD patients and their caregivers are well trained in exercising control and managing the ever-present risk of metabolic decompensation. As our research shows (Rajtar 2021), IMD patients and/or their caregivers practice self-care through "developing an awareness of the body" (Bates 2019: 46). Generally, after vigilantly observing their children for years, many caregivers, primarily mothers, could "read" the first symptoms of metabolic crisis, such as lack of appetite, vomiting, and muscle pain. Moreover, they knew what would precipitate metabolic decompensation: skipped nightly feedings, stress, too much exercise, and fever. The mother of a LCHADD child expressed this sense of generalized attentiveness on her Instagram account as follows:

Rising CK[3] may lead to damage of the muscles and organs (including vision, liver, heart); [it may lead to] severe hypoglycemia at any time. This may result in coma, which is a straight path to the patient's death. ... Now, [regular] vaccination has led to elevated CK levels; this could have easily been caused by infection, too much physical activity, and even severe stress. An intravenous glucose infusion is the only medicine in the ward. There is no other cure. This disease cannot be cured. It accompanies the patient for their entire life. You have to learn to live with it.

Many people with IMD and their caregivers practice "hygienic vigilance," what, in different research contexts, Alex Nading (2014) and Cheryl Mattingly et al. (2011) called "chronic work" and "chronic homework" respectively. This chronic work of *vigilancia* (surveillance) employed in Nicaragua was to "create a sense of generalized alertness to the ever-present danger of dengue" (Nading 2014: 166). Like dengue, IMDs and metabolic decompensation "could only be controlled, contained, and managed" (Nading 2014: 167). The notion of "chronic homework" highlights that patients and their caregivers are to carry out this "kind of work ... in their home contexts in the treatment of their chronic conditions" (Mattingly et al. 2011: 348). As the father of a MCAD child argued on an Internet support group in early 2021:

[MCAD] is a genetic defect; [it's] life-threatening no doubt. Like diabetes, cancers, and viruses (e.g., COVID) and many other ailments in this world. If we were to panic because of each of those ailments, we would have to hurt our children by locking them up in a sterile room and not letting them out. This is pointless.

From this perspective, C-19 is a potentially life-threatening infection, though it is far from unique. Neither does it require appropriating new skills and competences for the people in these groups.

Conclusion: Chronic Living in the Context of the Coronavirus Pandemic

In this chapter, we have focused on the "chronic living" (Manderson and Wahlberg 2020) of people with rare inherited metabolic diseases and their caregivers in the context of the C-19 pandemic. We recognize that infectious diseases, such as C-19, and pre-existing medical conditions, such as rare inherited metabolic diseases, "do not cancel each other," but rather "coexist" (Manderson and Wahlberg 2020: 430). While biomedical and social science scholarship tends to foreground the ways in which C-19 inhibits the management and treatment of IMDs, in this chapter we have offered a different perspective. We have utilized the concept of "vulnerable articulations" (Trundle et al. 2019), which emphasizes the dynamic interrelatedness of diverse vulnerabilities and ways in which "positive vulnerability" allows us to address the effects of its negative counterpart. IMD as a negative "pre-existing vulnerability" (Adams 2020) requires patients and/or their caregivers to practice what we have called "hygienic vigilance" in order to ward off metabolic decompensation and other negative consequences of the medical condition. Along with adhering to dietary regimens, patients and/or their parents had been trained in and mastered handwashing, self-isolation, and shielding well before the arrival of the coronavirus pandemic. These strategies have become resources or "positive vulnerabilities" that have allowed IMD people and their caregivers to address the negative vulnerabilities that result from their rare genetic condition and weakened immunity. Thus, practicing "hygienic vigilance," as they have always done, contributes to the resilience of people with rare inherited metabolic diseases during the C-19 pandemic, and in fact, has rendered them much better prepared to deal with this pandemic than generally healthy people whose children are also generally healthy.

Acknowledgments

Our thanks go to all research participants as well as project researchers Anna Chowaniec, Jan Frydrych, Anna Kwaśniewska, and Filip Rogalski. We also thank the National Sciences Center in Poland for funding this project via grants no 2017/26/E/HS3/00291 and 2015/17/B/HS3/00107.

Notes

1 This Lampe et al. 2020 article presents data obtained in two surveys carried out by the European Reference Network for Hereditary Metabolic Diseases (MetabERN). MetabERN is a non-profit European network that connects specialized centers that focus on rare IMDs. It is considered "the main reference point and cluster of expertise for the rare metabolic community in Europe" (Lampe et al. 2020: 2).

2 Along with the authors of this chapter, two other researchers have been involved in gathering data within our ongoing project on an anthropology of rare diseases. Led by Rajtar, this project aims at comparing the situation of people with IMDs and their families in Finland, Poland, and Sweden. Additionally, Rajtar carried out an earlier project on LCHAD deficiency, an FAOD, in Poland and Finland between 2016 and 2019. The outbreak of the C-19 pandemic has negatively impacted the possibility of conducting ethnographic research, especially our ability to travel to Finland and Sweden. Even before the C-19 pandemic, however, our meetings and conversations with interlocutors involved practicing the "hygienic vigilance" described in this chapter. All interlocutor names used are pseudonyms.

3 An elevated plasma creatine kinase (CK) level is considered "the most sensitive measurement for diagnosis" of rhabdomyolysis (RM) (Hannah-Shmounti et al. 2012: 427). Rhabdomyolysis is a "a potentially life-threatening syndrome characterized by the breakdown of muscle fibers" (Basheer, Mneimneh, and Rajab 2017: 1). Metabolic and genetic disorders along with strenuous exercise are among the numerous causes of rhabdomyolysis.

References

Adams, V. 2020. Disasters and capitalism... and COVID-19. *Somatosphere*, March 26, 2020. Available at: http://somatosphere.net/2020/disaster-capitalism-covid19.html/

Basheer, N., Mneimneh, S., and Rajab, M. 2017. Seven-digit creatine kinase in acute rhabdomyolysis in a child. *Child Neurology Open* 4: 1–4.

Bates, C. 2019. *Vital Bodies. Living with Illness*. Bristol: Policy Press.

Caduff, C. 2020. What went wrong: Corona and the world after the full stop. *Medical Anthropology Quarterly* 34(4): 467–487.

Centers for Disease Control and Prevention. 2020. People with certain medical conditions. Available at: www.cdc.gov/coronavirus/2019-ncov/need-extra-precautions/people-withmedical-conditions.html (Accessed August 14, 2020).

Council of the EU. 2009. Council Recommendation of 8 June 2009 on an action in the field of rare diseases (2009/C 151/02). *Official Journal of the European Union* 52(3): 7–10. https://eurlex.europa.eu/LexUriServ/LexUriServ.do?uri=OJ:C:2009:151:0007:0010:EN:PDF (Last accessed March 29, 2021).

Coyle, L.A., and Atkinson, S. 2019. Vulnerability as practice in diagnosing multiple conditions. *Medical Humanities* 45(3): 278–286.

Curtis, V.A. 2007. Dirt, disgust and disease: a natural history of hygiene. *Journal of Epidemiology and Community Health* 61: 660–664.

Elmonem, M.A., Belanger-Quintana, A., Bordugo, A., Boruah, R., Cortès-Saladelafont, E., Endrakanti, M., et al. 2020. The impact of COVID-19 pandemic on the diagnosis and management of inborn errors of metabolism: A global perspective. *Molecular Genetics and Metabolism* 131: 285–288.

EURORDIS. 2020. People living with a rare disease were severely impacted during first COVID-19 wave: 30 million people in Europe must not be forgotten once again. Available at: http://download2.eurordis.org/rbv/covid19survey/PressRelease_ COVID19surveyresults_Final2.pdf (Last accessed March 15, 2021).

Hannah-Shmounti, F., McLeod, K., and Sirrs, S. 2012. Recurrent exercise-induced rhabdomyolysis. *CMAJ* 184(4): 426–230.

Honkasalo, M.-L. 2018. Guest Editor's Introduction: Vulnerability and inquiring into relationality. *Suomen Antropologi: Journal of the Finnish Anthropological Society* 43(3): 1–21.

Katz, A.S., Hardy, B-J., Firestone, M., Lofters, A., and Morton-Ninomiya, M.E. 2020. Vagueness, power and public health: Use of "vulnerable" in public health literature. *Critical Public Health* 30(5): 601–615.

Lampe, C., Dionisi-Vici, C., Bellettato, C.M., Paneghetti, L., van Lingen, C., Bond, S., et al. 2020. The impact of COVID-19 on rare metabolic patients and healthcare providers: results from two MetabERN surveys. *Orphanet Journal of Rare Diseases* 15: 341.

Mackenzie, C. 2013. "The Importance of Relational Autonomy and Capabilities for an Ethics of Vulnerability." In C. Mackenzie, W. Rogers, and S. Dodds (eds.), *Vulnerability: New Essays in Ethics and Feminist Philosophy*, 34–59. Oxford: Oxford University Press.

Manderson, L., Wahlberg, A. 2020. Chronic living in a communicable world. *Medical Anthropology* 39(5): 428–439.

Mattingly, C. 2016. "Resilience, Disparity, and Narrative Phenomenology: African American Families Raising Medically Vulnerable Children." In C. DeMichelis and M. Ferrari (eds.), *Child and Adolescent Resilience Within Medical Contexts*, 37–49. Switzerland: Springer.

Mattingly, C., Grøn, L., and Meinert, L. 2011. Chronic homework in emerging borderlands of healthcare. *Culture, Medicine and Psychiatry* 35: 347–375.

Metabolic Support UK. n.d. Social Distancing, Self-Isolation and Shielding. Available at: www.metabolicsupportuk.org/the-difference-between-social-distancing-and-self-isolation/ (Last accessed March 13, 2021)

Metabolic Support UK. 2020. Inherited Metabolic Disease & Coronavirus (COVID-19) Webinar. 23.03.2020. Available at https://metab.ern-net.eu/wpcontent/uploads/2020/04/COVID-Webinar-Slide-Template_Version-FINAL-23Mar-1.pdf (Last accessed March 29, 2021).

Ministry of Health. 2020. Rozporządzenie Ministra Zdrowia z dnia 13 marca 2020 r. w sprawie ogłoszenia na obszarze Rzeczypospolitej Polskiej stanu zagrożenia epidemicznego. Dziennik Ustaw poz. 433. Available at: https://isap.sejm.gov.pl/isap.nsf/download.xsp/WDU20200000433/O/D20200433.pdf (Last accessed March 29, 2021).

Ministry of the Interior and Administration. 2020. Rozporządzenie Ministra Spraw Wewnętrznych i Administracji z dnia 11 czerwca 2020 r. zmieniające rozporządzenie w sprawie czasowego zawieszenia lub ograniczenia ruchu granicznego na określonych przejściach granicznych. Dziennik Ustaw poz. 1030. Available at: https://isap.sejm.gov.pl/isap.nsf/download.xsp/WDU20200001030/O/D20201030.pdf (Last accessed March 29. 2021).

Nading, A.M. 2014. *Mosquito Trails. Ecology, Health, and the Politics of Entanglement*. Berkeley, CA: University of California Press.

Oge-Enver, E., Hopurcuoglu, D., Ahmadzada, S., Zubarioglu, T., Aktuglu Zeybek, A.C., and Kiykim, E. 2021. Challenges of following patients with inherited metabolic diseases during the COVID-19 outbreak. A cross-sectional online survey study. *Journal of Pediatric Endocrinology and Metabolism* 34(1): 103–107.

Ołtarzewski, M. 2018. Badania przesiewowe noworodkow w Polsce, 2018 rok [Newborn screening in Poland – 2018]. *Postępy Neonatologii* 24(2): 111–122.

Oudshoorn. N. 2020. "On Vulnerable Bodies, Transformative Technologies, and Resilient Cyborgs." In *Resilient Cyborgs. Living and Dying with Pacemakers and Defibrillators*, 37–55. New York: Palgrave Macmillan.

Palmboom, G., and Willems, D. 2014. "Dealing with Vulnerability: Balancing Prevention with Resilience as a Method of Governance." In A. Hommels, J. Mesman, and W.E. Bijker (eds.), *Vulnerability in Technological Cultures. New Directions in Research and Governance*, 267–283. Cambridge, MA: MIT Press.

Panter-Brick, C. 2014. Health, Risk, and Resilience: Interdisciplinary Concepts and Applications. *Annual Review of Anthropology* 43: 431–448.

Plan. 2021. *Plan dla Chorób Rzadkich* [Plan for Rare Diseases]. Available at: www.gov.pl/web/zdrowie/projekt-uchwaly-rady-ministrow-w-sprawie-przyje ciadokumentu-plan-dla-chorob-rzadkich---pre-konsultacje

Pugliese, M., Tingley, K., Chow, A., Pallone, N., Smith, M., Rahman, A., et al. 2020. Outcomes in pediatric studies of medium-chain acyl-coA dehydrogenase (MCAD) deficiency and phenylketonuria (PKU): a review. *Orphanet Journal of Rare Diseases* 15: 12.

Quesada, J., Hart, L.K., and Burgois, P. 2011. Structural vulnerability and health: Latino migrant laborers in the United States. *Medical Anthropology* 30(4): 339–362.

Rajtar, M. 2020a. The concept of vulnerability within research ethics and health policies on rare diseases. *Przegląd Socjologiczny* [Sociological Review] 69(3): 107–127.

Rajtar, M. 2020b. The Pre-Existing Vulnerabilities of Patients With Rare Disorders in Poland During a Global Pandemic (#WitnessingCorona). *Medizinethnologie Körper, Gesundheit und Heilung in einer globalisierten Welt*. 6.05.2020. Available at: www.medizinethnologie.net/the-pre-existing-vulnerabilities-of-patients-with-raredisorders-in-poland-witnessing-corona/ (Last accessed March 29, 2021).

Rajtar, M. 2021. Between Two "R"s: Caring for eyes and muscles in those with a rare metabolic disorder. Paper presented at the Chronic Living Conference 2021, Copenhagen, March 4–6.

Rare Diseases Act of 2002. 2002. Public Law 107–280, 6. November 2002. Available at: www.congress.gov/107/plaws/publ280/PLAW-107publ280.pdf (Last accessed March 29, 2021)

Siddiq, S., Wilson, B.J., Graham, I.D., Lamoureux, M., Khangura, S.D., Tingley, K., et al. 2016. Experiences of caregivers of children with inherited metabolic diseases: A qualitative study. *Orphanet Journal of Rare Diseases* 11(1): 168.

Soncco, R. 2020. Lessons for self-isolation from chronically ill patients. *Somatosphere* 29.03.2020. Available at http://somatosphere.net/2020/lessons-for-self-isolation-fromchronically-ill-patients.html/ (Last accessed March 26, 2021).

Sykut-Cegielska, J. 2020. Zalecenia postępowania z pacjentami z wrodzonymi wadami metabolizmu w związku z epidemią COVID-19. Available at: http://pediatriametaboliczna.pl/zalecenia-postepowania-przy-wrodzonych-wadachmetabolicznych-w-zwiazku-z-epidemia-covid-19/ (Last accessed March 29, 2021).

Timmermans, S., and Buchbinder, M. 2013. *Saving Babies? The Consequences of Newborn Genetic Screening*. Chicago, IL: University of Chicago Press.

Trundle, C., Gibson, H., and Bell, L. 2019. Vulnerable articulations: The opportunities and challenges of illness and recovery. *Anthropology & Medicine* 26(2): 197–212.

Von der Lippe, Ch., Diesen, P. S., and Feragen, K. 2017. Living with a rare disorder: A systematic review of the qualitative literature. *Molecular Genetics & Genomic Medicine* 5(6): 758–773.

WHO [World Health Organization]. 2010. Birth Defects—Report of the Secretariat. 3rd World Assembly. Geneva: WHO. https://apps.who.int/gb/ebwha/pdf_files/WHA63/A63_10-en.pdf (Last accessed March 29, 2021).

WHO [World Health Organization]. 2020. Coronavirus. Available at: www.who.int/health-topics/coronavirus#tab=tab_1 (Accessed March 29, 2020).

9 Negotiating COVID-19 in Russia on the Eve of the Introduction of Social Restrictions

Tatiana O. Novikova, Dmitry G. Pirogov, Tatyana V. Malikova, and Georgiy A. Murza-Der

Introduction: Anxieties, Stress, and the Initial Alarm Phase of Negotiating COVID-19 in Russia

In this chapter, we turn to existential questions about and negotiations with C-19 in Russia at the end of March 2020. We chose this time period for our research because of the uniqueness of the situation at that time: it was a life in-between. The number of C-19 cases was still minimal, but it was clear that more would come. The number of government documents designed to support the economy and to advocate preventive measures grew rapidly during this time (Government.ru 2020). Some federal districts were put on standby. The main recommendations and restrictions in March 2020 concerned:

- Prevention of the entry of the coronavirus into Russian territory:
  - Suspension of transport connections with several countries;
  - Suspended access for citizens of all foreign countries.
- Detection of cases of infection in Russia and prevention of the spread of the disease within the country:
  - Isolation and strict medical supervision of those who arrived before the travel ban, Russians coming back from other countries, and those in contact with them;
  - Mandatory quarantine for persons with coronavirus infection and those who had contact with them;
  - Recommendation for persons over 65 years not to leave their home unless necessary. In some federal districts of Russia, this was more than a recommendation; it was a complete prohibition;
  - Observance of the anti-epidemic regime in educational institutions, including, if necessary, the transition to distance education and work;
  - Employers should consider transferring employees to work remotely;

DOI: 10.4324/9781003187462-12

- Abolition and prohibition of mass cultural sports, events, and so on;
- Mandatory disinfection of contact surfaces in all working spaces during the day.

Thus, since the beginning of March 2020, Russia had been in a situation of change and of expectations of more severe transformations of social life. People were aware of the situation abroad. It was a period of massive informational overload and uncertainty, of great activity on the parts of the Russian government and media, and of the interiorization of these actions into the lifeworlds of ordinary Russians. At the end of March 2020, there was a dismantling of the psychological spaces in which Russians lived. The predictability of the environment and the ability to manage one's schedule and personal time shifted to uncertainty. People lost their sense of agency and control over their lives.

Long before the concept of "stress" was widely understood, Hans Selye (1976) identified stress as a major factor in health and developed the concept of the "stress response." According to Selye, the stress response is triphasic, involving an initial "alarm phase," followed by a stage of resistance or adaptation, and finally, if the stress continues for too long and/or the organism (human or animal) does not sufficiently adapt, a stage of exhaustion or even death. This "in-between" period in Russian life may be characterized as the "alarm phase" or the "anxiety phase" of the stress generated by the coronavirus pandemic. In March 2020, we had an opportunity to explore this initial alarm phase as it took place in our country. We believed such an exploration to be important because understanding cultural and other factors influencing people's abilities to cope with a stressful situation can mitigate its potentially negative effects.

Methods and Materials

For this study, we posted notifications on social networks such as Facebook, Vkontakte, and WhatsApp asking people to fill out our questionnaire. We also sent the link for participation to the entire St Petersburg State Pediatric Medical University community. We used only one inclusion criterion: participants had to be 18 years of age or older. Our total data sample on which this chapter is based includes 1,108 respondents.

Participants were asked to complete the questionnaires in Russian through Google Forms. We informed potential participants of the objectives and goals of the study before starting the survey. We also informed them that their participation was anonymous, confidential, and voluntary. We collected data from March 21 to March 27, 2020 in order to capture this transitional and transformational Covidian movement—after the disease had entered Russia and before it became widespread.

We divided our 1,108 respondents into three age groups (please note: all percentages are rounded off):

- Group 1 (G1) contained 497 respondents aged 18–29; 384 (77%) of whom were women, and 113 were men (23%);
- Group 2 (G2) contained 441 respondents aged 30–49; 347 (79%) were women and 94 (21%) were men;
- Group 3 (G3) contained 170 respondents over 50 years of age, 130 (76.5%) of whom were women and 40 (23.5%) were men.

The educational level of the respondents was:

- 58% – higher education
- 19% – incomplete higher education
- 10% – specialized (professional) secondary education
- 12.5% – secondary education
- 1% – incomplete secondary education.

The main activities engaged in by our respondents were: 65% – work; 26% – education; 8% – currently not engaged in any activity. 66% of respondents had a permanent partner, and 28% had underage children. All respondents were more likely to live in cities with a population exceeding 1 million. At the end of March 2020, most respondents had not personally encountered C-19. Only seven respondents in G1 and one in G2 had tested positive for COVID. Three respondents in G1 and 2 in G2 mentioned that they had relatives or friends who were C-19 positive. In G3, there were no respondents personally faced with C-19. In all three groups, around 75% knew about the coronavirus from the media; and around 46% regularly kept track of statistics on C-19 in the country and abroad. So, as elsewhere, the end of March 2020 saw the beginning of the breakdown of Russia's social reality, which this chapter will both describe and analyze. Again, we chose this particular period to study because it is a snapshot of a society in transition—"in-between" pre-pandemic life and the full establishment of the new life order; therefore it was full of the ambiguity we will discuss in the following section.

Ambiguity in Public Awareness of COVID-19

The alarm phase of stress experienced by Russians at the end of March 2020 correlates with the concept of "ambiguity," meaning doubtfulness or uncertainty, a lack or fragmentation of information in human experience (Budner 1962; Vives & Feldman Hall 2018). The key dissociative source of ambiguity is intolerance of ambiguity (Kornilova 2015): the awareness of uncertainty involves the multipotency of the future and too many possible bifurcation points. The picture of the future is fragmented, and the familiar vision of it is blurred.

We stress that coping with uncertainty consists of three components—cognitive, emotional, and behavioral. Factual knowledge about C-19 provides the cognitive component of coping. The overall understanding of C-19 in Russia was complicated by conflicting views and the need to form a personal opinion about it to guide one's actions. The emotional component of coping is based on assessing the degree of threat to one's life. This assessment also depends to a large extent on the volume and nature of the information provided. Cognitive and emotional components underlie the behavioral components, which in Russia are implemented in terms of strict adherence to official recommendations and complicated by regressive coping measures such as denying, minimizing, or trying to avoid stressful situations. Russians have historically been characterized by this duality, which is constituted by the ambivalent combination of following official positions on specific issues while also following spontaneous popular traditions. For one brief example, Russian culture is characterized by the coexistence of the Orthodox Church and the ancient pagan traditions within it (so-called *Dvoeverie*—"double faith").

The specificity of C-19 is that it is a new disease (or rather was during the time period of our study). So, it is possible to spread questionable and sometimes false information about this disease regarding, for example, the factors related to viral transmission, the duration of the incubation period, what its symptoms are, and how likely it is that someone will die from it (Ornell et al. 2020). In our view, and as also shown in other chapters in this volume, the dissemination of misinformation about C-19 frequently contributes to more significant and troubling ambiguities and uncertainties that heighten anxieties in the "alarm phase." The "Scale of Information about COVID-19" parameter (see Table 9.1) allowed us to determine our respondents' then-current knowledge about and perceptions of C-19, and the degree of their understanding, or lack thereof, about coronavirus infection. The basis for this scale was constituted by the most critical aspects of the WHO's prevention guidelines (WHO n.d.). The WHO "Scale for Receiving and Exchanging Information" inquired about the specifics of the information disseminated about COVID-19. Understanding "exposure to information about the impending threat" (Mertens et al. 2020) as a predictor

Table 9.1 Respondents' Awareness of COVID-19 and Evaluation of Subjective Knowledge of and Satisfaction with Their Knowledge about COVID-19*

Parameter	G1	G2	G3
General Awareness	3.9	3.8	3.9
Believing misinformation about C-19	2.1	2.2	2.4
Subjective knowledge	7	6	5.5
Awareness satisfaction	6	6	5

Note: * Table 9.1 presents average values; for "General awareness" and "Believing misinformation about C-19" min=1, max=5; for "Subjective knowledge" and "Awareness satisfaction" min=1, max=10.

of uncertainty, we expanded on this parameter. We included the level of awareness and subjective satisfaction with the information available on the disease. The results showed a high level of awareness among respondents (see Table 9.1); there are no statistical differences among the groups. However, respondents in G3—the older group—were more likely to create their own theories about C-19 than other age groups. This may indirectly indicate a tendency for G3 respondents to use pre-existing, cognitively stabilizing coping patterns under conditions of information stress (see Davis-Floyd 2018).

As Table 9.1 shows, respondents assessed their awareness of C-19 and their satisfaction with this awareness as "average." Views on the accessibility, completeness, and quality of the information differed among the three groups, as did the degree of subjective satisfaction with the awareness of C-19. The G1 respondents indicated more awareness than respondents of other groups, and were satisfied with the available information. The higher informational satisfaction in G1, in our opinion, is based on the facts that young Russian people (persons under 30) use a wide range of information sources—a perceived necessity to them—and that young people's attitudes around C-19 are generally based on statements from their peers and social media, often ignoring expert assessments and opinions.

For G3, their critical attitude towards the available information may be related to the fact that these older respondents have more experience and knowledge. Their level of satisfaction depends on the degree to which the information satisfies their need for depth of knowledge, and on the reliability of the information source. Respondents from G2 take in information according to their current needs. For them, the information is crucial when it affects the main areas of their day-to-day operations: their salaries, other aspects of their jobs, and their children's education.

The media consumption associated with obtaining information about COVID-19 is multimodal (see Table 9.2). The Internet was one of the most popular sources of information about COVID-19 for all age groups. In a situation of uncertainty and anxiety, respondents felt a need to have 24/7 access to up-to-date information. Internet news channels best meet these requirements. However, the information provided is not always reliable and is often contradictory. Mertens et al. (2020) note the significance of frequency of access to information sources, stating that repeatedly engaging with trauma-related media content shortly after traumatic events may prolong acute stress experience (ibid; see also Holman, Garfin, and Silver 2014), especially when the threat is of personal importance, as with COVID-19.

As shown in Table 9.2, G3 more often relied on TV information than respondents from other groups. Respondents of G1 are more likely than others to seek C-19 information on social media. The digital environment is that space where young people check their perceptions and assessments.

All respondents preferred to share information in person. It was common for respondents of all groups to share about how C-19 was

Table 9.2 COVID-19 Information Exchange, %*

Parameter	G1	G2	G3
Sources for Obtaining Information:			
Social Networks	27%	19%	16%
Internet news channels	23%	26%	25%
TV, radio	8%	16%	23%
Newspapers	0.8%	1.4%	2.3%
Conversations with colleagues and friends	17%	14%	13%
Official sites of the city administration	10%	10%	9%
Websites of health organizations	13%	12.5%	11%
Other	0.7%	0.6%	0.8%
Channels for Information Exchange:			
Private Conversations	42%	48%	49.5%
Forums and Social Nets	29%	26%	24%
Messengers (WhatsApp. Viber. пр) and SMS	29%	26%	24%
Other	0.6%	0.6%	2.3%
Preferred Categories for Information Exchange:			
Relatives	36%	33%	31%
Friends	36%	31%	31%
Work/study colleagues	24%	28%	26%
Fiduciary relationships	3%	7%	10%
Little-known people	1%	1.2%	2.%
Strangers	0.2%	0.5%	0.5%
Information to Be Exchanged:			
Personal anxieties and fears	18.5%	18%	13%
Information on acquaintances and friends	13%	13%	14.5%
Broadcast of official news and media reports	30%	32%	41%
Videos and photos of people at the epicenter of the epidemic.	6%	10%	12%
Memes about C-19	30.5%	24%	17%
Other	1.4%	3.4%	3.5%

Note: * For clarity, these percentages are rounded off, as they are in all the Tables in this article.

affecting their friends and relatives. There is a statistical difference in how often respondents shared their own experiences and fears about C-19. Respondents of G1 and G2 were more likely to share those fears and anxieties than G3, as shown in Table 9.2. The members of G3 seem to have felt the need to share with others information broadcast on TV news and media. As these respondents tended to be oriented towards official information channels, we assume that they preferred to report information they believed to be reliable.

The Changing of Everyday Activities in the Pandemic Situation

Given that everyday life practices had to change dramatically as a result of the pandemic, we wished to identify and analyze those changes via

Table 9.3 Daily Routine Changes, %

Parameter Group	No Changes			More Frequently			Less Frequently		
	G1	G2	G3	G1	G2	G3	G1	G2	G3
Hygiene and PPE	62%	58%	61%	37%	42%	39%	0.9%	0.3%	0.2%
Healthcare	87%	86%	85%	12%	13%	15%	1.2%	0.9%	0.5%
Indoor Living	74%	69.5%	75%	25%	30%	25%	1.1%	0.5%	0%
Food Shopping	83%	80.5%	86%	15%	19%	14%	2%	0.9%	0%
Social Activity:	50%	51%	54%	44%	41%	37%	6%	8%	8%
Self-Isolation	40%	47%	49%	51%	41%	38%	9%	12.5%	13%
Limitations on Interpersonal Interactions	61%	55.5%	60%	36%	41%	36%	3%	4.1%	4.6%

two specific questions: (1) Did Russians' way of life change on the eve of the introduction of the restrictive measures? (2) Were our respondents psychologically prepared for the changes in social reality? (See Table 9.3.)

To answer the questions posed above, as shown in Table 9.3, we used the scale "Changes in Daily Routines." We asked about any changes in the respondents' day-to-day functioning, such as: hygiene and use of personal protective equipment (PPE); healthcare; indoor living; grocery shopping; social activities; and interpersonal interactions. We included a scale to examine the respondents' willingness to abide by social restrictions. Respondents were asked to note their psychological readiness for possible limitations on their daily activities: 1 = minimum preparedness and 10 = maximum preparedness.

In general, most respondents (more than 50% of each group) reported no changes in their daily living (see Table 9.3). This lack of change can be captured in Holavin's model of "social inaction." His analysis of his respondents' diary entries from March to April 2020 noted that the absence of changes could often be described through the prism "should have done, but didn't do" (Holavin 2020: 143). These cases of non-compliance with the new social norms opened a window of opportunity for non-response and for rethinking official and/or media claims about COVID-19. Holavin described this non-compliance as an escape from restrictions against the spread of the coronavirus, a way of preserving autonomy and freedom in a new, highly regulated reality in which people may disagree with those regulations and refuse to follow them.

When respondents did change their routine practices, these changes followed the proposed new regulations to limit the spread of C-19. Yet only about 1% of respondents in all groups reported a decline in some of their routine practices. The exception is the parameter "Social Activity and Interpersonal Interactions." The percentage of people less likely to limit some forms of social interaction due to C-19 was low, ranging from

6% to 9% (see Table 9.3). The major changes in these Russians' habitual lifestyles as shown in Table 9.3 were in hygienic routines, social activities, and interpersonal interactions.

The changes within the "Hygiene and PPE" parameter are paradoxical. They entailed simultaneous disbelief that their everyday practices had to change and an increase in self-protective practices. From early childhood, everyone knows that it is imperative to wash hands to protect oneself from infection. Yet the face mask does not belong to ordinary life. So the start of its everyday use was the start of a new kind of life for which people—as represented by our respondents—were not yet prepared.

The same dynamic can be seen in the parameter "Social Activity and Communication." In Table 9.3, we can observe a tendency to increase various types of social distancing. Within this parameter, more than for others, we can detect the effects of what we are terming *Covidian dissidence*. Table 9.3 shows that it is possible to identify a group of people who have actually increased their social activity in spite of C-19. We will discuss the changes within this parameter in more detail below.

The parameter "Healthcare" is about how typical for Russians are such procedures as:

- nasal irrigation—a personal hygiene practice through which the nasal cavity is washed with water or a saline nasal spray.
- taking antiviral and immuno-stimulating drugs and nutritional supplements;
- regular (once or twice a day) temperature measurement, and so on.

Among those who noted no change in this parameter, about 90% reported that they "never" do these things in their everyday lives. Yet in March 2020, doctors recommended these activities as preventive of COVID-19. We felt it essential to know whether our respondents actually followed the recommendations or ignored them, as the percentage of those who had become more aware of these activities does not exceed 15% in all groups. Table 9.3 shows that the percentage increases with age. In addition, the older respondents were much more likely to make use of traditional medicine practices. Traditional Russian methods of preventing viral infection include wearing garlic amulets, drinking tea made from *tinder fungus*, drinking vodka with red pepper, spending time in a sauna, and putting dry mustard in socks. We found a firm belief among our respondents that drinking tea infused with ginger and lemon and eating garlic and onions provide good protection against C-19. Significant changes in behavioral practices within this parameter likely occurred later. Public demand for different drugs and medical supplies had increased by September 2020, by which time many Russians would routinely take their temperatures and use pulse oximetry to measure the levels of oxygen in their blood, ingest various supplements, and engage in other health-protective practices.

Within the "Indoor Living" parameter, most Russians already did regular wet cleaning and ventilation in normal times. The majority of respondents did not use antiseptics to clean surfaces or treat rooms. In all groups, those who did implement such practices were generally women, as they tend to be more careful about cleanliness and order. This disproportion results from existing gender stereotypes about men's and women's roles in Russia and the extent to which people's behaviors follow these stereotypes. Those who did make changes within this parameter—again mostly women—were more likely to use antiseptics for cleaning (37%–44%) and to ventilate apartments (21%–26%). Some male respondents did become more active in ventilating the premises. We speculate that the older the men, the more rigid they tend to be regarding their habitual behaviors, as the most minor changes in the "Indoor Living" parameter were among the men of G3. In Russian culture, changes in behavior in caring for the home in a pandemic situation must not appear to infringe upon men's dignity.

We included the "Food Shopping" parameter because Russians' experiences of various socio-economic difficulties have always been accompanied by changes in the population's purchasing behaviors. Around the world, stores emptied out as people rushed to buy essential items after COVID struck. However, around 80% of our respondents in all groups reported that they had not begun to buy food and necessities in bulk (as shown in Table 9.3), and the percentage of those who had started to buy more goods does not exceed 20% in all groups. On one hand, we suppose that respondent's answers may be socially desirable: they likely did not want to be seen as engaging in irrational practices that are ridiculed in society, yet implemented nevertheless. On the other hand, analysis of the growth of consumer demand (Bulletin on Current Trends in the Russian Economy 2020) showed that purchasing activities peaked in the first quarter of 2020, during which the largest trading networks showed an acceleration in revenue growth, mainly due to increased demand in March 2020. From the second week of March to the first week of April 2020, there was an increased demand for essential goods that could be stored for long periods. As early as the second week of April 2020, consumer shopping began to decline, with supermarkets and hypermarkets (supermarkets combined with one or more department stores) suspending their operations—mainly due to the closure of the malls and a sharp drop in traffic (The State of the Russian Consumer Market n.d.). Therefore, we assume that the mentioned percentage of increased food shopping represents the peak in purchasing activity due to the boom around C-19.

As we noted above, one of the most changed parameters was "Changes in Social Activity." We have considered these changes within two contexts, both shown in Table 9.3:

• Different self-isolation practices
• Limitations on interpersonal interactions

We can find significant changes in both of these aspects. Our respondents became more likely to avoid public places. They used public transport more rarely, and began to avoid leaving their homes except in cases of emergency.

To understand the response "No changes" despite restrictions on visits to various public places, it is necessary to note that the younger the respondents were, the more likely they were to visit public places, and vice versa. Yet interestingly, in this alarm phase of social changes, the percentage of those who had made more visits to various public places and events is higher in G2 and G3. We can interpret these findings in the following ways: Respondents over 30 perceive visits to public places as having some subjective value above and beyond everyday routines. For example, G2 may wish to take their children to their favorite park. G3 may perceive going to a restaurant or visiting exhibitions as meaningful events that they do not wish to live without. Yet, as we will see below, even though G1 participants made fewer visits to public places than G2 and G3, GI participants found it hardest to give up visiting public places.

We note that the changes affected interpersonal interactions somewhat less than the parameter "self-isolation." On average, 30–40% of all respondents had started to restrict different types of social contacts more frequently. Respondents became warier of people with pronounced symptoms of respiratory diseases (G1–44%; G2–42%; G3–37%) and much more frequently avoided tactile contact (G1–37%; G2–47%; G3–41%).

Russians in general do not distance themselves from foreigners or from those who have returned from abroad. However, at the end of March, the number of those who began to be cautious increased: all age groups kept more distance from returnees from other countries. This may be related to the fact that, as previously noted, there were already regulations on compulsory self-isolation of returnees from abroad in March. Moreover, the media had been active in broadcasting information about COVID-19. We assume that elements of stigmatization of infected persons who had returned from abroad and those living with them had begun to emerge. By the end of March 2020, our respondents had started to restrict contact with their loved ones more often (G1–35%; G2–34%; G3–33%). We associate this restriction with the concerns of respondents for older relatives and relatives with chronic diseases.

Subjective Willingness to Follow Social Restrictions

Respondents in all groups reported a high level of subjective willingness to follow almost all restrictions asked about in our survey (see Table 9.4). The highest degree of preparedness in all groups related to the possibility of canceling mass events. Respondents of G3 were subjectively more prepared for such cancellations. For this older age group, attending cultural events is more related to realizing internal interests and values, and a way to vary

Table 9.4 Subjective Willingness to Follow Social Restrictions (M)**

Parameter: Social Restrictions	G1	G2	G3
Cancellation of mass events*	7.8	7.8	8.4
Disinfection of public and working spaces	8.7	8.7	8.9
Forced examination of somatic state	7.7	7.7	7.95
Prohibition to leave home	5.5	5.6	6.1
Remote work from home*	7.4	7.6	7.9
Closure of kindergartens. schools*	7.8	8.3	8.2
Ban on traveling abroad	7.7	7.9	7.8
Ban on leaving/entering other parts of the country	6.3	6.5	6.5
The imposition of a curfew	4.7	4.95	5.1

Notes:
* $p \leq 0,05$
** Table presents average values; min=1, max=10.

their leisure activities. For young people, participation in cultural and social activities is an integral part of their self-identification. For them, "to be" seems to entail an urgent need for participation in social life. We suggest that is why, despite the inadequate preparedness of respondents in all three groups for a possible lockdown, it is G1 respondents who were least prepared to be "locked inside four walls."

All respondents reported a high level of preparedness for disinfection in public areas, such as restaurants, and felt ready for the mandatory health checks that they expected to come. At the beginning of March 2020, the Chief State Physician of the Russian Federation issued several decrees concerning additional preventive measures. It then became necessary to organize daily thermometry of employees, to prevent patients with signs of viral respiratory illness from entering a work environment, and to disinfect workplace equipment, including telephones, computers, and other office equipment. In educational institutions, it was decreed that there should be mandatory daily morning thermometry for students and staff. The implementation of these decrees was entrusted to the regional authorities. In most of Russia, these measures were introduced at the end of March 2020. We suppose that this readiness was high among our respondents because some of these activities had already been implemented much earlier in March. For example, the Moscow metro had already been carrying out remote thermometry using thermal imaging cameras. At catering facilities, staff members had to process tables with additional sanitizers.

As Table 9.4 shows, respondents from all three groups were relatively prepared to accept the restrictions imposed on the items "Readiness to send employees to work remotely from home" and "Readiness to close kindergartens and schools." However, there were statistical differences among these groups. G3 respondents were more likely than G1 and G2 to work remotely from home. We interpret this finding as follows: at the end of March 2020, the media broadcast that self-isolation and limitations of interpersonal interaction would primarily affect persons of pensionable age (65+) and those with chronic diseases. Also, some organizations had already introduced restrictive measures for these categories of citizens. Some staff had already been transferred to remote working arrangements.

All respondents were the least prepared for such restrictions as "Ban on leaving home," "Imposition of curfew," "Ban on leaving/entering other regions of the country" (see Table 9.4). These limitations were related to a fundamental change in the way Russians think about freedom of movement and everyday space. Such restrictions may generate fears of existential isolation—fear of being alone with oneself—and these experiences may generate trauma. Lack of willingness to follow such restrictive measures may be associated with a lack of awareness or denial of the gravity of the situation. Many of our respondents at that time had not yet accepted that the world had changed.

Expected Negative and Positive Impacts of COVID-19

Positive expectations about life are essential to peoples' sense of wellbeing, whereas negative expectations can negatively affect psychological health, and their effects can work to actualize and intensify loss. Table 9.5 shows the possible negative effects of COVID-19, while Table 9.6 shows its possible positive effects.

The average number of expected negative impacts of C-19 in the three groups varied slightly, between 4.71 and 5.08. The number of possible positive effects (3.3–3.7) from the spread of C-19 was almost equal in the age groups studied (see Table 9.5). There are statistical differences in the numbers of negative and positive effects chosen in the questionnaire.

Table 9.5 The Possible Negative Effects of COVID-19

Negative effects	G1	G2	G3
Negative effects (M. points*)	4.7	4.9	4.5
Death	30%	33%	35%
Loss of health	40%	46%	49%
Death of loved ones	56%	67%	69%
Difficulties in obtaining medical care	49%	55%	65%
Economic instability	69%	66%	77%
Job loss	21%	26%	28%
Restriction on movement	57%	60%	70%
Decline in social activity	37%	43.5%	55%
Feelings of helplessness	18%	28%	30%
Reduction of interpersonal contacts	33%	34%	45%
Decline in quality of life	58%	56%	72%

Note: * M – the average number of chosen negative effects.

All respondents reported that they expected more negative impacts of C-19 than positive, leading to anxiety and the possibility of protests to changes and attempts to recapture the normality of pre-COVID life (see below).

For G1, there was either a wide variability in the choice of possible adverse effects, or respondents barely noted possible negative effects of C-19. We link those findings to the broadcasting of information that C-19 was a lesser threat to youths and a greater threat to older people. Also, the members of this group may have lower levels of health literacy and of critical thinking for assessing possible threats.

In G3, more than 70% of respondents identified risks such as loss of economic stability, loss of quality of life, and reduced mobility (see Table 9.5). With age, there appears to be a greater homogeneity of choices (as listed on the questionnaire) of possible negative consequences. This may be because the most severe social restrictions were more likely to have affected the older age group, reducing their self-confidence, raising the level of anxiety within the scope of the possibilities of exercising their professional activities, and increasing the objective risk of job loss.

As Table 9.5 shows, the majority of respondents were frightened by the potential decline in economic stability; this fear was probably the result of the information pressure from the mass media, which catastrophized the economic development of Russia due to the pandemic. The fear of economic instability might also be a reflection of the national memory of the post-Soviet experience of the early 1990s, during which citizens' incomes and savings were devalued.

The lowest number of respondents in all groups chose "job loss" as a possible adverse effect of C-19. We suppose that, for many Russians, there is no relation between the country's economic situation and their occupation, as the majority work in state-owned enterprises. Confidence in job security may stem from confidence in the protection and support of the State. However, more than 50% of respondents reported expectations of reduced quality of life during the pandemic, influenced by restrictions on movement, reduced social activity, loss of direct interpersonal contact, and limited access to necessary medical care.

The least reported expected adverse effects in all groups were death, unemployment, and feelings of helplessness. The more positive expected effects of C-19 were the opportunities to develop better personal hygiene skills and to take care of one's health and that of loved ones (see Table 9.6).

As Table 9.6 shows, between 30% and 40% of respondents reported an expected increase in leisure time as a positive possible impact of C-19. Also, respondents indicated the ability to gain new knowledge and experience during the pandemic, yet did not interpret this as a positive effect. But according to the reports of search services such as Google and Yandex, it is possible to identify a significant change in Russian search requests in March

Table 9.6 The Possible Positive Effects of COVID-19

Positive effects	G1	G2	G3
All positive effects (M, points*)	3	4	4
Increased attention to healthcare	40%	41%	46%
Increased attention to hygiene	52%	54%	50%
Increased attention to close relationships	43%	42.5%	49%
Increased self-testing	22%	22%	31.5%
Engagement in behavior training for emergencies	38.5%	37%	36%
Increased soul-searching	28%	36.5%	38%
Increased budget planning skills	20%	17.5%	18%
Additional income	3%	5%	7%
Increased social activity	4%	6%	7%
Increased interpersonal contacts	4%	6%	4%
More free time	30%	42%	35%
Increases in knowledge and experience	37%	39%	32%
Improving quality of life	4%	6%	13%

Note: * M – the average number of chosen positive effects.

2020. The most numerous searches in the second half of March 2020 on the Yandex search service contained the words "without leaving the house." Users asked what to read and were looking for online music concerts. In April, there was a decrease in such requests, as many had already learned more or less how to deal with the new conditions (ibid. 2020). Also, the acquisition of new knowledge was realized through increased understanding of the disease. Among the possible benefits of the pandemic's spread, respondents pointed to an improved environmental situation due to reduced business hours. Some respondents (only 1.8%) made misanthropic remarks in their comments about possible positive effects, such as "It's natural selection"; "Decreasing number of people"; "Rejuvenation of society." All respondents noted possible adverse effects of C-19; and 3.7% did not see any possible positive effects of the pandemic.

Conclusion: Action and Inaction

We have considered the period covered in this chapter within the context of social action or inaction in the first, "alarm phase" of the stresses generated by the coronavirus pandemic. Based on the ideas of Bykhovets and Cohen-Lerner (2020) and Mertens et al. (2020), we have identified three predicates of a changing socio-psychological space:

- The level of informational awareness of COVID-19;
- The realization of behavioral changes in everyday cultural life (Petukhov and Pirogov 2018);
- The emotional impacts of C-19.

Our respondents' "average" level of knowledge and satisfaction with the ever-flowing information about C-19 indicates that there was no one reliable (valid) source of information. Respondents compensated for this lack by turning to many different sources, mostly involving the media but also including conversations with colleagues and friends. It is clear how and through which channels age-specific information should be provided—social media for younger people, TV and print newspapers for older ones. Information is vulnerable to inaccuracy and misinterpretation, yet it is impossible to control the policies of and the information provided by mainstream social media networks. These provide a wide field for manipulating consciousness by interested parties in a situation of ambiguity and uncertainty via the provision of fake news. The group of respondents under 30 years of age appeared to be particularly vulnerable to (mis) information impact, most likely due to their lack of health literacy and critical thinking and their socio-psychological characteristics.

The pandemic disruptions of the regular order of life forced people into action or inaction. "Action" entails a conscious change in activity in the context of a particular parameter of everyday functioning. "Inaction" is the conscious refusal to engage in a conscious activity; it can also be seen as an unconscious passivity (Holavin 2020). We invoke these concepts of action and inaction to analyze the differences in individual behavior in a situation of the breakdown of normality, which can include a conscious (or unconscious) strategy of continuing to act in habitual ways despite the pandemic and its disruptions of normality (Belinskaia 2014). Regarding the perceptions of pandemic-related constraints and restrictions, we can say that the pandemic itself was perceived in varying ways by our respondents— some positive, most negative. Among our respondents, major changes in everyday functioning were associated with limited social activities and communications. Physical and social exclusion were reported to be the most frustrating factors. The respondents in G1 and G2 were the most frustrated by the restriction of freedoms. This topic was quite sensitive for them; it later turned into a tipping point that triggered waves of protest, such as refusals to wear masks or gloves and to engage in social distancing or self-isolation. Our data indicate that the seeds of these later waves of protest were sown during the period of our research, which, again was from March 21–March 27, 2020—precisely located in the early "alarm phase" of the pandemic.

Expectations for the future among our respondents blurred from openly optimistic scenarios to deeply pessimistic ones. We interpret these via Hobfolls' and Lilly's (1993) notion of the need to balance between loss and resourcefulness. Simultaneously, the main factor that emerged as significant was not the cognitive processing of verifiable information, but rather believing misinformation. We conclude by suggesting that truthful and comprehensive information on COVID-related restrictions, and on COVID-19 itself, could reduce the intense stresses of fear and anxiety by reducing ambiguity and uncertainty.

References

Belinskaia, E.P. 2014. Uncertainty as a category of modern social psychology of personality. *Psihologicheskie issledovaniya* 7(36): 3.

Budner, S. 1962. Intolerance of ambiguity as a personality variable. *Journal of Personality* 30: 29–50.

Bulletin on Current Trends in the Russian Economy. 2020. Consumer demand: Regional differences. 63. July.

Bykhovets, Y.V., and L.B. Cohen-Lerner. 2020. Pandemic COVID-19 as a multifactorialtraumatic situation. *Institut Psikhologii Rossiyskoy Akademii Nauk. Sotsial'naya I Ekonomicheskaya Psikhologiya* 5(2(18)): 291–308.

Davis-Floyd, R. 2018. Open and closed knowledge systems, the 4 stages of cognition, and the cultural management of birth. *Frontiers in Sociology* 3: 23. doi:10.3389/fsoc2018.2018.0023

Government.ru. 2020. *Health and epidemiological safety*. Accessed April 26, 2021. http://government.ru/rugovclassifier/667/events/

Hobfoll, S.E., and R.S. Lilly. 1993. Resource conservation as a strategy for community psychology. *Journal of Community Psychology* 21: 128–148.

Holavin, A.O. 2020. Social inaction at early stages of the COVID-19 pandemics. *Sotsiologicheskie Issledovaniya* 11: 139–148.

Holman, E.A., D.R. Garfin, and R.C. Silver. 2014. Media's role in broadcasting acute stress following the Boston Marathon bombings. *Proclamation of the National Academy of Science USA* 111(1): 93–98.

Kornilova, T.V. 2015 The principle of uncertainty in psychology of choice and risk. *Psikhologicheskie Issledovaniya* 8(40): 3. http://psystudy.ru

Mertens, G., L. Gerritsen, S. Duijndam, E. Salemink, and I.M. Engelhard. 2020. Fear of the coronavirus (COVID-19): Predictors in an online study conducted in March 2020. *Journal of Anxiety Disorders* 74:102258.

Ornell, F., J.B. Schuch, A.O. Sordi, and F.H.P. Kessler. 2020. "Pandemic fear" and COVID-19: mental health burden and strategies. *Brazilian Journal of Psychiatry* 42(3): 232–235.

Petukhov, A.S., and S.V. Pirogov. 2018. Practice theories as a methodology for everyday life studies *Vestnik Tomskogo Gosudarstvennogo Universiteta. Filosofiya. Sotsiologiya. Politologiya* 41: 159–167.

Selye, H. 1976. Stress without distress. In Serban G. (ed.), *Psychopathology of Human Adaptation*. Boston, MA: Springer, 147–183.

The State of the Russian Consumer Market and the Rating of FMCG Trade Networks. n.d. Accessed April 22, 2021.https://inforetail.ru/

Vives, M.L., and O. FeldmanHall. 2018. Tolerance to ambiguous uncertainty predicts prosocial behavior. *Nature Communications* 9(1): 2156. doi:10.1038/s41467-018-04631-9. PMID: 29895948; PMCID: PMC5997641.

World Health Organization (WHO). Coronavirus disease (COVID-19) advice for the public: Myth busters. n.d. Accessed March 24, 2021. www.who.int/ru/emergencies/diseases/novel-coronavirus-2019/advice-for-public/myth-busters.

10 The Quest for a Cure for COVID-19

Controversies and Negotiations Around Biomedical Treatments and Traditional Asian Medicines

Danuta Penkala-Gawęcka

Introduction: Unpreparedness, Global Health, and the Quest for a Cure

The coronavirus pandemic has provoked, from the very beginning, an intense search for an effective treatment, especially desired because the prospects for speedy vaccine development were then uncertain, and because governments, healthcare systems and societies were not adequately prepared for this global threat. In *Unprepared*, published three years before the coronavirus pandemic struck, Andrew Lakoff (2017) prophetically pointed to deficiencies in the politics of global health that contribute to the lack of global institutional preparedness to prevent or deal with pandemics. In his critical analysis of the concept of "global health," Fassin (2012) described the expansion of Western biomedical models of health and disease and the influence of social inequalities on people's health and access to healthcare. He addressed, among other topics, the politics of the production and distribution of pharmaceuticals, which still limit access to basic treatments in the countries of the Global South. In Fassin's view, the idea of global health has not been put into practice and "health remains largely seen as a national affair rather than a global question" (2012: 99). The ongoing pandemic has revealed the challenges that Lakoff (2017) had predicted of achieving a global emergency response to a catastrophic global health crisis.

Unpreparedness, on both macro- and micro-levels, has intensified perceptions of risk and uncertainty in the face of this new global health threat. People's responses to this threat are emotionally charged—although they approach COVID-19 risk differently, it commonly induces, in various sociocultural contexts, uncertainty, fear and anxiety, and even panic (Lupton 2013; Brown 2020).[1] Many place their hopes on the discovery of an effective treatment that would prevent severe cases of disease and deaths.

In this chapter,[2] I focus on the quest for drugs—possible tools to fight COVID-19—that began in biomedical research just after the first announcements of the epidemics, and on the search for non-biomedical treatments, especially those stemming from various types of traditional

DOI: 10.4324/9781003187462-13

medicine, such as Chinese, Tibetan, Ayurvedic, and Siddha (see below). I utilize specific examples to examine the issues of biomedical knowledge production and circulation, and contestations and negotiations around certain drugs, clinical trials, and "emergency use." I also highlight the strengthening of Asian traditional medical systems during the pandemic and describe some of the controversies around the use of their treatments. These controversies stem from major differences in biomedical and traditional medicine epistemologies. I base my analysis on available documentation, ranging from academic articles to short pieces in special "COVID-19 forums" at universities or in scholarly journals, blogs, and media reports.

Mediatizing the Pandemic: Biocommunicability and the Infodemic

It is important to highlight the role of mediatization in the spread of information about the pandemic, including the ever-unfolding news on drugs and preventive measures against COVID-19. Mainstream media reports on the pandemic and social media debates often fuel uncertainty and fear, which contribute to the circulation of rumors and conspiracy theories (Ali 2020b). The roles of social media in the dissemination of false information are widely acknowledged. In the Covidian context, UN Secretary-General António Guterres called this dissemination a "pandemic of misinformation" (Pazzanese 2020). The World Health Organization (WHO) repeatedly warns of an "infodemic" (the proliferation of information during an epidemic—both accurate and inaccurate), offers advice on how to manage this threat, and alerts the public that "misinformation or mixed messages can cost lives" (WHO 2020b). A special WHO initiative, "Myth Busters," seeks to debunk common misconceptions about the novel coronavirus, its spread, and methods of COVID-19 prevention and treatment. Myth Busters refutes, among others, false beliefs that eating garlic, drinking alcohol, spraying or drinking bleach (as suggested by the former president Trump) or any other disinfectant can protect against COVID-19, or that antibiotics and mineral supplements can prevent or treat the disease (WHO 2020a). Interestingly, this WHO campaign uses infographics with questions that repeat the misinformation and then refute it. Partington (2020) discusses this strategy and concludes: "Like the virus itself, the infodemic seems to call for vaccination."

Mediatization is closely connected with "biocommunicability," understood as multiple ways of production, circulation, and reception of health knowledge (Briggs 2011). Briggs notes that biocommunicability is characterized, first of all, by the proliferation of health issues within news coverage. In his words:

> biocommunicable cartographies link researchers, clinicians, reporters, health educators, medical journals, state officials, publics, HMOs,

insurers, corporations, and communicative and biomedical technologies
in vast networks that seem to constantly shift as new knowledge emerges.
(Briggs 2011: 471)

As Berlivet and Löwy (2020: 536) point out, biocommunicability has become
even more complex because of the growing roles of social media. These
phenomena and processes strongly influence perceptions of the pandemic,
uncertainties, fears and hopes for finding an effective[3] and safe treatment.

The Quest for Effective Pharmaceutical Cures for COVID-19

A telling example that illustrates the ongoing search for treatments against
COVID-19 is the "Coronavirus Drug and Treatment Tracker" provided
by *The New York Times* (Wu, Zimmer, and Corum 2021). This Tracker
presented "an updated list of 24 of the most-talked-about treatments for the
coronavirus," stipulating that "most are still at early stages of research." In
addition to recent updates, it provides brief information about "promising"
and "not promising" treatments, statements about "mixed evidence" and
"insufficient data," and reiterates warnings issued by the FDA (US Food &
Drug Administration) and the WHO against the use of several specific drugs.
The data presented often change as a result of the continuous search for
proofs of efficacy of particular drugs and therapies. From the perspectives
of those who are infected and those at high risk of infection, such "updated
lists" may represent subsequent waves of hope and disappointment, revealing
that the belief that a "magic bullet" will be discovered is unfounded. For
specialists, this is not surprising in the case of viral infections, and hope is
rather placed in a combination of medications, especially those developed
previously to combat other viruses (Greshko 2021).

According to Berlivet and Löwy (2020), the process of the
pharmaceuticalization of public health favors technological solutions
for health crises, without the participation of the lay public. However, as
these authors note, the quest for effective therapies for COVID-19 has led
some experts to contest the rules of clinical research, to discuss evidence of
effectiveness, and to claim for greater involvement of lay people in treatment
decisions. Addressing UK Government policymaking during the pandemic,
Hammersley (2020) highlighted the complexities of scientific evidence,
such as uncertainty and fallibility, a multiplicity of sources, and varying
views among scientists. He examined blurred boundaries between evidence
and advice and the role of ideology, and special, often political, interests,
which lead some decision-makers to act on the basis of uncertain evidence.
Differences in interests lead to difficulties in communication between
scientists and politicians; such difficulties are also visible in the controversies
around the effectiveness of particular drugs and therapies for COVID-19.

It is important to understand that risk assessment of newly introduced
treatments is difficult, due in part to still-inadequate knowledge of the

coronavirus. Grimen (2009: 21) rightly stated that "health care is often based on uncertain and contested knowledge," and this has been clearly revealed by the current pandemic. Biomedical authority may be easily weakened; such weakening is contributed to not only by rumors and conspiracy theories, but also by media hype surrounding the appearance of "new," "miraculous" drugs, followed by the next waves of disappointment. In the face of the pandemic, it has become common to treat patients with some "classic" drugs used off-label, which may blur the notions of evidence and proof. In the following analysis, I focus on two biomedical drugs used by many around the world to prevent or treat COVID-19—hydroxychloroquine and amantadine. In the case of amantadine, I give special attention to relevant examples from Poland, since this drug was first proposed as a treatment for COVID-19 by Polish doctors.

Negotiating, Contesting, and Repudiating Hydroxychloroquine

The career of chloroquine (a drug long used against malaria) and especially its derivative—hydroxychloroquine (used mainly for treating autoimmune diseases and promoted as an anti-COVID-19 treatment) is narrated in an in-depth study by Berlivet and Löwy (2020). They highlight the role of French microbiologist Didier Raoult, who has strongly advocated the use of hydroxychloroquine since March 2020 on the basis of a non-randomized clinical trial, and describe world campaigns in favor of this drug that have been greatly influenced by social media support.

Hydroxychloroquine, praised in March and April 2020 as a very promising or even effective treatment for COVID-19, was used in many countries, such as China, Italy, Spain, France, and the USA. However, therapeutic recommendations differed in particular countries; in Sweden, for instance, this drug was not recommended for COVID-19 patients due to its unproven effectiveness and risk of severe side effects. In Poland, the Office for Registration of Medicinal Products, Medical Devices and Biocidal Products published, on April 24, 2020, information based on the article "COVID-19: Reminder of Risk of Serious Side Effects with Chloroquine and Hydroxychloroquine," which had been issued one day earlier by the European Medicines Agency (EMA). According to this information, chloroquine and hydroxychloroquine, which have been introduced in specialized hospitals for COVID-19 patients, should be used with careful consideration of possible side effects, especially heart rhythm problems, which are sometimes fatal (Cessak 2020). Nevertheless, the decision to use Arechin (the brand name for chloroquine) and Plaquenil (hydroxychloroquine) as "supplementary drugs for SARS-CoV-2 infections" dramatically limited their availability for those who really needed them—patients with lupus and other autoimmune diseases (Rajtar 2020).

In May 2020, the WHO announced that hydroxychloroquine had turned out to be ineffective in treating or preventing COVID-19, and then decided to stop its clinical trials among hospitalized patients (WHO 2020c). In the USA, it was widely used until mid-June, when the FDA admitted that the drug's potential benefits in cases of COVID-19 did not outweigh its health risks (Huizen 2021). Since December 2020, the WHO has been creating a "living" guideline containing accurate, up-to-date information on COVID-19 management; among the first entries were strong recommendations against the use of hydroxychloroquine in patients with COVID-19 and for prophylaxis (WHO 2020d, 2021; Huizen 2021).

From the perspectives of medical anthropology and its branch, pharmaceutical anthropology, it is interesting to observe the trajectories of hydroxychloroquine and other drugs, following Whyte's et al. (2006) argument that the "social lives" of pharmaceuticals should be carefully studied. The race to find an effective treatment for COVID-19 generated interrupted life trajectories of drugs that were originally developed for other diseases, in the course of randomized controlled trials (RCTs) grounded in evidence-based medicine (EBM). In the fight against SARS-CoV-2, these drugs are used as "emergency tools" without required long-lasting tests, and their new lives usually end in failure or only partial success. In the pandemic situation, the epistemic certainties of EBM have been mitigated and distorted.

In the face of emergency, as noted by Berlivet and Löwy (2020) for hydroxychloroquine, discussions on the value of RTCs and on proofs of effectiveness have rapidly intensified. These controversies have led to challenges to the authority of experts and to "debates on the role of the lay public in decision-making that concerns them directly" (Berlivet and Löwy 2020: 526). The case of chloroquine and hydroxychloroquine also highlights the significant roles played by some prominent politicians, who entered into these debates in the name of defending people's interests. In May 2020, the Presidents of Brazil (Jair Bolsonaro) and the United States (Donald Trump) promoted the use of these drugs despite the numerous warnings issued by medical experts.[4] Such populist, anti-expert political activities, together with social media propaganda, have influenced people's individual searches for effective anti-COVID-19 drugs and have often caused them to resort to self-medication.

Contesting Amantadine: A "Promising" Treatment for COVID-19?

While chloroquine and hydroxychloroquine became the "heroes" of the first months of the pandemic, amantadine made its entrance as an anti-COVID-19 treatment a bit later. This drug had been used against influenza A, but was withdrawn due to subsequently recognized viral resistance. At present, amantadine is mainly used to treat Parkinson's disease. In spring 2020, Polish doctors and researchers from the Department of Neurology, Medical University of Lublin, and the Department of Experimental Pharmacology,

Polish Academy of Sciences in Warsaw—professors Rejdak and Grieb with their teams—observed that none of their 22 patients with Parkinson's and other neurological disorders who were taking amantadine and caught COVID-19 developed its most severe symptoms. The researchers published this observation in April 2020 and then, while admitting that it was too early to advocate amantadine as a treatment for COVID-19, suggested a controlled trial of this drug to discover whether it is effective against the novel coronavirus (Grieb et al. 2021—Letter to the Editor submitted in November 2020).

Meanwhile, Dr. Bodnar, a pulmologist from Przemyśl, Poland, self-treated with amantadine for COVID-19 and, since March 2020, has treated many coronavirus-infected patients with success, according to his statements and his patients' responses. Dr. Bodnar published guidelines with dosing recommendations online, adding a warning against taking this drug without a doctor's advice (Derza 2021). He has strongly advocated including amantadine into standard medications for COVID-19; however, several influential doctors, such as Professor Simon, an infectious disease specialist, have severely criticized its off-label use and have warned that it may be harmful for patients and can lead to the development of drug-resistant strains of SARS-CoV-2 (Mazur-Puchała 2021). Professor Flisiak, Chair of the Polish Association of Epidemiologists and Infectionists, also claimed that there were no scientific grounds for the use of amantadine against SARS-CoV-2 infections; therefore it was not recommended by this Association (Mikołajska 2020). These controversies and debates among specialists reveal differing approaches to the question of the need for and the validity of scrupulous clinical tests, as outlined above. In the view of Dr. Bodnar and his supporters, satisfying results of treatment, although scientifically unproven, should be regarded as a sufficient test of drug effectiveness when human lives are at stake. Importantly, there are also differences between Bodnar's claims that at least 99% of severe cases of COVID-19 can be stabilized with amantadine and Rejdak's cautious statements about using the drug at an early stage of the disease as the primary condition of its effectiveness (Mazur-Puchała 2021).

A significant increase of interest in amantadine has been observed in Poland since an announcement of its use in self-treatment for COVID-19 by the Vice-Minister of Justice in December 2020, which caused a political scandal and accusations of breaking the law by the state's top law officer. The Vice-Minister admitted to using this drug, which was not recommended and available only by prescription, on the basis of the information on Dr. Bodnar's experimental treatments. The Vice-Minister was enthusiastic about the effects of amantadine and added that he would demand that the Ministry of Health "work on this drug." The first response of the Polish Ministry of Health referred to the lack of recommendations for the use of amantadine, since its effectiveness and safety had not been tested. Shortly afterward, the Minister of Health announced that he had asked the Polish

Agency for Medical Research to start a clinical study on the use of this drug in preventing the progression of and treating COVID-19. It is noteworthy, however, that it took about seven months from the first information about amantadine as a promising treatment to commissioning its research (Mikołajska 2020).

Extensive media coverage of the "amantadine case" and social media interest resulted in increased demand in Poland for the drugs Viregyt-K and Amantix (brand names for amantadine), which quickly limited their accessibility at pharmacies (again, they are only available by prescription). Yet it is easy to receive prescriptions for these drugs from several "Internet clinics," which advertise their services with such messages as "You can get an e-prescription in five minutes" following an online consultation with a doctor. According to a Polish journalist who checked this possibility, the whole procedure took 15 minutes and this paid e-consultation consisted only of filling out a form by providing some personal data and information about one's health (Grzęda-Łozicka 2021). In addition, an illegal trade in these drugs flourishes on the Internet. Hence, self-medication with amantadine became quite widespread in Poland during the third and fourth wave of the pandemic, despite specialists' warnings of the potentially dangerous side effects of its use without a doctor's recommendation. In fact, a Polish doctor cannot legally recommend amantadine for COVID-19. Specialists often point out that until the results of the clinical study launched by the Agency for Medical Research are known, this drug should not be used to treat patients (Grzęda-Łozicka 2021).

Amantadine may now be considered a "promising" treatment for COVID-19. It does not promise a cure, but only to alleviate viral progression when used at an early stage, or to "contribute to mitigation of COVID-19 in infected patients" (Grieb et al. 2021: 412). According to the April 2021 statement of the Polish Agency for Medical Research, the results of the amantadine tests, under the project led by Professor Rejdak, should be known in a few weeks, and even if this drug "does not significantly affect the course and severity of the acute phase of infection, it will still have an important impact on the severity and course of neurological complications" (Polish Agency for Medical Research 2021). During a press conference on April 14, 2021, the Minister of Health announced that the results would be available in two weeks. He also warned against self-treatment with amantadine and said that many patients who had taken that risk were admitted in bad shape to hospitals, and some deaths had been recorded. The next statements by Prof. Rejdak revealed that final results of the tests might be expected at the end of May; however these predictions also turned out to be much too optimistic. According to the information of May 22, 2021, the main obstacle has been an insufficient number of participants; only when a minimum of 100 and ideally 200 patients would be gathered and tested—which was expected to occur in the summer of 2021—might the final results be available (Zdziebłowski 2021). However, on December

7, 2021, in response to the Vice-Minister of Justice's (mentioned above) query about the very slow progress in the amantadine tests, the Ministry of Health spokesman announced that so far, the trial did not confirm the effectiveness of amantadine, but preliminary results could be presented only after "achieving a statistically significant number of recruited and tested patients" (Lechowicz-Dyl 2021).

Importantly, observations similar to those of Rejdak and Grieb were made by a group from Cambridge University, and some clinical studies on amantadine for the prevention of SARS-CoV-2 symptomatology have been launched in Spain and Mexico (Cortés-Borra and Aranda-Abreu 2021). An international consortium for studying amantadine as a promising anti-COVID-19 drug, with the membership of Prof. Rejdak's team, has been organized, and other tests have started in Denmark. Thus, we may follow the life trajectory of this drug over time, and hope for its at least partial success, although its testing on patients is a slow, arduous process.

Having described a few of the many biomedical efforts to find a cure for COVID-19 and the negotiations around them, I now turn to an examination of several traditional Asian medical systems, the roles these systems are playing in relation to COVID-19, and their contestations by and negotiations with biomedical systems.

Traditional Asian Medicines and COVID-19

Amidst the pandemic, given that the search for an effective biomedical treatment for COVID-19 has not brought great success (as described above), it is not surprising that the use of traditional medicines has been increasing around the world. Traditional and complementary medicines (T&CM) have been continuously used in many countries, sometimes for thousands of years, and the phenomenon of medical pluralism/medical diversity—the coexistence of dominant biomedicine with various forms of non-biomedical treatments—can be found almost everywhere (WHO 2019). (The fact that such ancient medical systems are now called "alternative" or "complementary" to biomedicine indexes its growing global hegemony.) The pandemic situation has enhanced this trend, especially in areas with weak biomedical healthcare systems such as Asia, Africa, and Latin America (Muhammad 2020; Ali 2020a). Researchers (e.g. Nguyen 2020) highlight the role of the Internet, and particularly social media, in disseminating information about the use of traditional remedies recognized as possible treatments against COVID-19, and promoting various new "miracle" cures. The WHO has generally endorsed T&CM and has supported efforts to integrate their services into national healthcare systems, provided that the quality, safety and efficacy of the therapies are proven (WHO 2013). In the quest for anti-COVID-19 treatments, the WHO has started working with some local research institutions to identify potentially useful traditional remedies and to confirm their efficacy and safety (Muhammad 2020).

Here I focus on Asian "great medical traditions," including traditional Chinese medicine (TCM) and Tibetan medicine, discussing their roles in the search for effective treatments for COVID-19. Since the start of the epidemic in Wuhan, TCM remedies have been used in China to alleviate COVID-19 symptoms, often in combination with biomedical drugs; according to the official reports, more than 90% of patients across the country have received such treatment (Jakhar 2020). The National Hygiene and Health Committee of the People's Republic of China issued recommendations for the use of TCM formulas in February 2020, and their region-specific versions were published online (Xin and Hsu 2020). Among the compound medications recommended in "early observational phases" of SARS-CoV-2 infection, when a patient is expected to self-medicate at home, were *Huoxiang zhengqi* and *Lianhua qingwen*, with 13 herbal components including forsythia (*Forsythia suspensa*) and rhodiola (*Rhodiola rosea*). Other formulas have been used in four "clinical phases" of the disease when an infected person was treated in a hospital (Jakhar 2020; Xin and Hsu 2020). Interestingly, the Wuhan Institute of Virology and the Shanghai Institute Materia Medica issued, at the end of January 2020, a statement that a TCM medicine called *Shuang huang lian* (with three main plant ingredients: forsythia, honeysuckle and Chinese skullcap) could hinder the progression of SARS-CoV-2. This statement resulted in an immediate rush to pharmacies, so this medicine was out of stock in China within a couple of hours (Cai 2020). This herbal remedy was then chosen for one of the large clinical studies that have been launched since February 2020 in China, with the assistance of WHO experts working with Chinese scientists to standardize this research (Maxmen 2020).

The Chinese government support for TCM during the COVID-19 pandemic has been much stronger than it was during the SARS epidemic in 2002–2003; nevertheless, almost 60% of SARS patients in mainland China received TCM remedies, usually combined with biomedical drugs (Hanson 2010: 236). Such combinations reflect the ongoing negotiations between the biomedical and traditional medical systems, showing that in China they sometimes manage to work in tandem with each other. Several Chinese studies claim that the use of TCM as a supplement to conventional biomedical treatments had beneficial effects in SARS treatment and dramatically reduced fatality from the disease, which can be an inspiration for using TCM in patients infected with SARS-CoV-2 (Yang et al. 2020). In her article on TCM and SARS, Hanson (2010: 237) thoroughly analyzed reports on the use of TCM medicines during the epidemic, and quoted the WHO's experts' opinion that both Western antiviral and anti-inflammatory drugs and Chinese herbal formulas "should be systematically tested in clinical trials during the next comparable epidemic." She also identified blind spots and media "blindfolds" that had hindered recognizing TCM contributions to the management of the SARS epidemic. Thus it is arguable that such trials should have been conducted during that crisis, in preparation for the next "comparable epidemic," which we now experience in heightened form as the COVID-19 pandemic.

TCM has become an important actor in Chinese government politics, intended to obscure their faults at the first stages of the epidemic and to demonstrate the superiority of China's anti-COVID therapies. TCM healing methods and remedies have been heavily promoted at home and abroad; President Xi Jinping called them a "treasure of Chinese civilization" and assured that China is eager to make them available to the world (Mai and Lo 2020; Jakhar 2020). TCM remedies have been sent from China together with "conventional" medicines and equipment to several countries of Africa, Asia, and Europe. While TCM practitioners felt empowered by this official support and promotion, some biomedical Chinese scientists and doctors urged caution and advised careful testing in line with the WHO's recommendations. However, skeptical voices have been largely muted as opposing the national Chinese policy (Mai and Lo 2020; Jakhar 2020).

It is informative to examine the debates around "scientific evidence" and "rigorous trials" in the context of TCM promotion. Arguments about a lack of evidence for TCM efficacy are put forward by its adversaries on the grounds of biomedical science and a paradigm of evidence-based medicine. Yet, as already indicated, discussions and negotiations around the validity of the randomized controlled trial versus empirical experience have gained momentum amid the current pandemic. In the case of TCM and other Asian medical traditions, these controversies are even more vivid. The value of the clinical trials aiming to evaluate the efficacy and safety of TCM medicines for COVID-19 patients, launched in China (Yang et al. 2020), is often contested by biomedical specialists (Cyranoski 2020). While critics argue that there has been no good evidence for TCM, since "there are no rigorous trial data that the remedies work" (Cyranoski 2020), adherents maintain that EBM trials, well-tailored to Western pharmaceuticals, are not applicable to traditional medicines. For example, as one Chinese expert said, every patient treated with TCM remedies "may require different medications and different dosages every day, and that has rendered a fair comparison impossible or meaningless" (Mai and Lo 2020). Undoubtedly, basic differences between the ontologies and epistemologies of biomedicine, which tend to be standardized and designed to cure illness after it happens, and those of traditional medical systems, which tend to be individualized and designed to prevent illness or to cure it holistically, by supporting the body's immune system, are at the root of these discrepancies (see Davis-Floyd 2018).

In addition to TCM, traditional Tibetan medicine (*Sowa Rigpa*) has gained a stronger position in China during the pandemic. Tibetan Sowa Rigpa doctors had helped their Chinese colleagues before the COVID-19 outbreak reached Tibet, and licensed formulas were sent by Qizheng, China's biggest producer of Tibetan medicines, to several Chinese hospitals where COVID-19 patients were being treated (Tidwell 2020). This mobilization of Sowa Rigpa resources has contributed to increasing its status in China, including

Tibet, where, as Tidwell states, "access to healthcare provided by Tibetan medical institutions now outnumbers that of biomedical clinics across the province" and many Tibetan Sowa Rigpa doctors cooperate with, instead of contesting, their "biomedical colleagues." Although mutual influence and knowledge flow between Tibetan medicine and biomedicine had been previously observed (see Adams, Schrempf, and Craig 2011), the current health crisis has stimulated their further development, resulting in positive and effective negotiations between the two medical systems.

The position of Tibetan medicine in India, as anthropological studies reveal (Gerke 2020a, b), is not so satisfactory. During Gerke's field trip to Dharamsala in February 2020, where no COVID-19 cases had yet been reported, the first public health preventive initiatives were being introduced. However, members of the local Tibetan community tended to rely on the traditional protective measures of Tibetan medicine and were convinced, in particular, of the efficacy of *rimsung* pills, worn as amulets. These protective "pills" are based on Tibetan classical medical formulas and contain written mantras together with 7–9 substances (garlic, sulfur, myrrh, musk and aconite, among others). Their potency is believed to come from the strong smell, considered efficacious against infection (Gerke 2020b: 197). Rimsung pills enjoyed extensive popularity during the initial stages of the pandemic, but the local medical administration ordered the halting of their distribution by Tibetan clinics "because they were causing anxiety and panic among the people" (Gerke 2020b: 206). From an anthropological perspective, it was just the opposite: these early responses of the Tibetans to an emerging epidemic could have helped to ease the shared emotions of fear and anxiety (ibid.: 207).

Gerke (2020a) and Banerjee (2020) highlight the politics of India towards its local traditional medical systems, which are acronymized as "AYUSH" (Ayurveda, Yoga, Unani, Siddha (see below), Sowa Rigpa (Tibetan medicine) and Homeopathy[5]). These politics have been entangled in frictions and a longstanding antagonism between AYUSH and the hegemonic biomedical system. This antagonism is seen as the main obstacle to using the potential of Ayurveda and other traditional medicines to fight COVID-19 in India. Banerjee (2020) addresses the politics of knowledge systems, pointing out that their complexities and contradictions have been exacerbated during the current pandemic. She argues that biomedicine has tried to position Ayurveda as the "Other," whereas Ayurveda proponents have made efforts to bring it closer to the standards set by biomedicine. Yet the continued dominance of biomedicine has led to the marginalization of Ayurveda, the core focus of which is on gaining and maintaining health via strengthening the immune system—an upstream, preventive approach—while biomedicine is centered in the downstream approach of fixing problems after they happen via curative interventions. Due to these fundamental epistemic differences, trial protocols established in biomedical pharmaceutical research are inappropriate for testing Ayurvedic medicines. According to

Banerjee (2020), "[Ayurveda's] epistemology allows for a different etiology of disease and treatment," and its strength lies in its emphasis on prevention, which might complement biomedical measures to fight the pandemic. Craig, Gerke, and van der Valk (2020) wrote in a similar vein, calling for critical reflection on the power dynamics and the "epistemic violence implicit in the application of biomedically based 'evidence-based medicine' to Asian scholarly medicines."

In this regard, it is worth noting that the Prime Minister of India, who met with representatives of the AYUSH sector in March 2020, urged them to start evidence-based research on traditional remedies. Consequently, the AYUSH Ministry has implemented some research projects designed to evaluate the impact of AYUSH interventions/medicines in the prevention and clinical management of COVID-19 (Rajalakshmi et al. 2020). The Ministry also established a COVID-19 input portal, where registered AYUSH practitioners can submit treatment suggestions for scientific validation (ibid.). According to Gerke (2020a), 2,000 proposals were submitted by April 14, 2020, but "it remains unclear how and when these suggestions will be 'scientifically validated.' " However, despite these controversies around EBM trials, AYUSH treatments have been used in India to fight COVID-19. For example, the government of Tamil Nadu has opened 29 special care centers in which COVID-19 patients are given Siddha medicines, which are the only treatments provided for those with mild symptoms, and in biomedical hospitals, patients receive integrated treatments (Rajalakshmi et al. 2020). Siddha is a traditional medical system that originated and evolved in South India, and is particularly popular in Tamil Nadu. It focuses on specific yoga practices and certain types of breathing, and also on mineral and herbal remedies; to treat COVID-19, mainly herbal remedies are used (Rajalakshmi et al. 2020).

Conclusion: The Need for Broad and Inclusive Approaches to Health Emergencies

In this chapter, I have focused on the quest for an effective COVID-19 treatment, addressing both biomedical tools against the novel coronavirus and the remedies of Asian traditional medical systems, including traditional Chinese medicine (TCM), Tibetan medicine, and Ayurveda. In the context of the uncertainty and fear surrounding the emergence of this new global health crisis, which has revealed insufficient preparation on the parts of governments, healthcare systems and societies, the efforts to fight it have led to the "emergency use" of a number of existing antiviral and other biomedical drugs. Most of these, after initial hopes and expectations, did not prove to be efficacious. Due to increasing mediatization and biocommunicability, closely linked to the current infodemic, self-medication with biomedical drugs and various traditional (or self-invented) treatments has become widespread. In some medically pluralistic regions of Asia, traditional medical systems have been strengthened, and new and positive negotiations and collaborations with biomedical practitioners have been established, despite the disputes and controversies highlighted herein.

In addition, practitioners and researchers of these traditional systems have been attempting to study them via the biomedical gold standard of the randomized controlled trial. Yet, since treatments within these systems tend to be highly individualized, many traditional medical practices cannot be studied in this way. That does not mean that they do not work, but rather that they often conflict with evidence-based medicine. Thus, biomedicine continues its boundary work (Gieryn 1983) and guards its epistemic borders, as is apparent in the (often unattainable) demand for the application of strict EBM trials to traditional medicines, even in a state of emergency. However, amidst the emergency of the coronavirus pandemic, biomedicine itself does not comply with all of its own rigorous standards, as I have shown. I conclude by noting that I agree with Gerke (2020a), who maintains that "epidemic emergencies demand broad and inclusive approaches," and that traditional medical systems in Asian and other countries can effectively contribute to public health efforts, especially in times of crisis.

Notes

1 Lupton (2013: 9) suggests the term "emotion-risk assemblage" to describe complex interconnections between risk and emotions; Brown (2020) draws attention to different approaches to COVID-19 risk in particular countries (and social groups) depending on the level of trust in the institutions and experts.
2 This text is partly based on my article published in Polish in 2020: COVID-19, niepewność, lęk i nadzieja. W poszukiwaniu skutecznego leku. *Lud* 104:185–212. doi: http://dx.doi.org/10.12775/lud104.2020.08. I substantially revised and updated this article for this chapter.
3 I cannot address here debates on the issue of efficacy/effectiveness of medical interventions, which are understood in medical anthropology differently than in biomedicine. However, in the next section, this notion is used in accordance with the biomedical approach.
4 President Trump announced that he was taking hydroxychloroquine for prevention. Then he began to praise another drug, remdesivir, as a new hope for COVID-19 patients and a great success for the US pharmaceutical industry (Berlivet and Löwy 2020: 535). Remdesivir has been, so far, the only drug fully approved by FDA (in October 2020) as a treatment for COVID-19, although "research suggests it may provide only a modest benefit to patients" (Wu, Zimmer, and Corum 2021). In November 2020, the WHO recommended against using remdesivir in patients with COVID-19 on the basis of a global randomized trial; however it is still routinely used in the USA and many other countries.
5 Homeopathy, although invented in Germany, has become very popular and almost "naturalized" in India.

References

Adams, V., Schrempf, M., and Craig S.R., eds. 2011. *Medicine Between Science and Religion: Explorations on Tibetan Grounds*. New York and Oxford: Berghahn Books.

Ali, I. 2020a. *Constructing and Negotiating Measles: The Case of Sindh Province of Pakistan*. PhD dissertation. Vienna, Austria: University of Vienna.

Ali, I. 2020b. The COVID-19 pandemic: Making sense of rumor and fear. *Medical Anthropology* 39(5): 376–379. doi: 10.1080/01459740.2020.1745481

Banerjee, M. 2020. Ayurveda and Covid-19: The Politics of Knowledge Systems, Yet Again. Hot Spots, *Fieldsights*, June 23. https://culanth.org/fieldsights/ayurveda-and-covid-19-the-politics-of-knowledge-systems-yet-again (accessed June 30, 2020).

Berlivet, L., and Löwy, I. 2020. Hydroxychloroquine controversies: Clinical trials, epistemology, and the democratization of science. *Medical Anthropology Quarterly* 34(4): 525–541. doi:10.1111/maq.12622

Briggs, Ch.L. 2011. "Biocommunicability." In M. Singer and P.I. Erickson (eds.), *A Companion to Medical Anthropology*. Malden, MA, Oxford, and Chichester: Wiley Blackwell, 459–476.

Brown, P. 2020. Studying COVID-19 in light of critical approaches to risk and uncertainty: Research pathways, conceptual tools, and some magic from Mary Douglas. *Health, Risk and Society* 22(1): 1–14. doi:10.1080/13698575.2020.1745508

Cai, Y. 2020. Extraordinary medicine. *Medical Anthropology Quarterly*, Rapid Response Blog Series, April 13. http://medanthroquarterly.org/rapid-response/2020/04/extraordinary-medicine/ (accessed May 15, 2020).

Cessak, G. 2020. Informacja Prezesa Urzędu z dnia 24 kwietnia 2020 r. w sprawie komunikatu Europejskiej Agencji ds. Leków dot. COVID-19. Urząd Rejestracji Produktów Leczniczych, Wyrobów Medycznych i Produktów Biobójczych. www.urpl.gov.pl/pl/informacja-prezesa-urz%C4%99du-z-dnia-24-kwietnia-2020-r-w-sprawie-komunikatu-europejskiej-agencji-ds (accessed April 30, 2020).

Cortés-Borra, A., and Aranda-Abreu, G.E. 2021. Amantadine in the prevention of clinical symptoms caused by SARS-CoV-2. *Pharmacological Reports*, February 18. doi:10.1007/s43440-021-00231-5

Craig, S.R., Gerke, B., and van der Valk, J.M.A. 2020. Asian Medicines and Covid-19: An Introduction. Hot Spots, *Fieldsights*, June 23. https://culanth.org/fieldsights/asian-medicines-and-covid-19-an-introduction (accessed June 30, 2020).

Cyranoski, D. 2020. China is promoting coronavirus treatments based on unproven traditional medicines. *Nature*, May 6. www.nature.com/articles/d41586-020-01284-x (accessed March 12, 2021).

Davis-Floyd, R. 2018. "The Technocratic, Humanistic, and Holistic Paradigms of Birth and Health Care." In R. Davis-Floyd (ed.), *Ways of Knowing about Birth: Mothers, Midwives, Medicine, and Birth Activism*. Long Grove IL: Waveland Press, 3–44.

Derza, B. 2021. Evaluating Amantadine as a Potential Treatment for COVID-19. *Pharmacy Times*, January 25. www.pharmacytimes.com/view/an-update-on-covid-19-vaccine-pause-variants-and-booster-shots (accessed March 12, 2021).

Fassin, D. 2012. "That Obscure Object of Global Health." In M.C. Inhorn and E.A. Wentzell (eds.), *Medical Anthropology at the Intersections: Histories, Activism, and Futures*. Durham, NC, and London: Duke University Press, 95–115.

Gerke, B. 2020a. Sowa Rigpa in Lockdown: On the Potency and Politics of Prevention. Hot Spots, *Fieldsights*, June 23. https://culanth.org/fieldsights/sowa-rigpa-in-lockdown-on-thepotency-and-politics-of-prevention (accessed June 30, 2020).

Gerke, B. 2020b. Thinking through complex webs of potency: Early Tibetan medical responses to the emerging coronavirus epidemic: Notes from a field visit to Dharamsala, India. *Medicine Anthropology Theory* 7(1): 188–209. doi:10.17157/mat.7.1.789

Gieryn, T.F. 1983. Boundary-work and the demarcation of science from non-science: Strains and interests in professional ideologies of scientists. *American Sociological Review* 48: 781–795.

Greshko, M. 2021. New Drugs Identified as Possible Tools to Fight COVID-19. *National Geographic*, February 24. www.nationalgeographic.com/science/article/new-drugs-identified-as-possible-tools-to-fight-covid-19 (accessed March 3, 2021).

Grieb, P., Świątkiewicz, M., Prus, K., and Rejdak, K. 2021. Amantadine for COVID-19. *The Journal of Clinical Pharmacology* 61(3): 412–413. doi:10.1002/jcph.1802

Grimen, H. 2009. Power, trust, and risk: Some reflections on an absent issue. *Medical Anthropology Quarterly* 23(1): 16–33. doi:10.1111/j.1548-1387.2009.01035.x

Grzęda-Łozicka, K. 2021. Kupiłam amantadynę w 15 minut. *WP abcZdrowie*, 9.04. https://portal.abczdrowie.pl/coraz-wiecej-osob-probuje-sie-leczyc-na-wlasna-reke-amantadyna-lek-jest-dostepny-na-recepte-ale-jak-sie-okazuje-to-nie-problem (accessed April 10, 2021).

Hammersley, M. 2020. Did Behavioural Science Cost Lives? Some Thoughts on UK Government Policymaking During the Pandemic. https://martynhammersley.files.wordpress.com/2020/11/did-behavioural-science-cost-livesf.pdf (accessed March 12, 2021).

Hanson, M.E. 2010. "Conceptual Blind Spots, Media Blindfolds. The Case of SARS and Traditional Chinese Medicine." In A.K. Ch. Leung and C. Furth (eds.), *Health and Hygiene in Chinese East Asia: Policies and Publics in the Long Twentieth Century*. Durham, NC, and London: Duke University Press, 228–254.

Huizen, J. 2021. WHO "Strongly" against the Use of Hydroxychloroquine for COVID-19 Prevention. *Medical News Today*, March 4. www.medicalnewstoday.com/articles/who-strongly-against-hydroxychloroquine-use-for-covid-19-prevention (accessed April 10, 2021).

Jakhar, P. 2020. COVID-19: China Pushes Traditional Remedies amid Outbreak. *BBC News*, June 29. www.bbc.com/news/world-asia-53094603 (accessed July 2, 2020).

Lakoff, A. 2017. *Unprepared: Global Health in a Time of Emergency*. Oakland, CA: University of California Press.

Lechowicz-Dyl, K. 2021. MZ: badania kliniczne nad amantadyną trwają. *Medycyna Praktyczna*, 07.12. www.mp.pl/covid19/covid19-aktualnosci/286591,mz-badania-kliniczne-nad-amantadyna-trwaja (accessed December 8, 2021).

Lupton, D. 2013. Risk and emotion: Towards an alternative theoretical perspective. *Health, Risk & Society* 15(8): 634–647. doi:10.1080/13698575.2013.848847

Mai, J., and Lo, K. 2020. Beijing Pushes Traditional Chinese Medicine as Coronavirus Treatment despite Questions over Benefits. *South China Morning Post*, March 23. www.scmp.com/news/china/society/article/3076500/beijing-pushes-traditional-chinese-medicine-coronavirus (accessed March 27, 2020).

Maxmen, A. 2020. More than 80 clinical trials launch to test coronavirus treatments. *Nature*, February 15. www.nature.com/articles/d41586-020-00444-3 (accessed February 2, 2021).

Mazur-Puchała, A. 2021. W aptekach brakuje amantadyny. Trwają badania nad skutecznością. *Medonet*, 12.02. www.medonet.pl/koronawirus-pytania-i-odpowiedzi/leczenie-koronawirusa,polacy-wykupuja-amantadyne--czy-jest-skuteczna-na-covid-19-,artykul,89570180.html (accessed February 13, 2021).

Mikołajska, M. 2020. Amantadyna lekiem na COVID-19? *Medonet*, 18.12. www.medonet.pl/koronawirus/koronawirus-w-polsce,koronawirus-w-polsce--amantadyna-w-terapii-covid-19--badania--decyzje-mz,artykul,02812179.html (accessed December 20, 2020).

Muhammad, F. 2020. COVID-19 pandemic: The role of traditional medicine. *International Journal of Infection* 7(3): e107090. doi: 10.5812/iji.107090

Nguyen, D. 2020. Traditional Medicine and Quest for Covid-19 Cure. *Yale Global Online*, April 28. https://yaleglobal.yale.edu/content/traditional-medicine-and-quest-covid-19-cure (accessed February 10, 2021).

Partington, G. 2020. Infodemic. *Polyphony*, April 29. https://thepolyphony.org/2020/04/29/infodemic/?utm_source=rss&utm_medium=rss&utm_campaign=infodemic (accessed May 20, 2020).

Pazzanese, Ch. 2020. Battling the "Pandemic of Misinformation." *The Harvard Gazette*, May 8. https://news.harvard.edu/gazette/story/2020/05/social-media-used-to-spread-create-covid-19-falsehoods/ (accessed August 23, 2020).

Polish Agency for Medical Research. 2021. We'll Know the Results of the Amantadine Study in a Few Weeks. https://abm.gov.pl/en/news/58,We039ll-know-the-results-of-the-amantadine-study-in-a-few-weeks.html (accessed April 14, 2021).

Rajalakshmi, S., Samraj, K., Sathiyarajeswaran, P., and Kanagavalli, K. 2020. Preparedness of Siddha System of Medicine in Practitioner Perspective during a Pandemic Outbreak with Special Reference to COVID-19. *CellMed* 10(4): 29.1–29.6. doi: 10.5667/CellMed.2020.0029

Rajtar, M. 2020. The Pre-existing Vulnerabilities of Patients with Rare Disorders in Poland during a Global Pandemic. *Boasblog. Witnessing Corona*, 5.06. https://boasblogs.org/witnessingcorona/the-pre-existing-vulnerabilities-of-patients-with-rare-disorders/ (accessed June 9, 2020).

Tidwell, T. 2020. Covid-19 and Tibetan Medicine: An Awakening Tradition in a New Era of Global Health Crisis. Hot Spots, *Fieldsights*, June 23. https://culanth.org/fieldsights/covid-19-and-tibetan-medicine-an-awakening-tradition-in-a-new-era-of-global-health-crisis (accessed June 30, 2020).

Whyte, S.R., Van der Geest, S., and Hardon, A. 2006. *Social Lives of Medicines*. Cambridge: Cambridge University Press.

World Health Organization (WHO). 2013. *WHO Traditional Medicine Strategy 2014–2023*. Geneva: WHO.

World Health Organization (WHO). 2019. *WHO Global Report on Traditional and Complementary Medicine*, Geneva: WHO.

World Health Organization (WHO). 2020a. Coronavirus Disease (COVID-19) Advice for the Public: Mythbusters. www.who.int/emergencies/diseases/novel-coronavirus-2019/advice-for-public/myth-busters (accessed May 28, 2020).

World Health Organization (WHO). 2020b. Infodemic Management. www.who.int/teams/risk-communication/infodemic-management (accessed March 20, 2021).

World Health Organization (WHO). 2020c. WHO Discontinues Hydroxychloroquine and Lopinavir/Ritonavir Treatment Arms for COVID-19, 4 July. www.who.int/news/item/04-07-2020-who-discontinues-hydroxychloroquine-and-lopinavir-ritonavir-treatment-arms-for-covid-19 (accessed July 5, 2020).

World Health Organization (WHO). 2020d. *Therapeutics and COVID-19: WHO Living Guideline*, 17 December. https://apps.who.int/iris/handle/10665/337876 (accessed February 12, 2021).

World Health Organization (WHO). 2021. *WHO Living Guideline: Drugs to Prevent COVID-19*, 2 March. https://apps.who.int/iris/handle/10665/339877 (accessed April 12, 2021).

Wu, K.J., Zimmer, C., and Corum, J. 2021. Coronavirus Drug and Treatment Tracker. *New York Times*, March 22. www.nytimes.com/interactive/2020/science/coronavirus-drugs-treatments.html (accessed April 9, 2021).

Xin, S., and Hsu, E. 2020. Translation of Beijing's Recommendations for Traditional Chinese Medicine (TCM) Treatment of Covid-19. Hot Spots, *Fieldsights*, June 23. https://culanth.org/fieldsights/translation-of-beijings-recomendations (accessed June 30, 2020).

Yang, Y., Islam, M.S., Wang, J., Li Y., and Chen, X. 2020. Traditional Chinese Medicine in the Treatment of Patients Infected with 2019-New Coronavirus (SARS-CoV-2): A Review and Perspective. *International Journal of Biological Sciences* 16(10): 1708–1717. doi:10.7150/ijbs.45538

Zdziebłowski, S. 2021. Brakuje osób do badań nad amantadyną. *Medonet*, May 22. www.medonet.pl/koronawirus/koronawirus-w-polsce,badania-nad-amantadyna-brakuje-chetnych-do-badan,artykul,00945944.html (accessed May 25, 2021).

11 How Do Small-to-Medium Enterprises (SMEs) Negotiate the COVID-19 Pandemic in Indonesia?

Santirianingrum Soebandhi, Kristiningsih, and Ira Darmawanti

Introduction: The Impacts of COVID-19 on Indonesian SMEs

In Indonesia and around the world, the COVID-19 pandemic has affected all areas of business—not only large companies, but also small and medium enterprises (SMEs). Indonesian SMEs have experienced their third crisis in the last 25 years. The first and second crises in Indonesia were caused by the global economic crises of 1998 and 2008 (Sahir et al. 2020). At that time, SMEs were still able to survive, and even become pillars of economic growth, whereas in the third crisis, which was caused by the COVID-19 pandemic, SMEs in most countries, including Indonesia, have been significantly and negatively affected (Mulyaman 2020; Sahir et al. 2020). Based on the existing data, the Indonesian Ministry of Cooperatives and SMEs noted that 43% of SMEs stopped operating due to this pandemic and its resultant changes in social and shopping behaviors (Fajar 2020). A survey conducted by Katadata (2020), a media and research company related to the Indonesian economy and businesses, showed that in June 2020, more than 200 SME entrepreneurs in Jakarta, Bogor, Tangerang and Bekasi (*Jabodetabek*), constituting 82.9% of Indonesian SMEs, had experienced negative impacts; 63.9% had more than a 30% turnover decrease. However, this survey also found that a small minority of SMEs experienced an increase in product turnover (ibid.).

Several SMEs, especially those in tourism, food and beverage, accommodation, sports sectors, and other sectors such as cellular phones, health logistics, and laundry, have been greatly and often positively affected by this pandemic. For example, a business such as a cellular phone shop or stall that provides top-up *pulsa* (phone credit) on a prepaid SIM card can gain opportunities, since most activities—such as school attendance, office meetings, shopping, and reciting the Qur'an in a group or mosque service—are now conducted online. This pandemic has forced people to change their habits and behaviors. Previously, Indonesians went to stores to shop for

DOI: 10.4324/9781003187462-14

their daily needs; now they are much more likely to buy online. Given these drastic changes in consumer behaviors, this study aims to understand how COVID-19 has affected SMEs in Indonesia and how they are negotiating this pandemic. Taken together, the results provide important insights into strategies that can be used by SMEs to make it through this pandemic and perhaps others to come. We conclude this article with a summation of these strategies and with practical suggestions for their implementation.

Methods and Materials

For this study, we employed a qualitative research method with a phenomenological approach (Creswell and Creswell 2018) that facilitated our explorations and descriptions of the conditions faced by SME entrepreneurs during the pandemic. We used purposive sampling (Fura and Negash 2020), which helped us to obtain relevant information from experienced and information-rich SME entrepreneurs. The criteria to participate in this study were that the SMEs had been established for at least three years and are domiciled in Indonesia, especially in the big city areas most affected by the COVID-19 pandemic. We conducted this research in December 2020 and between March and April, 2021. We applied primary and secondary data for the purposes of our study. We derived our primary data from the 20 in-depth interviews we conducted with SME owners or managers. Our interview questions dealt with how their business conditions were affected during the COVID-19 pandemic. Some of these interviews were conducted in person and, due to the pandemic, others were conducted by phone or online, according to interlocutor preference. We conducted our interviews in the Indonesian language, which was understood by all study participants. We then manually transcribed and coded all interviews. The questions asked included information about: company characteristics and location; the conditions they experienced as a result of the pandemic; the difficulties they encountered; how they dealt with these difficulties; the adaptions they had made; any new business strategies they had implemented or planned to implement; and their expectations for the future. We obtained secondary data from previous studies by others, news from the media, and information from official government agencies.

COVID-19 in Indonesia: A Situational Analysis

The first case of COVID-19 in Indonesia was reported on March 2, 2020 (Nuraini 2020). As of April 6, 2021, Indonesia had reported 1,542,516 positive cases; of these, 1,385,973 had recovered, and 41,977 had died (KPCPEN 2021a). To prevent further transmission, the Indonesian Government issued a regulation to limit public interaction by implementing large-scale social restrictions (*Pembatasan Sosial Berskala Besar*, or PSBB) in some regions (Cabinet Secretary of the Republic of Indonesia 2020). The implementation of PSBB differed among regions, depending on their situation (Hakim 2020). Many Indonesians rejected these preventive measures—some because of their need to make a living; others because they wished to continue their education, their religious activities, and/or their social activities; and because the government provided no assistance to individuals of any kind (Purnamasari 2020).

The Indonesian Government conducted massive COVID testing on traditional market traders, because the traditional market is a place where multiple physically close interactions take place. Yet the rapid and/or swab test was not easily accepted. Dozens of the sellers in Cileungsi Market (Bogor), Abian Timbul Market (Bali), Kahayan Market (Palangkaraya), and Pinasungkulan Market (Manado) were reported to be resisting the tests because they did not want to know the results. Testing positive would mean that they had to be hospitalized or in self-isolation, which meant that they could not sell in the markets to earn their daily livelihoods (Wiyanto 2020; Berutu 2020; Kompas 2020; Sata 2020).

As Ali (2021) argues, there are many COVID-19 pandemics (see Introduction); these include an economic pandemic, as COVID-19 has critically affected the economic system worldwide. Similarly, the pandemic in Indonesia has not only significantly impacted the health sector, but also the economic sector. The SME entrepreneurs we interviewed experienced a significant decrease in purchases, which negatively affected their business sustainability. A survey conducted by the LIPI (*Lembaga Ilmu Pengetahuan Indonesia*) Economic Research Center May 1–20, 2020 on the performance of Indonesian SMEs showed that 94.69% of these businesses experienced a decline in sales (Nugroho 2020). Meanwhile, a survey conducted by the Mandiri Institute in August 2020 showed that 66% of SMEs were still operating on a limited basis; 28% were operating normally; and 6% had stopped operating (Trimahanani 2020). Without a backup plan for the SMEs' economic crisis, it began to endanger the national economy (Handoko 2020).

One of the efforts to increase public and business optimism for economic recovery is now the COVID-19 vaccination program, which is expected to boost economic growth (KPCPEN 2021c). The first phase of COVID-19 vaccination started on January 13, 2021; the President of the Republic of Indonesia, Joko Widodo, was the first person to receive the shot, as a symbolic statement that all Indonesians should be vaccinated (KPCPEN 2021e). This first stage targeted health workers and showed satisfactory results (KPCPEN 2021b). The second phase of COVID-19 vaccination ran from the third week of February to May 2021; its vaccination targets were Public Service Officers, including market traders, teachers, public transportation officers, and elderly community groups (60 years and over) (ibid.). The SME entrepreneurs, especially in the retail and tourism sectors, have also been prioritized for receiving the COVID-19 vaccine (KPCPEN

2021d). As of June 2021, around 12 million Indonesians had been fully vaccinated, and another 18 million had received their first dose, out of a population of around 270 million. Although the government has carried out a massive vaccine promotion campaign, many Indonesians still reject the vaccination due to fears around vaccine safety and side effects, doubts about vaccine efficacy, and feelings of distrust in vaccines in general. In addition, rumors and hoaxes about the "illegality" of vaccines and their contradictions of certain religious principles also contribute to this mistrust (Fisipol 2021). For example, one such rumor holds that the vaccine contains ingredients that are *Haram* (forbidden) for Muslims.

SMEs in Indonesia: Obstacles to Sustainability

The COVID-19 crisis has had a devastating effect on the global economy (Eggers 2020). SMEs as drivers of a country's economy are the most vulnerable sectors compared to other businesses because of their limited resources (Winarsih, Indriastuti, and Fuad 2020; Saturwa, Suharno, and Ahmad 2021). SMEs in Indonesia have faced the same conditions as in other countries during this pandemic. In this section, we present the results of several studies on how COVID-19 has affected Indonesia SMEs' sustainability and how they can overcome this crisis.

Lutfi and colleagues (2020) examined the impacts of physical distancing policies on SMEs. The results indicate that these policies have resulted in decreased product demand and income, and some even had no income at all. SMEs have also experienced an increase in raw material and production costs due to supply chain problems. This study also revealed that one of the most important strategies that SMEs needed to implement was the utilization of information technology. It further showed that government economic stimulus policies could help SMEs to survive.

Research conducted by Tairas (2020) found that SMEs engaged in food and beverage services and other business that rely on people's mobility and activities have been the most impacted. This study involved 34 SMEs representing 34 Indonesian provinces. The results show that there are five primary obstacles faced by SMEs during the pandemic: (1) funding or financial access to loans to survive the crisis; (2) the availability of raw materials, as these can affect product quality; (3) labor as the main input in the production process, since most Indonesian SMEs still utilize manual production techniques; (4) obstacles in marketing efforts due to restrictions on physical mobility during the pandemic; and (5) designing attractive packaging. This research suggests three ways to overcome the impact of the COVID-19 pandemic on SMEs: first, by providing education about sustainable business to help SMEs keep up with the economic challenges; second, training in creative economic strategies and products to help them to compete with other countries; and third, assistance in marketing, both for the domestic and overseas markets. A study by Winarsih, Indriastuti, and Fuad (2020) proposed a sustainability framework for SMEs in facing the pandemic. According to this study, the restrictions on outdoor activities cause SMEs to need to change their business strategies, in particular via digital transformation.

Muditomo and Wahyudi's (2020) research revealed that the policies imposed during the COVID-19 pandemic are a momentum for SMEs to accelerate digital transformation. This research developed a reasonable digital transformation model by mapping Indonesian SMEs' digital transformations. This study concluded that the main triggers for SMEs to adopt digital transformation are external factors, meaning that they tend to only follow digital strategies implemented by other SMEs. In so doing, they fail to show their own uniqueness and might lose their competitive advantage. Although many Indonesian SMEs have implemented digital transformations, most have not set an instrument to measure their digital transformation achievements. And they only apply partial digitization of their business functions, especially in their sales functions.

Hidayati and Rachman (2021) conducted a literature review on government policies and business strategies for SMEs in Indonesia in the midst of the COVID-19 pandemic. The results indicate that the Indonesian government has responded to the crisis faced by SMEs with several strategic approaches, which include:

1. Social support such as food packages, reduced electricity rates, and cash assistance;
2. Tax incentives for SMEs with an annual turnover of below IDR (Indonesian Rupiah) 4.8 billion (approximately $330,742 US);
3. Credit relaxation and restructuring, which include postponement of installment payments and interest subsidies for credit and capital assistance recipients;
4. Working capital stimulus;
5. Cooperation with state-owned enterprises to facilitate SMEs to continue operations;
6. Creating innovative products in order to increase online sales;
7. Maintaining good relations with suppliers and distributors;
8. Strengthening collaborations with partners;
9. Utilizing technology and e-commerce in marketing and distribution; and
10. Developing the flexibility to quickly respond to changing environments.

Research Findings: The Conditions of SMEs during the COVID-19 Pandemic

We interviewed entrepreneurs in the fields of food and beverage, construction, beauty salon/skincare, barbershop, souvenir/gift shop, and garments, as they represent the goods and services industry. Table 11.1 is a summary of the data we obtained from our interviews with SME entrepreneurs.

Table 11.1 Summary of Interviews on the Conditions of SMEs during the COVID-19 Pandemic

Business Field	General Condition	
Food and Beverage	Food business has experienced losses due to restrictions on the number of visitors and opening hours, excepting those that offer online delivery.	Because online sales have increased, the shipping costs have increased as well.
Barbershop	Both the number of customers and sales had initially decreased, but after 3 months, the customers started to return.	The income is low but there was no change in the monthly operational expenses or in employee salaries.
Construction	There was a drastic decrease in construction projects, especially because many middle-class people postponed these to wait for better conditions. However, small projects such as private renovations or residential home constructions were ongoing.	The news about the COVID-19 pandemic reported in the media contributed to the downturn in the construction service business.
Beauty salon/ skincare	There was a large decrease in sales and visits. Consumers rarely came to beauty salon and skincare services for treatment.	Consumers visit the beauty salon/skincare services only as needed, and many stopped going to them out of fear of contagion.
Garment	There has been a large decrease in the number of orders.	People tend to prioritize the need for food, so garment product sales decline.
Souvenirs/Gift shop	There was a large decline in sales due to the prohibitions on birthday parties, weddings, and office events.	The absence of orders from parties and celebrations.

Our interviews show that SMEs in both the goods and services industries faced a decline. As a result of the government-imposed restrictions described above, most Indonesians have tended to limit their outdoor activities (Cabinet Secretary of the Republic of Indonesia 2020). Therefore, SMEs that want to survive this crisis have had to understand and adapt to the changing habits of society and discover or generate new possible business opportunities.

Business Adaptations

"Adaptation" can be defined for our purposes here as an action taken by entrepreneurs and their teams in responding to environmental changes and making necessary adjustments (McKee, Varadarajan, and Pride 1989). The

Table 11.2 Summary of the Interview Results about SMEs' Business Adaptations

Business Field	Adaptation
Food and Beverage	Generating online sales/orders and delivery services to consumers. Digitizing food ordering and delivery.
Barbershop	Doing offline and online promotion, digitizing promotion services, implementing health protocols such as cleaning and sanitizing for services, providing in-home service.
Construction	Expanding the projects to fight against the pandemic, such as building disinfectant booths and providing medical equipment. Expanding renovating housing projects in suburban areas where COVID outbreaks have been minimal.
Beauty salon/ Skincare	Selling the beauty products through online marketing, implementing strict health protocols for customers coming to the salon or clinic.
Garment	Selling pandemic necessities such as masks that are designed using beautiful fabrics.
Souvenirs/Gift shop	Giving discounts for those who buy in bulk, combining the primary products with the additional products needed in the pandemic (e.g. hand sanitizer, masks, etc.).

table above shows a summary of the interview results with SMEs on how they have adapted to the pandemic situation.

As Table 11.2 shows, the SMEs in our study made adaptations by accomplishing digital transformations in their product sales and promotion strategies. They also shifted to projects or products demanded by the pandemic. SMEs in the service sectors implemented strict health protocols for customer service; these work not only to prevent viral spread, but also to generate confidence among their customers.

Business Opportunities

Besides the ability to adapt, SMEs also have had to become innovative and thorough in identifying possible new business opportunities. Based on our data and literature review, here we provide examples of some business opportunities that can or have been achieved by Indonesian SMEs:

*   Indonesia has a wealth of extraordinary spices and traditional drinks that can boost the body's immune system. Having good immunity is believed to be one of the ways to prevent coronavirus infection (UNMUL 2020). Many food and beverage SMEs added new variants to their products, especially herbs or bottled immune booster drinks, or sell spice mixes called *empon-empon*, which can boost the body's immune system.
*   Given that more people are working from home and it is not possible for them to go a coffee shop or café, SMEs can adjust by making coffee by the liter to drink at home.

- Masks are not only necessities during the pandemic; they can also be part of fashion and thus can serve as expressions of individual styles in the way that clothing does. Within Indonesia's rich and varied cultures, each region has its own characteristics. SMEs in the garment sector have innovatively produced masks using fabric motifs from various Indonesian regions, such *batik* and *tenun* (a woven fabric). They also design company masks that include the company logo or name.
- The garment industry can and is taking advantage of the online work and school from home policies by producing more fashionable home-dresses called *daster*. Daster is not a different type of mask; it is an informal home-dress or day dress made of comfortable thin fabric that is common for women to wear at home.

Indonesian SMEs' Expectations and Efforts to Meet Them

SMEs in Indonesia are major contributors to the economy and to individuals' needs (Saturwa, Suharno, and Ahmad 2021; Hidayati and Rachman 2021). They also contribute to creating more job opportunities. Yet, as previously noted, these SMEs have been greatly affected by the coronavirus pandemic, which resulted in a significant decline in sales for most. Thus, SMEs have needed support to stay afloat. Such support must (and has—see below) come from local and national governments, and from entrepreneurial associations in the particular SME's industry. SME entrepreneurs expect support in the forms of networking, promotion, and ease in financial bank transactions and loans.

Table 11.3 contains a summary of the results based on our data about what kind of support SME entrepreneurs have expected during the COVID-19 pandemic.

Table 11.3 Summary of the Interview Results Regarding SMEs' Expectations

Expectation	
For government	Providing training, financial assistance, ease of licensing, reducing taxes, supporting SMEs to open business opportunities to improve skills, affirming the health protocols, and helping the small business economy.
For SME entrepreneur associations	Assisting in integrated product promotion, increasing cooperation/mutual product purchase, and providing information about possible business opportunities.
For mass media	Preventing the dissemination of misleading information and frightening public broadcasts that worsen the situation.
For educational institutions	Providing proper training, such as in digital marketing, financial management, how to increase sales ratings, and online selling guidance.

In Table 11.3, it can be seen that our interlocutor SMEs expect support from the government, from associations related to their businesses, and from the media and educational institutions. This support can take the forms of trainings to improve skills, financial assistance, and clear guidelines from the government. SMEs also expect cooperation in terms of promotion and sales from other SME entrepreneurs. Meanwhile, the media is expected to convey accurate and balanced information that will not mislead the public.

Government and Private Types of Support

Responding to SMEs' expectations, from the initial months of the COVID-19 pandemic until the present (April 2021), governments, state-owned enterprises (*Badan Usaha Milik Negara*, or BUMN) and private companies in Indonesia have done many things to help keep the SMEs' businesses up and running. Those actions have included the following:

- The Ministry of Cooperatives and Small and Medium Enterprises, in collaboration with Food State-Owned Enterprises, has launched the *Belanja di Warung Tetangga* (Shopping in the Neighborhood) program. This program is a government effort to allow the traditional stalls to compete with modern retail. Thus, the traditional stalls (*warung*) can get easier access to competitive goods and connections to online platforms. In addition to strengthening the SME economy, especially that of the traditional stalls, this program also facilitates a sufficient supply of daily needs in the midst of the COVID-19 pandemic (Kementerian Koperasi dan UKM 2020).
- The Indonesian government also has a Productive Presidential Aid for Micro-Enterprises program for eligible SMEs. It was expected that this financial assistance would enable many SMEs to maintain their businesses (Wisnubroto 2020), and indeed, it has.
- Training, mentoring and business consultations are also provided by state-owned companies such as Pertamina, Bank Rakyat Indonesia, and others as a form of real support for SMEs amid challenging viral spread conditions (Pertamina 2020; Suheriadi 2020).
- Both public and private educational institution also take roles in supporting the sustainability of SMEs in the midst of the pandemic. Some activities are carried out in the form of assistance with financial reports, digital marketing, regional specialty product branding, etc. (Unair News 2020; UWKS 2020).
- Support systems from the private sector include #UnileverUntukIndonesia, which provides assistance and technology systems for the management of local minimarkets and traditional stalls (Unilever 2020); LocalsUnite from Tehbotol Sosro) to support Indonesian local brands in developing their businesses during COVID-19 (KumparanNews 2020); #TerusUsaha from Grab Indonesia, which has a program to upgrade skills and digitize

Indonesian SMEs (Grab 2020); and many other training and mentoring programs provided by the private sectors and the communities.

Discussion

The COVID-19 pandemic has affected SMEs in various sectors, not only in Indonesia but also globally (Tairas 2020; Parth 2020). The results of our study are in line with previous studies, which show that the COVID-19 pandemic and the implementation of social restriction policies to prevent its spread have impacted SMEs' revenue, cash flow, and profit (Tairas 2020: Parth 2020; Omar, Ishak, and Jusoh 2020). Moreover, declining household purchasing power due to massive layoffs has caused shifts in consumption patterns, some of which have resulted in decreased demand for particular SMEs' goods and services (Pakpahan 2020). Therefore, SMEs have needed to adjust their strategies in order to survive, recover, and even thrive during the pandemic (Winarsih, Indriastuti, and Fuad 2020). Our results have also shown that SMEs engaged in food, garment, and barbershop businesses can adjust their strategies through online sales or conduct their businesses with strict health protocols. However, SMEs in the construction sector have experienced difficulty in running their businesses, since their work requires physical presence at their work sites.

The coronavirus pandemic has accelerated the adoption of technology and e-commerce among SME entrepreneurs (Hidayati and Rachman 2021; Muditomo and Wahyudi 2020). The use of digital technology has increased the productivity of many SMEs during this pandemic (Papadopoulos, Baltas, and Balta 2020; Winarsih, Indriastuti, and Fuad 2020). The directive to keep physical distance and avoid crowds can be overcome by utilizing online transportation applications to deliver products (Lutfi et al. 2020) or by using e-commerce sites to boost sales (Winarsih, Indriastuti, and Fuad 2020). The conditions of the SMEs in our study are similar to those in other countries. SMEs worldwide are expected to adopt technologies and use e-commerce sites as a business strategy to survive. For example, research by Gray (2020) in Canada shows that food delivery services have increased during the implementation of social distancing policies. Other research has shown that the use of e-commerce sites in countries such as the United States, the United Kingdom, and the People's Republic of China has also increased significantly (OECD 2020).

Our study indicates that collaboration between the government, community, state-owned enterprises, and the private sector has been carried out to support SMEs in running their businesses. This collaboration is in line with the Indonesian government's policy of helping SMEs to overcome the pandemic (Kementerian PPN/Bapennas RI 2020; Hidayati and Rachman 2021). Such collaborations have also been activated in many other countries to aid in the pandemic sustainability of SMEs (United Nations Conference on Trade and Development 2020).

SMEs and the New Life Order

The challenges faced by SMEs during the COVID-19 pandemic are serious. The Indonesian government regulations on limiting people's activities to prevent viral spread severely impacted the sales of SMEs' products/services, as did media reports on COVID-19. The decline in various SME sectors required rapid remediation to ensure that these SMEs remain relevant to the new life order.

As we have shown, while many SMEs failed to adapt to pandemic conditions and therefore went out of business, others have generated creative and innovative adaptations, which we have detailed herein and which mostly involve digital and online activities. The entrepreneurs who keep running their businesses offline, such as barbershops and nail and hair salons, have developed and are developing effective marketing strategies such as in-home services while adhering to health protocols.

SMEs have expected to receive support from the government and from their professional organizations, and have indeed received many forms of support. This support has taken the forms of financial aid or business tools and training (especially relating to online sales). The communities served by particular SMEs can also serve as forums for sharing knowledge, increasing inter-business cooperation, and as a means of product promotion. The mass vaccination programs have resulted in optimism among SME entrepreneurs that soon they will be able to run their businesses under normal conditions. Yet it seems highly likely that many of the online strategies developed by SMEs to survive under pandemic conditions will be continued even after COVID-19 is no longer a threat. The lessons learned that we have provided in this chapter can serve to help Indonesian SMEs, and perhaps those in other countries, during this pandemic and any pandemics yet to come. Thus, in conclusion, we here provide a summary of those lessons.

Conclusion: Practical Suggestions

The following are some actions that SMEs can take to keep their businesses relevant to Covidian conditions and that can also work in post-Covidian times:

- Government regulations about restrictions on the number of restaurant visitors and opening hours can certainly reduce sales. To overcome this problem, culinary businesses can sell food in vacuum packaging (frozen food) that can be stored for a certain period. They can also collaborate with online applications such as GoFood or GrabFood to avoid dine-in activities.
- SMEs can also execute digital transformations by selling online and using digital payment methods to reduce physical contact.

- The social activity restriction on weddings, gatherings, and meetings have a large impact on the catering business. As a solution, such enterprises can offer a daily menu that can be selected individually. They can also offer boxed foods with a certain minimum order that can be consumed in offices and homes.

- For the souvenir/gift shop business, along with giving discounts, they can also combine their main products with products that are currently needed during the pandemic, such as masks, hand sanitizers, and disinfectants to attract more consumers.

- Businesses for which online adaptations are impossible, such as beauty salons and barbershops, can provide home treatment services with strict health protocols. Yet they can use online websites to promote such services.

- SMEs are required to apply health protocols, such as providing plastic barriers between the sellers and the buyers, using mask and face shields, and providing hand washing facilities and hand sanitizers. Taking these measures helps to increase public confidence in SMEs.

- Since one survey conducted by WeAreSocial (2021) reveals that YouTube is in the first rank of the most visited social media platforms in Indonesia, followed by WhatsApp, Instagram, Facebook, and Twitter, SMEs can use these social media platforms to sell their products. They can also use e-commerce platforms such as Shopee, Tokopedia, or Bukalapak. It is important to note that the SMEs need to pay significant attention to which platforms are most visited by consumers in order to be more effective and strategic in marketing their products.

- SMEs should implement a means of measuring and monitoring their digital transformation achievements, so that they can know the results of these online efforts.

- SMEs also need to pay attention to the potential number of people that marketers can reach via digital advertising. The potential number of people who can be reached using ads on Facebook are around 140 million, 107 million on YouTube, 85 million on Instagram, and 14.05 million on Twitter (WeAreSocial 2021). The cost for paid advertisements depends on the digital advertising scheme chosen and the size of the target audience (Hidayat 2021). In terms of e-commerce platforms, Shopee, Tokopedia, Bukalapak, and Lazada Indonesia are the top four most clicked on e-commerce sites in the country (Statista 2021). Regarding Internet use, the average Indonesian spends 9 hours a day on the Internet and uses 3 hours a day for social media (WeAreSocial 2021). This data is from a report in the second quarter of January 2021, one year after the COVID 19 outbreak began (ibid). It is quite possible that Internet use is higher due to more activities done at home. These phenomena represent strong potential for SMEs to grow their businesses.

References

Ali, I. 2021. Rituals of containment: Many pandemics, body politics, and social dramas during COVID-19 in Pakistan. *Frontiers in Sociology* 6(83). https://doi.org/10.3389/fsoc.2021.648149.

Berutu, S.A. 2020. Pedagang Pasar Cileungsi Tolak Tes Masif, Bupati Bogor: Ada Miskomunikasi. Accessed April 7, 2021. https://news.detik.com/berita/d-5050267/pedagang-pasar-cileungsi-tolak-tes-masif-bupati-bogor-ada-miskomunikasi.

Cabinet Secretary of the Republic of Indonesia. 2020. Health Minister Signs Regulation on Guidelines to Propose Large-scale Social Restrictions amid COVID-19 Pandemic. Accessed August 1, 2020. https://setkab.go.id/en/health-minister-signs-regulation-on-guidelines-to-propose-large-scale-social-restrictions-amid-covid-19-pandemic/.

Creswell, J.W., and J.D. Creswell. 2018. *Research Design: Qualitative, Quantitative, and Mixed Methods Approaches.* 5th ed. Thousand Oaks, CA: SAGE Publications.

Eggers, F. 2020. Masters of disasters? Challenges and opportunities for SMEs in times of crisis. *Journal of Business Research* 116: 199–208. https://doi.org/10.1016/j.jbusres.2020.05.025.

Fajar, T. 2020. 43% UMKM Tutup Akibat Covid-19. okezone. Accessed August 8, 2020. https://economy.okezone.com/read/2020/05/19/320/2216489/43-umkm-tutup-akibat-covid-19.

Fisipol. 2021. Beragam Survei Sebut Penolakan dan Keraguan Masyarakat Terhadap Vaksin COVID-19. Accessed April 7, 2021. https://fisipol.ugm.ac.id/beragam-survei-sebut-penolakan-dan-keraguan-masyarakat-terhadap-vaksin-covid-19/.

Fura, D.L., and S. Desalegn Negash. 2020. A study on the living experiences of people during the COVID-19 pandemic: The case of Wolisso Town home-stayed university students. *Journal of Psychology & Psychotherapy* 10(5): 384.

Grab. 2020. Ajak Jutaan UMKM Tingkatkan Keterampilan Digital, Grab Buka Kelas #TerusUsaha Mulai Hari Ini! Accessed December 5, 2020. www.grab.com/id/en/press/social-impact-safety/kelas-terususaha-umkm/#:~:text=dan%20naik%20kelas.-,Kelas%20%23TerusUsaha%20merupakan%20program%20pelatihan%20gratis%20bagi%20UMKM%20Indonesia%20untuk,dan%20kanal%20digital%20Grab%20Indonesia.

Gray, R.S. 2020. Agriculture, transportation, and the COVID-19 crisis. *Canadian Journal of Agricultural Economics/Revue canadienne d'agroeconomie* 68(2): 239–243. https://doi.org/10.1111/cjag.12235.

Hakim, R.N. 2020. Jokowi: PSBB Tidak Seragam di Seluruh Indonesia. Accessed April 6, 2021. https://nasional.kompas.com/read/2020/04/10/06010051/jokowi--psbb-tidak-seragam-di-seluruh-indonesia-.

Handoko, L.T. 2020. Membangkitkan UMKM di Masa Pandemi dengan Inovasi dan Teknologi. Accessed April 6, 2021. http://lipi.go.id/siaranpress/membangkitkan-umkm-di-masa-pandemi-dengan-inovasi-dan-teknologi/22212.

Hidayat, F. 2021. Bisnis Digital Advertising di Indonesia Menjanjikan. Accessed April 10, 2021. www.beritasatu.com/digital/729729/bisnis-digital-advertising-di-indonesia-menjanjikan.

Hidayati, R., and N. Megawati Rachman. 2021. Indonesian government policy and SMEs business strategy during the Covid-19 pandemic. *NIAGAWAN* 1(1): 1–9. https://doi.org/10.24114/niaga.v10i1.21813.

Katadata. 2020. Digitalisasi UMKM di Tengah Pandemi Covid-19. Accessed August 8, 2020. https://katadata.co.id/umkm.

Kementerian Koperasi dan UKM. 2020. Program "Belanja Di Warung Tetangga," Toko Tradisional Mampu Bersaing Dengan Retail Modern. Accessed November 27, 2020. www.depkop.go.id/read/program-belanja-di-warung-tetangga-toko-tradisional-mampu-bersaing-dengan-retail-modern.

Kementerian PPN/Bapennas RI. 2020. *Kajian Kebijakan Penanggulangan Dampak COVID-19 terhadap UMKM: Survei Kebutuhan Pemulihan Usaha Bagi UMKM Indonesia.* https://aptika.kominfo.go.id/wp-content/uploads/2020/12/BAPPENAS-Penanggulangan-Dampak-Covid-19-terhadap-UMKM-Final-v1_0.pdf.

Kompas. 2020. Tolak Rapid Test Massal, Pedagang Pasar Pinasungkulan Manado Rusak Pos Kesehatan. Accessed April 7, 2021. https://regional.kompas.com/read/2020/06/22/21233151/tolak-rapid-test-massal-pedagang-pasar-pinasungkulan-manado-rusak-pos.

KPCPEN. 2021a. Data Sebaran. Accessed April 6, 2021. https://covid19.go.id/.

KPCPEN. 2021b. Inilah Kelompok Masyarakat Sasaran Prioritas Vaksinasi COVID-19 Tahap Kedua. Accessed April 7, 2021. https://covid19.go.id/edukasi/masyarakat-umum/inilah-kelompok-masyarakat-sasaran-prioritas-vaksinasi-covid-19-tahap-kedua.

KPCPEN. 2021c. Kesuksesan Program Vaksinasi Akan Dorong Pemulihan Ekonomi. Accessed April 6, 2021. https://covid19.go.id/berita/kesuksesan-program-vaksinasi-akan-dorong-pemulihan-ekonomi.

KPCPEN. 2021d. Pelaku UMKM Dukung Vaksinasi Tahap Kedua Demi Percepat Pemulihan Ekonomi. Accessed April 7, 2021. https://covid19.go.id/p/berita/pelaku-umkm-dukung-vaksinasi-tahap-kedua-demi-percepat-pemulihan-ekonomi.

KPCPEN. 2021e. Program Vaksinasi COVID-19 Resmi Dimulai. Accessed April 7, 2021. https://covid19.go.id/p/masyarakat-umum/program-vaksinasi-covid-19-resmi-dimulai.

KumparanNews. 2020. Lewat #LocalsUnite, Teh Botol Sosro Berdayakan Produk UMKM Indonesia. Accessed December 5, 2020. https://kumparan.com/kumparannews/lewat-localsunite-teh-botol-sosro-berdayakan-produk-umkm-indonesia-1uTkM8hRPGy/full.

Lutfi, M., P. Chintya, D. Buntuang, Y. Kornelius, Erdiyansyah, and B. Hasanuddin. 2020. The impact of social distancing policy on small and medium-sized enterprises (SMEs) in Indonesia. *Problems and Perspectives in Management* 18(3): 492–503. https://doi.org/10.21511/ppm.18(3).2020.40.

McKee, D.O., P. Rajan Varadarajan, and W.M. Pride. 1989. Strategic adaptability and firm performance: A market-contingent perspective. *Journal of Marketing* 53(3): 21–35.

Muditomo, A., and I. Wahyudi. 2020. Conceptual model for SME digital transformation during the Covid-19 pandemic time in Indonesia: R Digital Transformation Model. *BASKARA: Journal of Business and Entrepreneurship* 3(1): 13–24. https://doi.org/10.24853/baskara.3.1.13-24.

Mulyaman, D. 2020. Collaborative Link & Match for SMEs as Solutions of COVID19 Pandemic. Accessed October 2, 2020. https://indonesiadevelopmentforum.com/2020/ideas/15619-collaborative-link-match-for-smes-as-solutions-of-covid19-pandemic.

Nugroho, A.E. 2020. Survei Kinerja UMKM di Masa Pandemi COVID19. Accessed April 7, 2021. http://lipi.go.id/berita/survei-kinerja-umkm-di-masa-pandemi-covid19/22071.

Nuraini, R. 2020. Kasus Covid-19 Pertama, Masyarakat Jangan Panik. Accessed April 5, 2021. https://indonesia.go.id/narasi/indonesia-dalam-angka/ekonomi/kasus-covid-19-pertama-masyarakat-jangan-panik.

OECD. 2020. E-commerce in the time of COVID-19. Accessed April 10, 2021. www.oecd.org/coronavirus/policy-responses/e-commerce-in-the-time-of-covid-19-3a2b78e8/.

Omar, A.R. Che, S. Ishak, and M. Abdullah Jusoh. 2020. The impact of Covid-19 Movement Control Order on SMEs' businesses and survival strategies. *Geografia Malaysian Journal of Society and Space* 16(2): 139–150. https://doi.org/10.17576/geo-2020-1602-11

Pakpahan, A.K. 2020. COVID-19 dan Implikasi Bagi Usaha Mikro, Kecil, dan Menengah. *Jurnal Ilmiah Hubungan Internasional: Edisi Khusus* 20: 1–6. https://doi.org/10.26593/jihi.v0i0.3870.59-64.

Papadopoulos, T., K.N. Baltas, and M. Elisavet Balta. 2020. The use of digital technologies by small and medium enterprises during Covid-19: Implications for theory and practice. *International Journal of Information Management* 55: 102192. https://doi.org/10.1016/j.ijinfomgt.2020.102192.

Parth, K. 2020. The economic cost of COVID-19: A potential pandemic impact on Indian economy. *International Journal of Advanced Science and Technology* 29(6s): 2182–2192. http://sersc.org/journals/index.php/IJAST/article/view/10931.

Pertamina. 2020. Pertamina Bangkitkan UMKM di Tengah Pandemi. Accessed December 5, 2020. www.pertamina.com/id/news-room/csr-news/pertamina-bangkitkan-umkm-di-tengah-pandemi.

Purnamasari, D.M. 2020. Survei: Sebagian Besar Warga Menolak PSBB karena Sulit Cari Nafkah. Accessed April 7, 2021. https://nasional.kompas.com/read/2020/04/23/13541671/survei-sebagian-besar-warga-menolak-psbb-karena-sulit-cari-nafkah.

Sahir, S.H., S. Patimah, Salmiah, Safriadi, and R. Sari. 2020. Discovering the Resilience of SMEs and Their Influencing Factors: North Sumatera's Evidence on Covid19 Crisis. Accessed October 2, 2020. http://sinta.ristekbrin.go.id/covid/penelitian/detail/449.

Sata, A. 2020. Tolak Rapid Test, Pedagang Pasar Kahayan Palangkaraya Kabur Tinggalkan Lapak. Accessed April 7, 2021. https://regional.inews.id/berita/tolak-rapid-test-pedagang-pasar-kahayan-palangkaraya-kabur-tinggalkan-lapak.

Saturwa, H.N., Suharno, and A. Aziz Ahmad. 2021. The impact of Covid-19 pandemic on MSMEs. *Jurnal Ekonomi dan Bisnis* 24(1): 65–82.

Statista. 2021. Top 10 e-commerce sites in Indonesia as of 4th quarter 2020, by monthly traffic (in million clicks). Accessed March 3, 2021. www.statista.com/statistics/869700/indonesia-top-10-e-commerce-sites/.

Suheriadi. 2020. 4 Program BRI Bantu UMKM Terdampak COVID-19. Accessed November 5, 2020. https://infobanknews.com/topnews/4-program-bri-bantu-umkm-terdampak-covid-19/.

Tairas, D.R. 2020. COVID-19 pandemic and MSMEs: Impact and mitigation. *Jurnal Ekonomi Indonesia* 9(1): 67–80.

Trimahanani, E. 2020. Outlook UMKM 2021, Pandemi Covid-19 Dorong Percepatan UMKM Go Digital. Accessed April 7, 2921. www.beritadaerah.co.id/2020/12/29/umkm-2021-tekanan-covid-19-dorong-percepatan-umkm-go-digital/.

Unair News. 2020. KKN Sampit Dampingi Masyarakat Berbisnis di Tengah Pandemi. Accessed August 17, 2020. http://news.unair.ac.id/2020/07/21/kkn-sampit-dampingi-masyarakat-berbisnis-di-tengah-pandemi/.

Unilever. 2020. #UnileverUntukIndonesia. Accessed December 15, 2020. www. unilever.co.id/about/unileveruntukindonesia/

United Nations Conference on Trade and Development. 2020. *COVID-19 and e-Commerce Impact on Business and Policy Responses.* United Nations Conference on Trade and Development.

UNMUL. 2020. UNMUL Produksi Minuman Daya Tahan Tubuh. Accessed December 15, 2020. https://unmul.ac.id/post/unmul-produksi-minuman-daya-tahan-tubuh-1585390272.html.

UWKS. 2020. Pengabdian Kepada Masyarakat Fakultas Ekonomi dan Bisnis (FEB) di UMKM Anggota Koperasi INTAKO Tanggulangin, Sidoarjo. Accessed December 21, 2020. https://uwks.ac.id/artikel/202056122010169536/625/penmas-feb-di-umkm-koperasi-intako-tanggulangin-sidoarjo.

WeAreSocial. 2021. *Digital 2021: Indonesia.* https://datareportal.com/reports/digital-2021-indonesia.

Winarsih, M.I., and K. Fuad. 2020. Impact of Covid-19 on Digital Transformation and Sustainability in Small and Medium Enterprises (SMEs): A Conceptual Framework. *Complex, Intelligent and Software Intensive Systems: Proceedings of the 14th International Conference on Complex, Intelligent and Software Intensive Systems (CISIS-2020)* 194: 471–476. https://doi.org/10.1007/978-3-030-50454-0_48.

Wisnubroto, K. 2020. Cara Dapatkan Bantuan Pemerintah untuk UKM. Accessed December 20, 2020. https://indonesia.go.id/layanan/keuangan/ekonomi/cara-dapatkan-bantuan-pemerintah-untuk-ukm.

Wiyanto, A. 2020. Sengit, 16 Pedagang Pasar di Denpasar Menolak Tes Swab karena Takut Positif. Accessed April 7, 2021. https://bali.inews.id/berita/sengit-16-pedagang-pasar-di-denpasar-tetap-menolak-tes-swab-karena-takut-positif.

Part III

Culturally Constructing and Negotiating COVID-19 in South Asia

12 Sri Lankans' Negotiations Around COVID-19

Can a Culture Control a Viral Outbreak?

Tharaka Ananda and Inayat Ali

Introduction

Herein we ask, are there any cultural traits within a given cultural system that can facilitate resistance to sudden viral outbreaks such as the coronavirus pandemic? During this pandemic, which is still ongoing in Sri Lanka as we write (May 2021), countries with diverse cultural systems have taken various measures to fight against the outbreak. However, it has become evident that technologically advanced countries could not control the outbreak, while some lower-resource countries, such as Bhutan, Taiwan, Vietnam, Micronesia, Samoa, the Solomon Islands, and Vanuatu engaged in engaged in successful controlling processes (NECSI 2021). When these countries are observed, one can see that the diversity and historicity of their cultural systems appear to have included various traits that worked successfully in controlling the coronavirus pandemic. Sri Lanka is one such country. In this chapter, we investigate the influential resistance traits of Sri Lankan culture that helped its people to successfully control the viral outbreak and to normalize daily life, while most of the other countries of the world are still fighting against this outbreak, often in inefficient and highly contested ways, as shown in other chapters in this volume—with the exception of Chapter 13 on Bhutan, which, as previously noted, also successfully controlled the coronaviral outbreak.

Although Sri Lanka is a multicultural and multiethnic country, we will focus on Sinhalese Buddhist cultural practices, as they represent the majority. Specifically, we will address cultural traits such as Sinhalese traditional rituals and customs; Sri Lanka's predominantly Buddhist belief system (which we will explore in terms of its flexibility and "middle path" observance); traditional medicines; traditional foods and beverages; family kinship and marriage (respect and obedience to elders, an elders-based kinship system); the extended family system; personality and socialization processes; the economy; the political culture; self-sustainability (most Sri Lankans have not become addicted to overconsumption and are satisfied with what they have); societal collectivity, collective endurance, and integrity; collectively

DOI: 10.4324/9781003187462-16

shared knowledge; cultural history; strong mental stability (health and balance); and collective endurance in crisis situations such as the 30-year Civil War. All of these elements play their parts in the development of cultural traits that can act as resistance factors against viral outbreaks, including the coronavirus and any other pandemics or other disasters that humans may confront in the future. This chapter aims to identify these traits in Sinhalese Buddhist culture and to explain how they work for viral resistance and control, as well as to keep the population calm and steady in the face of adversity.

Methods and Materials

This is an ethnographic study in which mostly participant observation and interview methods were used for data collection. As Tharaka Anand lives in Sri Lanka, she has been a participant-observer of the COVID-19 situation of the country from the first wave (March 2020) to the third wave (May 2021). Thus in this chapter, we draw heavily on her own personal experiences and understandings. We conducted interviews with 20 interlocutors to gather data on people's perceptions of the COVID-19 pandemic and their use of cultural practices, rituals, traditional medicines, and other herbs as preventive measures against both COVID-19 and other viral infections. Our interlocutors—12 women and 8 men—were between the ages of 50 to 80. We purposively focused on people aged 50 and above to gather precious data on the cultural traits that belong to the older generations of Sri Lankan culture. The interviews were conducted during periods of relative normalcy when no isolations nor curfews were activated. These interviews took place in the form of normal conversations. These types of conversations that include the older generations of families are common, as they generally welcome the opportunity to describe their memories to the younger generations of the family whenever they are together. We also relied on Internet resources, but to a much more minimal extent. We obtained additional data in early 2021 regarding laypeople's perceptions of COVID-19 (Ananda, Nahallage, & Ali nd). Since we consider our interlocutors to be highly representative of other Sinhalese Sri Lankans, we will speak of Sinhalese people in general rather than always specifically referring to our interlocutors.

COVID-19: The Sri Lankan Context and Response

A case of "pneumonia" in a Chinese tourist from unknown reasons was first reported in Sri Lanka on January 27, 2020. The first known coronavirus infection in a local person was reported on March 11, 2020. To prevent viral spread, the government banned the traditional April celebrations of the Sinhalese and Hindu New Year. By May 2021, nearly 18 months later, the total number of confirmed COVID-19 cases reported in the country was 109,862, including 687 deaths (Coronavirus Disease 2019 (COVID-19) – Situation Report, 2021). Of those who died, 63% were men and 37% were women. 42% of the total of deceased persons were 61–75 years old. Over 12,000 infected people were hospitalized (ibid.). The first wave of the pandemic continued until September 2020; the second wave commenced in October 2020 as COVID-19 clusters were reported in different parts of the country. In April 2021, the government did allow the celebration of the Sinhala and Hindu New Year, urging people to simply celebrate with their families. Nevertheless, the third wave occurred after this celebration, as for the first time in Sri Lanka, the infected cases reported per day jumped to over 1000 on April 28, 2021—to be precise, 1111 cases were reported on that day. (Before the New Year date, an average of 250 cases of infection was reported daily.)

From then on, COVID-19 cases were being reported at over 1000 per day; and from April 28 until May 2, 2021, a total of 7486 new cases were reported and their number is still increasing at this time of writing (May 2021) (Epidemiology Unit 2021). The government named this sudden rise in cases the "Post Sinhala and Hindu New Year Cluster." Government schools, universities, and other educational institutions were closed again on April 27, 2021. By the first week of May 2021, the government had isolated 77 *Grama Niladhari* (Administrative) Divisions that belong to 13 districts of the country (*Ada Derana 24*, 2021). In addition, those with known viral exposure were quarantined in their own homes for two weeks under the surveillance of Public Health Inspectors (PHI), and most of those who were actually infected were asked to stay in their homes until they could be hospitalized if needed when recovered patients were discharged from the hospitals.

During the pandemic's first wave, the government enforced a strict strategy for case detection by identifying contacts, implementing quarantine measures, imposing travel restrictions, and isolating small villages where the virus had been rapidly spreading (Ananda, Nahallage, & Ali nd). The countrywide mobility restrictions were the government's main pandemic containment measures. However, by early May 2020, the government had allowed the partial re-opening of private and government offices and businesses. During the first wave, the government also introduced a relief fund called the "COVID-19 Healthcare and Social Security Fund," which granted around US$25 per low-income family during April and May 2020. Yet, during the second wave, the Sri Lankan government was reluctant to enforce another lockdown, considering the escalating economic crisis (ibid.) By January 2021, the government-initiated vaccination program as a main preventive measure seemed to be the only way to finally and ultimately stop viral spread. Thus, as previously noted, when the Sinhala and Hindu New Year approached again, the government did not implement strict measures but simply asked people not to gather or to hold large celebrations.

Seeking to avoid the third wave, the government declared a single day—April 12, 2021—as a special holiday for the Sinhala New Year auspicious rites and celebrations, which normally were prescheduled from April 13–16. For the New Year celebrations, people usually get together, and markets and other shopping centers of the country are crowded. As people had not been allowed to officially celebrate the Sinhala New Year in 2020, people celebrated 2021's New Year with their relatives and families. Social and government media broadcast regular programs encouraging people to travel to celebrate to those areas of the country where most urban people go to be with their extended families for the New Year seasonal celebrations. The government did state that it was still important to follow the COVID-19 preventive measures. But it seems that people were misled by the existence of the vaccination and got the message that there were no more COVID-19 risks in the country. Even the daily reported cases were not highlighted during the Sinhala New Year season. This may be due to the significant decrease in the country's economy in 2020: the government seemed to be focused on this holiday as the most celebrated and economically advantageous yearly event in the country, and on this event-generated increase in economic exchanges among the citizens of new goods and other materials for household chores and other needs.

Nevertheless, transmission rates in the country have remained low compared to those of other countries. The total population of Sri Lanka is 21.8 million. The cumulative cases per 1 million people were 5039, and COVID-19 deaths per million were 31. For comparison, in India, the cumulative cases per million were 12,290 and the deaths per million were 139. In Singapore, the cumulative cases per million were 10,421 and deaths were 5. In the Southeast Asian region, the cumulative cases per million were 9877 and deaths were 126 (Epidemiology Unit 2021). (See Table 12.1.)

These figures show that viral spread and infection in Sri Lanka have been relatively well-controlled. This control was further intensified with the commencement of the vaccination program in April 2021. By the end of May 2021, around 1 million (total 996,575) people had been vaccinated with the Covisheild, Sinopharm, or Sputnik V vaccines (ibid.).

Table 12.1 Cumulative COVID-19 Cases and Deaths per Million

Countries/region	Cumulative cases per 1 million	Deaths per million
Sri Lanka	5039	31
India	12,290	139
Singapore	10,421	5
Southeast Asian Region	9877	126

The Cultural Background of the Country

Sri Lanka, located on an island near India, is a multi-ethnic, multi-religious country with a majority Sinhalese Buddhist ethnic population (75%). Among around 10 of the other ethnic groups that reside in the country, 11% are Sri Lankan Tamils and 9.2% are Sri Lankan Muslims; these are the second and third most prominent ethnic groups (Department of Census and Statistics 2012; Sri Lanka Demographics Profile 2019). Even though the Vedda people of the country represent only 0.05% of the country's population, they are considered to be one of its unique Indigenous groups with a specific cultural identity (Silva & Punchihewa 2011; Department of Census and Statistics 2012; Ananda 2019).

Buddhism has primarily shaped the belief system of the Sinhalese people. The Sinhalese Buddhist population observes and follows Buddhism as a philosophy and as a path shown by Lord Buddha around 2500 BCE. During the rule of King Devanampiyathisa in the *Anuradhapura* period (3rd century BCE), Buddhism had been introduced to Sri Lanka from India. From then onwards, the Sinhalese embraced Buddhism and considered it as their main religion; it became the specific basis of the entire Sinhalese cultural system. To be more precise, Buddhism is more of a philosophy than a religion, in which the main teachings include specific practices such as non-violence, relinquishment of worldly attachments, and the "middle path," so-called because it involves avoiding the extremes of self-indulgence and of total self-denial. The Buddha also taught the Eightfold Path: right view, right intention, right speech, right livelihood, right effort, right mindfulness, and right concentration. These teachings of the Buddha mainly shape Sinhalese behavioral and thinking patterns; thus they are traditionally a non-violent and self-sustaining group.

In addition, Hindu deities and regional deities (there are specific deities worshipped by people in specific regions, who are considered to be the guardians of these regions) are also given a considerable place in their belief system. *Yakshas* (demons) also have their special space, which has been passed down from the pre-Buddhist era.

The Sri Lankan economy is mainly based on the cultivation of the staple food, rice—in its traditional varieties. At present, most commonly red rice (*Rathu Kekulu*)[1] is cultivated and is grown in extensive paddy fields, while vegetables, greens, grains, and cereals are cultivated in rain-fed lands called *Chenas*. Rice (wet cultivation) is grown in two main seasons targeting monsoon rains. During the dry season, these rural agriculturalists shift to dry—or slash-and-burn—Chena cultivation by clearing an untouched forest area, setting it on fire, and cultivating it immediately after. As the area has not been tilled previously, the soil is very fertile and brings in a high crop yield. However, farmers refrain from cultivating too many of this type of chena, as it leads to a reduction in forest cover. Thus, such areas are abandoned after being tilled for two or three seasons to allow the forest to regenerate

(Ananda & Nahallage 2014). These patterns ensure a sufficient supply of healthy food until the next rice harvesting period.

The medicinal system of the Sinhalese, called *Hela wedakama* or *Deshiya Chikithsa* in Sinhala, and "Sinhalese Traditional Medicine" in English, has over 3000 years of history. Before the introduction of Ayurveda from India, this system was the most prominent and accepted healing method. Natural herbs, ritualistic performances, and healthy foods are the main medicines prescribed by Sinhalese Traditional Medicine practitioners (Ananda, Nahallage, & Ali nd).

The colonization of Sri Lanka began in 1505 and ended in 1948. During this period of 443 years, Sri Lanka was under the rule of the Portuguese (1505–1658), the Dutch (1658–1796), and the British (1796–1948), who granted it independence in 1948. A huge transformation of the Sinhalese cultural system took place during this lengthy colonial period. After independence, many Sinhalese could not continue their former ways of life and had to form new cultural traits as adaptations to the new socio-economic environment. Specifically, traditional society had turned into a capitalistic social system with newly introduced educational, legal, religious, language, political, agricultural, and legal systems. These types of external factors that were added during the colonial period caused adverse changes to the whole cultural system. For example, with the introduction of land policies, traditionally inherited lands were taken over by the government, as people had no legal documents to prove their ownership; and the traditional agricultural system of the upcountry and low country areas of the country had been shifted into tea, coffee, and rubber production for the benefits of the colonizers. During the transformation from a colonized to an independent country, the political and economic domains of the culture became more prominent and have come to dominate most of the traditional cultural domains. Yet the latter's influence remains; for example, for their most important decisions, political leaders always try to get the support of Buddhist monks, as that support indirectly signifies the approval of the Sinhalese Buddhist people, who obey and respect the decisions of the monks. Yet despite these major transitions in Sri Lankan society that resulted from the influences of Westernized and globalized cultural systems, the majority of the country's people, especially the rural villagers, still follow the traditional way of life.

The COVID-19 Pandemic and Cultural Responses

The Sri Lankan people have confronted various epidemics throughout their history; the most devastating were the Great Influenza pandemic and the malaria epidemic. Deaths from the influenza pandemic totaled 307,000. In Sri Lanka, it had peaked in two discrete (northern and southern) regions in early October of 1918 and in a second (central) region in early March 1919 (Chandra & Sarathchandra 2014). The most devastating malaria epidemics occurred during 1934–1935; they ravaged the entire island, infecting an estimated 5 million people and causing approximately 80,000 deaths (Wijesundere & Ramasamy 2017). Dengue, leprosy, measles, and chickenpox epidemics have also plagued this island nation. For preventive measures, the people drew from specific cultural methods that we will describe in detail below. In particular, Sinhalese people consider measles and chickenpox to be diseases imposed by deities that can be healed using traditional healing practices (see also Chapters 10 and 14, and Ali 2020.)

The Religious/Philosophical Belief System

As previously noted, the religious/philosophical belief system of the Sinhalese mainly developed based on Buddhism, yet it also includes Hindu and Sinhalese deities, demons, and other spiritual entities. Buddhism in its practical aspect is a flexible religion/philosophy that does not demand the kinds of offerings and observances that are required in other religions. Thus, a Buddhist can decide whether or not to follow the eight precepts of the middle path described above, and which is the most important determinant of morality for Buddhist laypeople. Therefore, Buddhism remains as a flexible religion that provides its adherents with the possibility of spiritual/metaphysical attainments. If an individual follows the middle path, the Four Noble Truths (see below), the Noble Eightfold Path described above, and other teachings of the Lord Buddha, he can attain the great *Nibbana* (Nirvana/enlightenment), which in Buddhism is believed to be achievable by anyone. In following the middle path, Buddhist Sri Lankans, as previously noted, tend to be satisfied with what they have and not lust for more.

Most Sinhalese Buddhists believe in Karma and say, "Everything happens for a reason and all are due to the Karma of the person." This thinking pattern has become a prime element in maintaining psychological stability in the face of possibly overwhelming events. They even consider the coronavirus pandemic to be the result of Karma, as most think of the pandemic as Karmic retribution for things they did in previous incarnations. Thus, most of those who had been practicing the Buddha's middle path and the traditional way of life did not become agitated when the government imposed curfews and isolation measures in response to the outbreak. Stories about the previous incarnations of Gautama Buddha and about various epidemics and how the Buddha successfully confronted such issues are often told as a means of providing solutions to the daily life issues of a Buddhist. Reasons and causes for various epidemics and pandemics are described as linked to Karma and the sinful acts of individuals. Family elders share these stories among the other family members, especially when they stayed together during the curfew period. Such comforting stories seemed to help in avoiding unnecessary panic. Middle path observances have also helped to maintain good mental health and stability during this pandemic. According to this teaching of the Lord Buddha, laypeople should practice the middle path in their every action without reaching the extreme ends of self-indulgence or self-denial. This middle path observance and the practice of contentment helped people to endure the pandemic with a balanced mentality—in sharp contrast to most of the other countries discussed in this volume, where fear and anxiety have heavily influenced behaviors.

Their Buddhism-centered belief system is the core of Sinhalese culture on which other cultural domains have been built. The responses of the Sinhalese to anything and everything are primarily based on this cultural background. When individuals became infected with COVID-19, they and their family members simply endured the pain without complaint. When those infected died, their families relied on the Buddhist teaching about the impermanent nature of the world for consolation. Therefore, in contrast to, for example, Pakistanis (see Chapters 16 and 17), Sinhalese people did not oppose the government COVID-19 death measures, which involved cremation of the body without the family present; thus the traditional Sinhalese death rituals could not be performed. Buddhists believe in the capability of the meritorious actions that an individual commits in a lifetime to provide a better life in their next incarnation.

Other practices followed by the Lord Buddha in his search for enlightenment include ascetic techniques in which he followed the very difficult path of the extreme self-denial end of the spectrum of suffering. This has become another of the ways in which Sinhalese manage difficulties in their life. If the Lord Buddha had to face these types of difficulties in search of Nibbana, then for a layperson, such difficulties are considered normal.

In Buddhism, the Four Noble Truths (*Arya Satyas*) are considered as the first teaching of Lord Buddha, comprising the essence of the Buddha's teachings. These are: (1) suffering is an innate characteristic of earthly existence; (2) suffering is accompanied by cravings, desires, and attachments to earthly things; (3) the end of suffering can be attained by the renouncement or letting go of these attachments; and (4) the eight-fold middle path leads to this letting go and the cessation of suffering (Basics of Buddhism 2019; Following the Buddha's Footsteps 2018). These teachings have for thousands of years formed the basis of the Buddhist belief system and have led to balance among the Sinhalese people and in their daily lifestyles, especially during crises such as the coronavirus pandemic.

Rituals, Rites, and Supernatural Entities

As in many other traditional societies, in Sinhalese culture certain rituals and associated customs serve as protective rites. Some of these rituals are performed individually and some are collective. Either way, these rituals are believed to help to solve various prevalent problems, such as generating protection from deities and demons for themselves, their cattle—which provide milk and help in plowing and paddy threshing—and their agricultural fields. In addition, these rituals are performed to prevent or heal diseases believed to be caused by deities and demons such as chickenpox, measles, and mental disorders. Among these rituals, the most common and famous are ceremonial dances that belong to three main traditions—the Upcountry, Lowcountry, and *Sabaragamwa*; these are sacrosanct performances to invoke blessings from the deities, so that the goodness that comes forth from them will overcome evil. When the month of April arrives, people join together to harvest their paddy cultivations. After the harvesting of the rice, the same paddy lands become the stages for these ritual performances. Entire villages get together to ask for the blessings of the deities and demons for themselves, their cattle, and the next harvest. Once these rituals are completed, the villagers believe that no harm can affect them until the next harvesting season.

During these ritual performances, participants should behave in the specific ways dictated by the ritual and how it is supposed to be performed. Most especially, they should avoid foods and behaviors that are considered impure and thus taboo. Offerings are made to multiple deities such as *Gambara, Suniyam, Saman, Kataragama, Ganesha, Dedimunda, Vishnu, Natha, Mangara,* and *Ishwara.* These are a few among the hundreds of deities included in the pantheon of ancient gods and goddesses. During these traditional ceremonial or "devil dances," offerings and worship are also dedicated to demons such as *Mahasohon, Riri, Kohomba,* and *Suniyam.* The collective behavioral patterns observable in these rituals have long been believed to serve as preventive measures against diseases and epidemics. The isolation and separation taboos imposed by the government seem to the villagers to relate to these rituals and to work in tandem with them. Therefore, the government's preventive measures against viral spread were accepted by the people in well-mannered ways, as they were able to perceive these measures as what Ali (2021) calls "rituals of containment" that fit well with their own longstanding "rituals of prevention."

Among the small Indigenous Vedda population of Sri Lanka, there are specific rituals called *Hathma, Kirikoraha,* and *Kowil.* These too are performed to protect their villages from diseases. The Vedda believe that if these rituals are not performed, their protective boundaries will be breached and diseases could enter their villages, harming the villagers and their cattle and lands. The habitats of the Vedda people are separated from "the outside" and are traditionally marked by specific boundaries. They never interact with outsiders, except in arrow blade exchanges with a Sinhalese blacksmith. In this way, they have purposefully isolated themselves throughout history, and these annual rites that enact their belief system have given them psychological and perhaps physical protection from diseases that come from outside. To date, none of the Vedda people in Sri Lanka have been reported to be seropositive for COVID-19.

Isolation and separation are not new concepts to the Sinhalese and Vedda people of the country. For example, when a Sinhalese girl reaches puberty, she is isolated and separated from her entire family for about three weeks until she bathes on an auspicious day. Also, when a villager is infected with chickenpox or measles, the entire house turns into a hospital with its own pharmacy—a small garden full of medicinal plants. The kitchen of a traditional Sinhalese house is called a "Medicinal Cottage" (*Veda Kutiya*), as many of the foods prepared there contain medicinal ingredients. When an individual of the house is infected with a communicable disease, he/she is quarantined in a new hut built separately from the main house, using threshed paddy leaves for the roof with the walls made of wattle and mud. A branch of the Neem tree (*Azadirachta indica*) is hung in front of the hut as a symbol that the person in this hut has a communicable disease. Then one individual of the house, usually the eldest child, brings healthy foods to the infected person's door. Food taboos are also observed: meat, eggs, and oily fish are considered impure foods and should be avoided, as those could attract devils and other supernatural entities to the house. Turmeric and neem leaves are always used to clean the floor of the house, the hut, and their surroundings. Fourteen days after the first contact with the virus, and before the sun rises, the infected individual is taken to a river or someplace where water flows to bathe. Before the bath, their body is covered with a turmeric and neem leaf mixture. After these rites, the formerly ill person is ready to reenter society.

During the treatments, special decoctions made of ginger, coriander, garlic, and lime are given to enhance immunity. *Kanda*, a mixture of varieties of herbs, is prescribed as an additional immune enhancer, is often eaten for breakfast, and is used as a treatment for various types of illness. To prepare Kanda, one or several herbal plants such as *Gotukola (Centella asiatica), Muguna Wenna (Alternanthera sessilis), Iramusu (Hemidesmus indicus)*, and *Haathawariya (Asparagus racemosus), Polpala (Aerva lanata), Karapincha (Murraya koenigii Spreng)* are ground and mixed with garlic and small portions of rice, salt, and coconut milk. Coconut milk enhances immunity and is good for detoxification. There is a saying that most Sinhalese are protected from external toxins due to their regular consumption of coconut milk, which is used in almost every Sinhalese meal. Even for people who are poisoned by serpent venom, herbal decoctions mixed with coconut milk are prescribed as treatments. In these and other ways, the traditional food practices of the Sinhalese people serve as protective agents against viruses and bacteria. Thus, Sinhalese traditional food practices and rituals were used locally as preventive methods against COVID-19 and other respiratory problems.

Instead of drinking regular black tea, the Sinhalese stick to their traditional drinks such as a coriander brew or tea made of various herbs mixed together. Coriander tea has been especially highlighted during the COVID-19 pandemic by Sri Lankan biomedical practitioners and Ayurvedic practitioners alike. Surprisingly, both systems also agreed on the value of breathing in the steam rising from a mixture of medicinal herbs boiled in water as a viable treatment for respiratory system-related issues such as those caused by COVID-19. In the absence of effective biomedical treatments for COVID-19, biomedical hospitals prescribe these treatments as effective methods for alleviating the symptoms of COVID-19 and as immunity enhancement techniques that every person should follow daily.

Kinship, Marriage, and Family

Due to the COVID-19 pandemic in Sri Lanka, people had to follow the physical distancing and curfew guidelines. The isolation regulations required people to stay inside their homes for over two months. One of the specific traits of the Sinhalese cultural system that has supported this isolation and social/physical distancing is its strong, patrilineal family and kinship pattern. Living in an extended family system supported most families to endure their isolation from others during this difficult period. In many other countries, as shown in other chapters in this volume, people who badly needed social contact became frustrated, anxious, lonely, and often depressed during isolation. These feelings were not predominant among the Sinhalese, as they received continuous support from their family members—very few Sinhalese live alone. Even younger children and teenagers were able to "balance their minds" despite missing seeing their friends. In the Sinhalese cultural system, unlike in the USA and other high-resource countries, teenagers do not tend to have separate lives. They and their younger siblings often appreciated the opportunity to spend much of their time with their grandparents and other family members. Even those without a large extended family tend to live with at least five family members representing two or more generations.

Because grandparents usually take care of their grandchildren, daycare centers are not available in most of the areas of the country. Associating with their grandparents tends to enhance children's happiness and active engagements with nature and with Buddhism. The stories that grandparents tend to tell their grandchildren are mostly "Jataka Tales"; these are parts of a voluminous body of stories about the previous incarnations of Guatama Buddha in both animal and human form. In these tales, the Buddha may appear as an outcast, an elephant, a king, or a god, but in whatever form, he exhibits some virtue that the story thereby inculcates into the children who listen to it. These stories help both children and adults endure life's difficulties with a balanced mentality and good health practices. In the Sinhalese cultural system, neighbors share their meals with each other. During the pandemic, wealthier neighbors continued to supply food to the less well-off, sometimes by hanging a bag of vegetables in front of their homes. Also, when families are quarantined, neighbors always take care of them through telephone conversations and by providing basic necessities.

These traditional patterns of hospitality and strong family and kinship patterns supported self-confidence and worked to prevent anxiety and stress among children and adults alike during the pandemic. The respect given to the elders helps to control the behaviors of the youngsters of the family. The extended family system also helps economically. If some family members lose their regular occupations due to COVID-19, others collectively support the entire family.

Society: Collective Integrity

People's patterns of thinking and behavior are shaped by the socialization process, as are their personalities. After independence in 1948, significant social phenomena that occurred in Sri Lankan society were Black July in 1983;[2] the Civil War (1983–2009);[3] and the JVP insurrection of 1987–1989.[4] These periods negatively affected the traditional harmonious social system of the country; people experienced social phobia due to the behaviors of the government and other parties. During the 30 years of the Civil War, most people lived with very limited resources under extensive curfew periods and other travel restrictions. These hard periods with limited freedom and extreme sociocultural conditions turned the Sinhalese into a strong group of people. Thus, the protests against COVID-19 curfews and enforced isolations that occurred in many other countries cannot be seen in Sri Lankan society, in which people had no problems with the preventive measures taken by the government. Compliance was given willingly and did not need to be government-enforced. Also, due to the 30 years of the Civil War, people tend to have more faith in the military than in the government. Therefore, the military has become a significant and socially accepted part of Sri Lankan culture, and people accepted any military interventions designed to control the pandemic. According to some, if the government would let the army control the pandemic, they would do a better job than the government is doing now. Nevertheless, people rarely protest government decisions, which also facilitated the government to take quick actions towards pandemic control.

As previously noted, the Sinhalese—especially the rural people—are not major consumers. This pattern of behavior also has been shaped according to Buddhism and the simple lifestyle that their forefathers had followed. Most of the rural Sinhalese grow their vegetables and grains on their lands. Even in the dry season, they cultivate vegetables and other necessary foods for their consumption. Also, using traditional food preservation practices, these people manage to supply food for their families throughout the year. The problems of food scarcity and high consumption are associated with the urban people of the country. The government had to take action to supply the needs of these metropolitans, especially for those who lived in the urban Colombo, Gampaha, and Kalutara areas; these were the areas at highest risk in all three waves of the pandemic.

Conclusion

In this chapter, we have described and discussed the specific traits of Sri Lankan Sinhalese Buddhist culture that were most helpful in controlling viral spread and in enabling people to deal calmly with the exigencies of the pandemic situation. To recap, these include their Buddhist beliefs; their multiple and varied confidence-inducing rituals and rites; their extended family system, which includes tremendous respect for their elders and a high valuation of their knowledge and experience; and the self-sufficiency of the rural population, their extensive knowledge of effective, non-biomedical medicinal remedies, and the high value they place on consuming only healthy foods that keep their immune systems strong. These cultural traits have been passed down through generations, especially those that give people a higher survival capacity during crises. Thus we have shown how and why the Sri Lankan Sinhalese have been able to deal with have been able to deal with the coronavirus pandemic more calmly and with far less anxiety than those in many other countries. As long as these cultural traits continue, Sinhalese Sri Lankans will remain well-equipped to deal with future pandemics and other disasters to come.

Notes

1 The kind of rice cultivated matters a great deal: red rice is full of nutrients, whereas white rice has no nutritional value. For example, when the island of Bali switched from red to white rice cultivation because white rice can be grown in three crops a year (whereas red rice can only be grown in two), its people rapidly became malnourished and remain so today (see Lim & Legett 2021).
2 "Black July" refers to a brutal state-sponsored genocide lasting from July 23–30 that killed at least 3000 Tamils, destroyed 5000 of their shops, and displaced over 150,000 Tamils.
3 Like Black July, this Civil War resulted from British-induced tensions between the majority Sinhalese and the minority Tamil. The Tamils had wanted to create their own independent nation-state, due to the continuous discrimination and violent persecutions against Sri Lankan Tamils by the Sinhalese dominated Sri Lankan Government. The Tamils did not succeed in this endeavor.
4 This was an armed revolt let by the Marxist group *Janatha Vimukthi Peramuna* (JVP)—the "People's Liberation Front"—against the Sri Lankan government.

References

Ada Derana 24. 2021. ADA DHERANA. http://sinhala.adaderana.lk/news/151967/ මගේ-දුක්වා-හුදකලා-කර-ඇති-ප්‍රදේශ

Ali, I. 2020. *Constructing and Negotiating Measles: The Case of Sindh Province of Pakistan.* PhD dissertation. Vienna, Austria: University of Vienna.

Ali, I. 2021. Rituals of containment: Many pandemics, body politics, and social dramas during COVID-19 in Pakistan. *Frontiers in Sociology* 6: 648149. doi: 10.3389/fsoc.2021.648149

Ananda, T., & Nahallage, C. 2014.   Traditional Agricultural Practices Unique to Meemure Village, Kandy District Sri Lanka. *International Journal of Multidisciplinary Studies* 1(1): 11–21. doi: 10.4038/ijms.v1i1.28

Ananda, T. 2019. *A Comparative Anthropological Study on Yakkure and Henanigala Indigenous Groups in Sri Lanka*. PhD dissertation. Nugegoda, Sri Lanka: University of Sri Jayewardenepura.

Ananda, T., Nahallage, C., & Ali, I. nd. "A Supernatural Medicine for COVID-19 in Sri Lanka: Medical Pluralism, Biomedical Hegemony, and Authoritative Knowledge." Unpublished ms, under review by *Frontiers in Sociology*.

Basics of Buddhism 2019. Public Broadcasting Service. www.pbs.org/edens/thailand/buddhism.htm

Chandra, S., & Sarathchandra, D. 2014. The influenza pandemic of 1918–1919 in Sri Lanka: Its demographic cost, timing, and propagation. *Influenza and Other Respiratory Viruses* 8(3). https://doi.org/10.1111/irv.12238

Coronavirus Disease 2019 (COVID-19) – Situation Report. 2021. www.epid.gov.lk/web/images/pdf/corona_virus_report/sitrep-sl-en-02-05_10_21.pdf

Department of Census and Statistics. 2012. *Census of Population and Housing 2012.*   www.statistics.gov.lk/Population/StaticalInformation/CPH2011/Census PopulationHousing2012-FinalReport

Epidemiology Unit. 2021. Ministry of Health, Sri Lanka. www.epid.gov.lk/web/index.php?lang=en

Following the Buddha's Footsteps. 2018. Instilling Goodness School. City of Ten Thousand Buddhas, Talmage, CA. https://online.sfsu.edu/rone/Buddhism/footsteps.htm

Lim, R., & Legett, S. 2021. "Bumi Sehat Bali: Birth on the Checkered Cloth." In B.A. Daviss and R. Davis-Floyd (eds.), *Birthing Models on the Human Rights Frontier: Speaking Truth to Power*, 55–74. Abingdon, UK: Routledge.

NECSI. 2021. *Some Are Winning – Some Are Not, Which Countries Do Best In Beating Covid-19?* Cambridge, MA: New England Complex Systems Institute. www.endcoronavirus.org/countries

Silva, P. D., & Punchihewa, A. G. 2011. Socio-Anthropological Research Project on Vedda Community in Sri Lanka.

Sri Lanka Demographics Profile 2019. 2019. IndexMundi.www.indexmundi.com/sri_lanka/demographics_profile.html

Wijesundere, D.A., & Ramasamy, R. 2017. Analysis of historical trends and recent elimination of malaria from Sri Lanka and its applicability for malaria control in other countries. *Frontiers in Public Health* 5. https://doi.org/10.3389/fpubh.2017.00212

13 Negotiating COVID-19 in Bhutan

Successfully Aligning Science, Politics, Culture, and Religion in a Unique Public Health Strategy

Mary Grace A. Pelayo, Ian Christopher N. Rocha, and Jigme Yoezer

Introduction: Bhutan and Its Demographics

Bhutan is a small, landlocked country located in the Eastern Himalayas in South Asia. It is bordered to the north by China and to the south by India. Although Nepal and Bangladesh are close to Bhutan, they do not share a geographical boundary. In 2020, the country had a population of 771,608 people in a land area of 38,394 square kilometers (National Statistics Bureau 2020). The country's government is a democratic constitutional monarchy and its state religion is Vajrayana Buddhism.

Bhutan's public healthcare system has long been admired by people globally as it embodies a healthcare ideal. Bhutan is known to provide free, medically pluralistic health care to its people; its constitution proclaims that "the State shall provide free access to basic public health services in both modern and traditional medicines." Thus, government revenue is the primary source of health financing in the country, wherein the total healthcare expenditure was 3.6% of the country's gross domestic product (GDP) in 2014 and has remained at around 4% until the present (Thinley et al. 2017).

The exponential rise in the country's hospitals from just two in 1961 to 55 in 2019 was impressive and is the country's testament to the efforts of the Ministry of Health (MOH) to intensify primary health care and keep up with global changes in health care (MOH 2020; National Statistics Bureau 2020). The country also now has 186 Primary Health Centers, 53 Subposts, 542 Outreach Clinics, three Thromde Health Centers, and five Health Information and Service Centers. As for the total number of the health workforce in the country, it was reported in 2019 to be at 5,901, of whom 376 are medical doctors; 1,187 are medical technologists and technicians; 620 are health assistants; 1,364 are nurses; 54 are *Drungtsho* (traditional Bhutanese medicine practitioners); 116 are therapy aides; and 2,184 are health administration and support officers.

Nonetheless, the doctor-to-patient ratio is still at 0.5, which means that it remains 50% below the ratio recommended by the World Health

DOI: 10.4324/9781003187462-17

Organization (WHO) 1:1,000 doctor-to-patient ratio by the World Health Organization (WHO). Moreover, the nurse-to-patient ratio of 18.4 per 10,000 people is still considered low compared with other South Asian countries. The number of hospital beds also decreased from 1.7 to 1.1 in 2012 and 2019 respectively (MOH 2020). Thus, due to the low doctor-to-patient and nurse-to-patient ratios, people with health conditions beyond the capacity or expertise of the Bhutanese healthcare system are flown out to hospitals in India at the government's expense.

Healthcare services are available in a three-tiered structure—primary, secondary, and tertiary levels—and traditional and allopathic medicine services are delivered side by side and are integrated into the system. Village health workers are also deemed as crucial practitioners in bridging health services and promoting them in communities. In the Kingdom of Bhutan, people's physical and mental faculties of health are given utmost regard, enacting WHO's definition of health as "a state of complete physical, mental and social well-being, and not merely the absence of disease or infirmity." A famous Bhutanese saying is "*lus lu natsha med, sems lu sdugsngal med,*" which means that "there must be no illness in the body and no stress in the mind" (Adhikari 2016).

As the world continues to be devastated by the challenges posed by the coronavirus disease 2019 (COVID-19) pandemic, the small Himalayan country of Bhutan has presented remarkably successful pandemic management as compared to the wealthy and significantly more technologically advanced countries of the world. In this chapter, we discuss the successful public health efforts of the Royal Government of Bhutan, together with its Ministries, its people, and its leading religious figures in responding to the coronavirus pandemic, and how an anthropological perspective was incorporated in their responses to this public health emergency, given that the culture of this tiny Buddhist country is deeply rooted in longstanding beliefs, customs, and traditions.

Bhutan's Successful and Commendable COVID-19 Responses: The Critical Importance of Preparedness

Bhutan is one of the few countries that has effectively managed COVID-19, with only 1,724 confirmed cases and just one fatality as of this time of writing (June 8, 2021). Among the total number of cases, only 307 are active, with daily cases of one to two digits only (WHO 2021). Despite being bordered by India, one of the pandemic's worst-affected countries, and China, the country where COVID-19 was originally detected, the total number of COVID-19 cases in Bhutan accounted for less than 1% of the country's population, demonstrating the success of the government's outbreak response (Lin 2021 et al. 2021; Rocha 2021; Rocha et al. 2021). Although Bhutan appeared to have little hope of escaping the pandemic's ravages, given that it is literally sandwiched by two giants with high cases of COVID-19, this tiny country has been able to successfully manage its fight against "coronaviral" spread. (The term "coronaviral" was coined by Robbie Davis-Floyd; see the Introduction to this volume.)

This success is attributed to many factors. Bhutan was able to act promptly and decisively, immediately putting in place critical public health strategies, such as identifying, testing, tracing, quarantining, and treating COVID-19 cases. The country also increased the capacities of health personnel and set up healthcare and testing facilities to ensure that basic health services would be delivered even during lockdowns (Turner 2020; Rocha 2021). These successful breakthroughs can be attributed to the first and foremost factor of the country's commendable outbreak response: their pre-preparedness for public health emergencies.

In November 2019, a month before COVID-19 was first detected in its neighbor China, and a few months before the pandemic reached this small kingdom, Bhutan was already engaging and collaborating with the WHO in simulating what a global public health emergency response should look like. In collaboration with Bhutan's MOH, the WHO conducted a simulation exercise at the Paro International Airport, wherein a passenger from abroad with a suspected and hypothetical contagious disease arrives in Bhutan. The armed forces, police, civil aviation, customs and food safety authorities, flight attendants, health officials, and the *Desuups*—the members of a national service volunteer group founded by the King—all cooperated and acted out their roles in this hypothetical scenario. In the event of a true pandemic, this highly prescient exercise allowed the participants to identify existing flaws and needs for improvement (Alaoui 2020; WHO 2020).

Clearly, the country's success in combating COVID-19 was due to meticulous planning and prompt response. In 2018, prior to the hypothetical pandemic scenario, the WHO had led an emergency readiness activity in which the country conducted a joint external evaluation of its emergency preparedness. The WHO and the Royal Government of Bhutan collaborated to establish a health emergency operations center and a WHO emergency operations center. Investing in equipment such as Medical Camp Kit tents, which can be deployed within hours if services are disrupted, is another form of readiness in which Bhutan engaged. By the time the coronavirus pandemic reached the country, these tents had already been utilized as flu clinics to manage patients with symptoms of pulmonary diseases, preventing them from mixing with other patients and spreading contagion. When the pandemic arrived, these tent clinics were presciently available to serve as COVID-19 screening facilities (Alaoui 2020; WHO 2020).

Additionally, the WHO and the country's MOH had also been working together to improve laboratory capabilities, including enhancing and advancing the biosafety level of the Royal Center of Disease Control (RCDC) by supplying equipment and providing personnel training. This early preparedness definitely assisted Bhutan's COVID-19 preparations and responses. Assessing the healthcare system's readiness and the availability of the healthcare workforce was another early essential action. The Bhutanese royal government, through its MOH, assigned and trained staff to lead the frontline response, utilizing and following the WHO protocols. Prior to the first case of COVID-19 in the country, the healthcare workers were also trained to don and doff personal protective equipment (WHO 2020).

Thus, when COVID-19 eventually did reach Bhutan, the country was already well-prepared. The first case of COVID-19 in the country, identified on March 5, 2020, was a tourist from the United States who had recently traveled to India. At first, he was asymptomatic, but after a few days, he experienced gastrointestinal symptoms, which led him to consult in a hospital in Thimphu (Kuensel 2020). After traveling to Punakha, returning to Thimphu, and developing flu-like symptoms, the tourist then went back to the same hospital. He was immediately isolated in an already prepared COVID-19 facility and his samples were sent to the RCDC. The patient's laboratory results came in rapidly, at midnight on March 6, 2020, and by exactly 6am, all of his primary contacts had been identified and quarantined (WHO 2020). Contact tracings were launched in accordance with the patient's travel itinerary, which included the airport and visits to some places in Thimphu and Punakha; he had also eaten at a café and in a high school park. The government authorities also immediately restricted foreigners' entry into Bhutan. Schools and institutes in 3 *Dzongkhags* (districts) were also closed for a few weeks to prevent coronaviral spread (Kuensel 2020). Although the country only had one case of COVID-19 at that time, the government responded very swiftly in an effort to prevent further cases.

We move now to August 11, 2020, when government officials launched a national lockdown after a woman who had been cleared from quarantine surprisingly tested positive for COVID-19. Contact tracing was immediately done. The government responded swiftly by closing schools, institutions, offices, and commercial establishments, and restricting vehicle movements. The people were encouraged to stay at home to protect themselves and their families from viral spread (Palden 2020a). In other words, Bhutan did everything possible to avoid community transmission. The country also documented a high rate of testing; people were encouraged to get tested, and the testing and quarantine facilities are free of charge (Turner 2020). These events and scenarios are just a few examples of the rapid and successful COVID-19 response of this small South Asian country.

In addition to their commendable public health measures and successful COVID-19 responses, Bhutan was also applauded for its rapid vaccination rollout. Although the country was late in establishing its vaccination program compared to other countries (see below for why), the program proved to be a huge success, with 93% of the adult population receiving vaccinations in less than two weeks (Rocha 2021). Consequently, as of this time of writing (June 2021), around 484,000 people have been inoculated with at least one dose of the COVID-19 vaccine, which accounts for approximately 63% of the overall population, putting the country on track to meet its objective of at least 70% coverage in order to achieve herd immunity (Mathieu et al. 2021; WHO 2021). Thus, Bhutan has become the fastest country to vaccinate a large portion of its population in just a few weeks, compared to other countries with successful vaccination programs, which took months to vaccinate the same percentage of their population as Bhutan (Rocha 2021). For example, it took at least six months for 50% of the US population to become fully vaccinated (Mathieu et al. 2021).

For COVID-19 preventive and control policies and protocols to be effective and successful, they must be implemented and promoted by effective leaders. These public health efforts in Bhutan are attributed to the leadership triad of King Jigme Khesar Namgyel Wangchuck, Prime Minister Lotay Tshering, and Health Minister Dechen Wangmo. Importantly, the 11-member cabinet of the current government of Bhutan comprises two physicians and two public health experts. Among them are the Prime Minister, who is a doctor, and the Health Minister, who is an epidemiologist and public health expert (Dorji and Tamang 2021). They both understand what is required for effective disease control, and thus they based their policy responses on science and evidence-based public health strategies. They spent significant amounts of time working with the National COVID-19 Task Force to control the outbreak. Additionally, the King has been quite visible and outspoken in supporting the efforts made by the Prime Minister and the Health Minister, and has heartily backed and praised their quick and well-informed decision-making. The King has also provided motivation, support, and leadership in addressing the country's Covidian concerns (Turner 2020; Dorji and Tamang 2021; Rocha 2021).

Bhutan's efficient COVID-19 responses hinge on community strength, with the King, the government, and the people working together. By distributing *kidu* ("wellbeing")—a system comprising the royal provision of resources to the poor—the King has displayed care and fulfilled his traditional responsibility as monarch. In the case of COVID-19, *kidu* took the form of economic assistance for 23,000 people. This touching and moving action by the King inspired others. As a result, members of the parliament contributed one month's salary to the *kidu* fund; hotel owners provided quarantine facilities for free; corporations donated cash; and farmers provided food (Turner 2020). Indeed, the leadership and governance of Bhutan's leaders greatly contributed to the effectiveness of the country's COVID-19 responses. In addition, and unlike in most of the other countries addressed in this volume, the government's communications with its citizens are always clear, straightforward, and decisive. Daily updates, contact numbers, and other particular information on COVID-19 from the government are always posted online for the general public, government entities, and private institutions. High levels of trust in the Royal Government and a track record of compliance with the Government's protocols have been major factors in the containment of COVID-19 in Bhutan (Turner 2020).

We highlight that health and happiness in Bhutan are considered as part and parcel of each other, and that Bhutan's pandemic resilience can be attributed to the people's selflessness and willingness to unite for the common good, as reflected in their Gross National Happiness Index; in 2015, a total of 91.2% of Bhutanese were narrowly, extensively, or deeply happy. Their spirit of compassion and altruism helps the population to address health and its negations from a holistic approach, and engraves in the people a sense of community and camaraderie in fighting public health and other emergencies. As noted by Kugelman (2021), it is common for communities to gather resources for the medical personnel who are serving in COVID-19 cases and facilities, but what makes the success story of Bhutan unique is the magnanimity of the people, who mobilized into one unified charity organization. This magnanimity is evident in the King's personal launching of a $19 million relief campaign for the citizens; the government's efforts to send care packages, especially to the elderly; the people's voluntary enlistments to assist the state in its fight against the pandemic; the parliament members' decisions to sacrifice their salaries for relief operations; the hotel owners' willingness to transform their facilities into quarantine sites; and the people's efforts to prepare, offer, and deliver food to their working legislators and to the health personnel taking care of patients infected with COVID-19. Bhutanese journalist Namgay Zam emphasized that it is their closeness that has kept the people together and that there may be no other country that exhibits this immense mutual trust between its leaders and ordinary people. This statement has also been supported by the editor of a Bhutanese newspaper, Tenzing Lamsang, who said that the country's greatest assets are its social cohesion and its people's ability to work as a team in times of crisis (Dasgupta 2021).

Aside from the efforts made by the royal government, much credit is due to the public health efforts of the Bhutanese healthcare professionals, who tirelessly treated and managed COVID-19 cases in the tents set up for that purpose. Credit is also due to the thousands of Desuups, also known as "guardians of peace," who selflessly volunteered to assist the medical workforce. Again, the Desuups are members of a volunteer organization founded by the King in 2011. These self-sacrificing and altruistic individuals played an essential role in the country's fight against COVID-19, especially given that the country has only 376 doctors and fewer than 3,000 healthcare professionals (National Statistics Bureau 2020; Rocha 2021). Aside from assisting the healthcare workforce, these volunteers were trained in disaster assistance and management and could be seen patrolling the southern border, monitoring lockdown compliance, and distributing necessary supplies. They have exemplified the national belief that COVID-19 management is a public obligation (Turner 2020).

Aligning Science, Medicine, and Religion: The Role of the Monks in Vaccination Launch Preparation

In the case of Bhutan, despite the fact that there were no actual anthropologists among the leadership, we suggest that there was commendable integration of *an anthropological perspective* into the country's pandemic measures, specifically concerning religion, culture, and tradition, and how these measures were negotiated, communicated, and implemented. For example, the government was careful to coordinate with the central monastic body in the highly successful launching of the vaccination rollout. In what Geertz (1973) called "thin description," we mentioned above that Bhutan's vaccine rollout was "late" compared to those of other countries. In fact, now layering in "thick" description (ibid.), we explain that Bhutan *purposefully* postponed the commencement of the vaccination launch. Some of the vaccines had arrived in the country two months before the vaccination campaign began. Yet the Minister of Health opted to delay the start of the immunization program across the kingdom, heeding the recommendation of the *Zhung Dratsang*—the central monastic organization. According to this group of Buddhist monks and astrologers, the stars were not yet in favor. Additionally, the *Dana*, which ran from February 14, 2021, to March 13, 2021, was an inauspicious and unlucky month that might jeopardize the kingdom's vaccination campaign. Since Bhutan is a profoundly religious country, the royal government and the MOH took the central monastic body's advice and vaccinated its citizens *after* the Dana, with the additional advantage that the Dana gave the government more time to plan their inoculation campaign so that it would be as well organized as possible (Rocha 2021).

The central monastic body of Bhutan, led by the *Je Khenpo* or Chief Abott, performed a three-day ceremony of *Sangay Menlha*, a medicinal Buddhist mantra, which was observed and joined in by thousands of Bhutanese via television and social media. This mantra, which many Bhutanese believe is a powerful prayer for keeping illness at bay, was performed a few days before the launch to coincide with the delivery of the additional needed doses of the COVID-19 vaccine. Even the first vaccine recipient was carefully chosen: a woman born in the Year of the Monkey, according to Buddhist astrology. On March 27, 2021—the Zhung Dratsang's chosen auspicious day, this first vaccine dose was administered in Thimphu at the fortuitous and favorable hour of 9:30 in the morning while prayers were performed with lighted butter lamps. For all Bhutanese, the occasion and ceremony called for a national feast, as it appeared to be the start of the final phase of their struggle against COVID-19. Since, as previously noted, most Bhutanese are exceptionally religious, the chosen occasion definitely improved vaccine acceptance in the country. Thus, we can say that Bhutan was successful in boosting COVID-19 vaccine uptake across the country by using a highly unusual and highly anthropological approach that incorporated science, religion, culture, and tradition (Rocha 2021).

In addition to the vaccination launch, the Je Khenpo has also played an essential role in the rest of the successful COVID-19 response. During the lockdown period, the Je Khenpo and the government urged the people to use their time for reflection and meditation. These involve reciting the *Chenrezi* and *Vajra Guru* mantras with utmost devotion, as mantra recitation is regarded as a powerful remedial practice for outer and inner illnesses in Buddhism (Palden 2020b). He also encouraged the public to be honest if someone were to exhibit the symptoms of the disease as a great service not only to others and the country but also to oneself. Since people worldwide seek to find meaning in the pandemic as they do in life, COVID-19 has been interpreted differently in various countries—for example, in Pakistan as a "supernatural test" or a "Western conspiracy" (see Chapter 17 of this volume and Ali 2021). The Je Khenpo had his own way of finding meaning: he explained that COVID-19 is a product of *lenchak*—karmic vengeance. For years, many people around the world have been continually killing animals for consumption and destroying their natural habitats, which are perfect examples of *lenchak* (Palden 2020b). As a result, humankind is facing the consequences of *lenchak* in the form of the pandemic, which is a manifestation of humanity's terrible deeds. This *lenchak* that the world is currently experiencing can be further explained by the *tendrel*—a Buddhist theory of causation that involves the interdependence and interconnectedness of all phenomena (Kuensel 2015). The karmic debt of past human greed and exploitation of other species was interpreted by the monks as a cause of the ongoing pandemic. Whether this is actually true or not is irrelevant because of its symbolic purpose—this interpretation gave meaning to the pandemic during a time when everything in the world seem to be in a state of limbo, and worked to encourage the Bhutanese population to act rightly and in symbiosis with their natural environment.

It is not surprising that the Buddhist monks have played a crucial role in the COVID-19 response and vaccination launch. As stressed by the MOH, monks always have the potential to play a significant role in advocating health behaviors at the grassroots level. In fact, the Je Khenpo has also been a vocal advocate for health concerns like salt iodization, the harmful effects of tobacco, and the prevention of sexually transmitted diseases (Thinley et al. 2017). Buddhist monks have a theocratic authority in the country's affairs, notwithstanding the formal establishment of democracy through the 2008 Constitution. This is because Buddhism is considered as the "spiritual heritage" of the constitutional monarchy, and the King, also known as *Druk Gyalpo* (Dragon King)[1] and Je Khenpo have shared authority over all matters of state and religion (Meier and Chakrabarti 2016).

From this viewpoint, given that Bhutan is the world's last surviving Vajrayana Buddhist kingdom, the Bhutanese consider their religion to be a cornerstone of their development and a vital element in shaping their social institutions, structures, lifestyles, and health. Monks playing a critical role in the vaccination preparation and rollout is therefore not a new scenario in the country, as this was also the case when the country pursued a tobacco-free nation (Thinley et al. 2017). Religion's widespread and exceptional influence on people's values and lives significantly enabled the smooth administration of the vaccination campaign and its acceptance in the country. Recognizing the importance of social as well as biomedical determinants of health is thus one of the most promising and effective methods of dealing with pandemics.

Conclusion: Bhutan as an Exemplary Precedent in Viral Containment and Vaccination Acceptance

Bhutan's unique—and uniquely successful—approaches to stopping the coronaviral spread and promoting vaccine acceptance in the country were successfully spearheaded by the country's leaders. It is anthropologically commendable that the Kingdom of Bhutan was able to successfully promote and carry out its vaccination campaign while fully respecting the cultural and religious traditions of its people. Additionally, the people respect and revere their King. They have deep trust in his governance, and in return, the King manifests himself as a prominent and central figure who has his people's best interests in mind, especially during this pandemic. This was perfectly depicted during his travels all over Bhutan to guide and support national efforts against the disease, and also during his presence in the launching of the nationwide COVID-19 vaccination program. Hence, not only were cultural traditions integrated into the science-based public health strategies of the country, but also the Kingdom of Bhutan provided an exemplary precedent of how effective leadership can play a significant role in health crisis mitigation. Bhutan's unique approach in addressing COVID-19, therefore, is a depiction of how appropriate planning, proper use of health resources, respect for the sociocultural, political, and religious aspects of the society, and strong central leadership worked together successfully to minimize and then stop viral spread.

The Bhutanese case attests to the material impacts of cosmology and to the articulations of multiple worlds. The ontological pluralism of practices to prevent viral spread also demonstrates the possibility in health care and policy of working together across worldviews, as the Bhutanese monks, traditional healers, and biomedical doctors do. In the time of COVID-19, this cosmopolitical economy and ontological pluralism rooted in interdependence have saved lives, as Bhutanese citizens have come together to universally implement preventive measures. Various challenges remain, yet the situation affords new possible futures as well. Renewed self-sufficiency efforts seek to encourage young people across classes to produce food and contribute physical labor for the country to address shortages in both.

In sum, the key factors for success in the Bhutanese case include the strong welfare state, high levels of health literacy and scientific fluency among political actors, high levels of public trust in the monarch, and the influential monks' active support of biomedical preventive measures. Again, these behaviors and discourses are rooted in *tendrel*: a cosmological theory unique to a Vajrayana Buddhist setting in which the central idea is the interdependence of phenomena as fundamental to existence. In addition to identifying the biomedical measures needed to address the virus as a medical problem, the monks also identify the root cause of this condition at the spiritual and ecological level through the concept of *lenchak*—the present karmic debt of past human greed and exploitation of other species and resources. Thus, political and religious actors, traditional medicine practitioners, and biomedical doctors simultaneously care for the population, and for each other.

Note

1 The current King of Bhutan, Jigme Khesar Namgyel Wangchuck, is the 5th *Druk Gyalpo*—the first was born in 1862. In the Dzongkha language—the official national language of the country—Bhutan is known as *Drukyul*, which translates as "The Land of the Thunder Dragon." Thus, while the Kings of Bhutan are known as *Druk Gyalpo* ("Dragon King"), the Bhutanese people call themselves the *Drukpa*, meaning "Dragon people."

References

Adhikari, D. 2016. Healthcare and happiness in the Kingdom of Bhutan. *Singapore Medical Journal* 57(3): 107–109. https://dx.doi.org/10.11622%2Fsmedj.2016049

Alaoui, S. 2020. Virus simulation helped Bhutan prevent COVID-19 deaths. United Nations Foundation. https://unfoundation.org/blog/post/virus-simulation-helped-bhutan-prevent-covid-19-deaths/

Ali, I. 2021. Rituals of containment: Many pandemics, body politics, and social dramas during COVID-19 in Pakistan. *Frontiers in Sociology* 6: 648149. doi:10.3389/fsoc.2021.6481

Dasgupta, D. 2021. Tiny Himalayan nation Bhutan shows how to fight COVID-19 pandemic. *The Straits Times.* www.straitstimes.com/asia/south-asia/tiny-himalayan-nation-shows-how-to-fight-pandemic

Dorji, T., and Tamang, S. T. 2021. Bhutan's experience with COVID-19 vaccination in 2021. *BMJ Global Health* 6(5). https://doi.org/10.1136/bmjgh-2021-005977

Geertz, C. 1973 *The Interpretation of Cultures*. New York: Basic Books.

Kuensel. 2015, February 19. Tendrel. https://kuenselonline.com/tendrel/

Kuensel. 2020, March 6. First confirmed Coronavirus case in Bhutan. https://kuenselonline.com/first-confirmed-coronavirus-case-in-bhutan/

Kugelman, M. 2021. The COVID-19 success story you never knew about. *Arab News.* www.arabnews.com/node/1817311

Lin, X., Rocha, I. C. N., Shen, X., Ahmadi, A., Lucero-Prisno, D. E. 2021. Challenges and strategies in controlling COVID-19 in Mainland China: Lessons for future public health emergencies. *Journal of Social Health* 4(2): 57–61.

Mathieu, E., Ritchie, H., Ortiz-Ospina, E., Roser, M., Hasell, J., Appel, C., et al. 2021. A global database of COVID-19 vaccinations. *Natural Human Behaviour.* https://doi.org/10.1038/s41562-021-01122-8

Meier, B.M., and Chakrabarti, A. 2016. The paradox of happiness: Health and human rights in the Kingdom of Bhutan. *Health and Human Rights Journal* 18(1): 193–208. www.hhrjournal.org/2016/04/the-paradox-of-happiness-health-and-human-rights-in-the-kingdom-of-bhutan/

Ministry of Health. 2020. Annual Health Bulletin. Thimphu: Policy and Planning Division, Ministry of Health. www.moh.gov.bt/wp-content/uploads/ict-files/2017/06/health-bulletin-Website_Final.pdf

National Statistics Bureau. 2020. *Bhutan at a Glance 2020*. www.nsb.gov.bt/publications/insights/bhutan-at-a-glance/

Palden, T. 2020a. March 21. Listen to health experts: His Holiness the Je Khenpo. *Kuensel*. https://kuenselonline.com/listen-to-health-experts-his-holiness-the-je-khenpo/

Palden, T. 2020b. August 12. Woman tests Covid-19 positive after five tests locking down entire country. *Kuensel*. https://kuenselonline.com/woman-test-covid-19-positive-after-five-tests-locking-down-entire-country/

Rocha, I. C. N., Pelayo, M. G. A., Rackimuthu, S. 2021. Kumbh Mela religious gathering as a massive superspreading event: Potential culprit for the exponential surge of COVID-19 cases in India. *The American Journal of Tropical Medicine and Hygiene* 105(4): 868–871. https://doi.org/10.4269/ajtmh.21-0601

Rocha, I.C.N., Hasan, M.M., Goyal, S., Patel, T., Jain, S., Ghosh, A., et al. 2021. COVID-19 and mucormycosis syndemic: Double health threat to a collapsing healthcare system in India. *Tropical Medicine and International Health*. https://doi.org/10.1111/tmi.13641

Thinley, S., Tshering, P., Wangmo, K., Wangchuk, N., Dorji, T., Tobgay, T., et al. 2017. The Kingdom of Bhutan health system review. *Health Systems in Transition* 7(2). https://apps.who.int/iris/bitstream/handle/10665/255701/9789290225843-eng.pdf?sequence=1&isAllowed=y

Turner, M. 2020. Bhutan's decisive response to COVID-19. *East Asia Forum*. www.eastasiaforum.org/2020/11/06/bhutans-decisive-response-to-covid-19/

World Health Organization. 2020. Invest in preparedness – Health emergency readiness lessons from Bhutan. www.who.int/news-room/feature-stories/detail/invest-in-preparedness-health-emergency-readiness-lessons-from-bhutan

World Health Organization. 2021. Bhutan: WHO coronavirus disease (COVID-19) dashboard with vaccination data. https://covid19.who.int/region/searo/country/bt

14 Negotiating India During the COVID-19 Crisis

Issues and Challenges

Suman Chakrabarty

Introduction: India's Second Wave

As I write (May 2021), India is experiencing its second wave of the coronavirus pandemic, with devastating public health crises occurring across its 29 states, unions and seven territories. The central as well as state bureaucracies completely failed to prevent this deadly second wave, due to a shortage of vaccines and other factors, even after giving a so-called "Best Effort" to contain the spread of this "unknown enemy of human existence" (Biswas 2021). It is evident that there can be phases of pandemic spread: a century ago, the influenza epidemic of 1918 caused more deaths in its second wave than in its first (Hardiman 2012). At the end of 2020, the Indian government insisted that the pandemic had been controlled, largely due to the government's preventive actions, which were taken before COVID-19 reached its more advanced stages (Sharma and Veer 2020). This overly optimistic belief proved to be unfounded: the new mutated variant B.1617, which originated in India, rapidly spread across the country and the world (Roberts 2021).

By May 3, 2021, the total number of COVID-19 cases in India had reached well over 20 million (as compared to 0.15 million total cases a year before, in May 2020), with over 16 million recoveries, a case fatality rate of 0.56%, and with 0.4 million cases occurring daily (GI 2021). India is the largest South Asian country by physical area and population—1.37 billion—with enormous ethno-linguistic and cultural diversities involving caste, religion, and multiple social groups (Joshua Project 2018). The impacts of the COVID-19 crisis on the different ethnic groups living in diverse geographical areas and their responses have varied significantly. In spite of this diversity, COVID-19 has created a common ground that has brought all sections of the Indian communities to the negotiating table to engage in crisis management (Alfredson and Cungu 2008). When I critically examined the crisis dynamics related to COVID-19 in India, I found that the issues and challenges are multidimensional in nature—as also suggested by Inayat Ali (2021). He noted that COVID-19 is far more than a medical pandemic; it has also created an "economic pandemic," a "social pandemic," a "structural pandemic," an "emotional/psychological pandemic," and a

DOI: 10.4324/9781003187462-18

"political pandemic." And in the Introduction to this volume, its editors added to these the "infodemic" and "the misinformation pandemic," which stem, as they note, "from the overwhelming amounts of information and misinformation spread daily through multiple types of media." All of these pandemics are at play in India.

The first COVID-19 reported case in India occurred on January 30, 2020 in Kerala. Thermal screenings in airports began on March 3, 2020; the first cancellation of railway services (the lifelines of India) was on March 22, 2020; and the first complete lockdown began on March 25, 2020 and was extended up to May 3, 2020. Therefore, as elsewhere, within 2–3 months of India's first case, serious and unexpected restrictions forced almost everyone to negotiate the risks of unfamiliar everyday life amid COVID-19. As an Indian myself, I feel that the strength of our people's fighting spirit comes not only from our multiple efforts to maintain our physical wellbeing, but also through practicing various overlapping stages of psychosocial and behavioral processes. An attitude of willingness to negotiate is one of these. Negotiations around COVID-19 have primarily occurred at the national level, and have also been active at regional and local levels through socio-cultural, economic, and political processes. Encompassing India's diversity, this present study aims to understand the issues and challenges of negotiated behaviors at both the macro and micro levels among various segments of the Indian population, including its "Scheduled Tribes," during the COVID-19 crisis.

Methods and Materials

For the study on which this chapter is based, I used both secondary and primary data. To obtain the secondary data, I carried out a literature review by using the key word "COVID-19," combined with "lockdown," "migration," "education," "poverty," "healthcare," "food security," "national health mission," "public health," "vaccination," and "India" on PubMed and Google Scholar from March 2020 to April 2021. I also carried out a manual search for relevant materials, and examined articles from several non-academic sources (e.g. news, websites, etc.). I collected qualitative primary data through telephone conversations and WhatsApp messaging with seven key interlocutors from April 9–22, 2020 (as used by Drabble et al. 2016). I obtained verbal consent from all interlocutors prior to this survey. I chose my key interlocutors on the basis of rapport from previous fieldwork that I had conducted for the last three years in the eastern and northeastern parts of India, mainly in tribal-dominated villages (Chakrabarty 2019a, b). Wishing to encompass at least some of India's diversity in my research for this chapter, I included interlocutors from Indian Indigenous groups called "Scheduled Tribes"—the *Santal* from *Purulia* district, the *Bodo* and the *Rabha* from the Alipurduar districts of West Bengal State, and the *Shabar* from rural areas of Odisha State. For northeast India, I interviewed representatives of the *Khasi* from Meghayala and the *Hmar* from the Dima Hasao district of Assam state.

These communities beg at least some brief descriptions here. The Santals constitute the largest Indigenous population in eastern India. They belong to the Austro-Asiatic language family and its Mundari-speaking group. They generally live in the forested mountainous and plateau areas of the Purulia District of West Bengal State. Their patriarchal society has its own distinct culture, traditions, religion, festivals, and a strong ethnic identity; their subsistence strategy is primarily agricultural. The Bodo, also agricultural and patriarchal, are the most populous Indigenous group in the Assam State of India; some also live in the northern part of West Bengal State. They have their own Bodo language, which belongs to Tibeto-Burman language family. They generally live in the foothills of the sub-Himalayan region of West Bengal and practice settled agriculture. The agricultural Rabha are likely the most autochthonous Indigenous group in India; they live in North and West Bengal. Their language is of the Indo-Mongoloid family, and they traditionally practice a matrilineal inheritance pattern and are relatively gender-egalitarian. In North Bengal, they occupy the forest fringe villages of Jaldapara and Buxa national parks. They have their own dialect and culture, yet at present their culture has greatly been influenced by Christianity. The Shabar are the most widely distributed Indigenous group in Eastern Odisha state in India. They speak the regional Oriya language and inhabit urban, rural, and forest areas. Most practice agriculture in rural areas. Linguistically, they belong to the Austro-Asiatic family; they traditionally practice a patrilineal inheritance pattern and thus are highly patriarchal.

The Hmar constitute a segment of the Chin-Kuki-Mizo group living in the Northeastern states of India, including Meghalaya, Mizoram, the Dima Hasao District of Assam, and Tripura. Hmars are of Mongoloid stock and are patriarchal. Though the Hmar tribal community is divided into exogamous clans, they do not strictly adhere to exogamy. In the Dima Hasao district, their culture is deeply influenced by Christianity. The Khasi are the best-known matrilineal Indigenous group in India. They live in Meghalaya State in northeast India and are the most populous group there. They mainly occupy West Khasi and the East Khasi hills. Despite their formerly strong cultural heritage, most of them have converted to Christianity. They speak a Mon-Khmer language of the Austro-Asiatic stock. They live on hilly slopes and depend primarily on cultivation. Later on in this chapter, I will describe the impacts of the multiple coronavirus pandemics on these particular groups. First, I begin with descriptions of COVID-related negotiations at the national and state levels.

Negotiations at the National Level

After the initial national lockdown was eased in early May 2020, due to the shortage of PPE (personal protective equipment) and ventilators, Indian officials negotiated the procurement of essential medical and protective supplies from China in hope of decreasing the rising infection rate (Aneja 2020). In contrast, although India had stopped the export of the anti-malaria drug hydroxychloroquine in the last week of March 2020, due to negotiations with high-resource countries such as the USA under President Trump, who widely promoted hydroxychloroquine (see Penkala-Gawęcka, this volume), India withdrew the restriction (Hindu 2020a). Meanwhile, border tensions between India and China remain unsolved even after well-meaning efforts and negotiations by both countries' diplomats (Levesques 2020).

Apart from negotiations through diplomatic relationships between India and other countries, the central government has also negotiated with different sectors of the Indian population who have been heavily burdened in their lives and livelihoods during the COVID-19 crisis. What I am calling the *culture of negotiation* between the government and its citizens started nationwide during lockdown with the televised lighting of a lamp on April 5, 2020 at 9pm for 9 minutes by Narendra Modi, the Prime Minister of India. This shared event was full of diversity: across religions (Hindu, Muslim, Christian, others) and castes in India, most citizens participated in that occasion, praying to their respective Gods and Goddesses in order to negotiate and mediate this crisis via their own religious beliefs and cultural constructions of COVID-19 (Hindu 2020b).

Regarding the "economic pandemic" generated by the coronavirus pandemic, the government negotiated the reform of the agricultural sector, and announced a COVID-19 economic relief package called *Atmanirbhar Bharat* (Self-Reliant India) totaling about $270 billion US, equal to 10% of the country's GDP in May 2020 (Dev 2020). Prior to that, on March 26, 2020, the Ministry of Finance announced a $1.7 trillion package under the *Pradhan Mantri Garib Kalyan Yojana* (PMGKY—the Prime Minister's Welfare Program for the Poor) for below-poverty-line families and other targeted groups, with an aim to provide cash incentives and free rations to them for the next three months (PIB 2020). Yet the economic crisis then started anyway, when approximately 120 million Indians lost their jobs in April 2020 alone due to lockdown, as noted by the Center for Monitoring the Indian Economy (Hindu 2020c). A survey conducted by the Statista Research Department showed that the average Indian household income dipped by a whopping 45.7% from February to April 2020 (SRD 2020).

Unfortunately, despite its efforts, India's response to the COVID-19-induced economic crisis is proving to be ineffective (Chandrasekhar 2020). Negotiation has fallen short in some specific vulnerable areas, such as the Indian textiles industry; e-learning education mainly for underprivileged and rural children; maintaining an appropriate food supply chain; informal workers; migrants in cities; farmers; and small businesses (see Chapter 11, this volume). There are also deficiencies in adequate salaries and trainings for approximately 900,000 community health workers, called Accredited Social Health Activists (ASHAs). India has also witnessed a great deal of gender-based violence and discrimination; the stigmatization of Muslims, doctors and medical staff dealing with COVID-19; and of *Dalits* (those who are considered to be "lower caste"), who are stigmatized and discriminated against for their "untouchable" occupational patterns. (They are often employed as sanitation workers, cleaners of drains, garbage collectors, and road sweepers.) Also vulnerable are India's insufficient basic infrastructure and its IT sector, among others (Singh et al. 2020; Bhamoriya et al. 2020; Jha 2020; Chinchwadkar and Kathuria 2020; Pandey et al. 2020; Swaroop and Lee 2021; Kanupriya 2021).

Therefore, I suggest that negotiations should be focused on strengthening multi-sectoral coordinations among home affairs, education, revenue, civil supplies, transport, water supply and sanitation, labor, agriculture, social welfare, information technology, and so on. In addition, negotiations should be strengthened at regional and state levels to improve healthcare resource availability and accessibility, and to create a robust surveillance system to monitor: multi-sectoral coordination; healthcare worker fatigue and burnout; the increased financial burdens and the other effects of lockdown on mental health status; dissemination of accurate information about effective COVID-19 preventive measures; the patient-bed ratio; and the costs of testing and treatment (Saya et al. 2020). Many who migrated for work internally from Uttar Pradesh, Bihar, Odisha, West Bengal (eastern and central Indian states) and northeastern Indian states to Delhi, Kerala, Maharashtra, Punjab, Gujarat and the Southern states faced problems such as lack of food, basic amenities, and health care; economic stress; and lack of transportation facilities to return to their native locales (Bhagat et al. 2020). India's population diversities and multidimensional resource problems have generated formidable challenges for effectively navigating and negotiating COVID-19 at the national level (Bajpai 2014).

Negotiations at the State Level

Within India, negotiation is an ongoing process between central and state governments, and negotiations regarding COVID-19 management among political powers vary by state. The supply of testing kits and other medical equipment, announcement of the duration of lockdown, selection of containment zones, and the online formal education system and its evaluation process remain major issues in which negotiations, as always, have played a vital role. Since the pandemic's beginnings, differences in political ideologies and pragmatic orientations have been generating mutual tensions between the central and most state governments. Kumar (2020) contested the excessive centralization, "lawless lawmaking," and non-consultative decision-making processes at the national government level of COVID-19 management. States have been disempowered and major decisions have been made by the national Ministry of Home Affairs (MHA) with little input from other Ministries, departments, or state governments.

Although public health management is a state responsibility, nevertheless, the central government has made itself solely responsible for designing health policy and planning in India during COVID-19. On the other hand, the central government did take advice from national agencies like the National Center for Disease Control, the National Health System Resources Center, and the Indian Council for Medical Research (ICMR). However, a World Bank report entitled "India's Public Health System: How Well Does It Function at the National Level?" (Das Gupta and Rani 2004) stated that implementation of the research findings of central agencies had become a challenge due to the lack of technical capacity at sub-national levels. This indicated that the benefits of health research are not effectively reaching those responsible for planning and implementation (ibid.). Thus, the COVID-19 situation has exposed the major shortcomings of the majority of Indian states in terms of budgetary deficits, lack of technical expertise for institutional management, and capacity constraints. The tension this situation has created between the central government and the states has often led to a culture of blame rather than to fruitful negotiation (The Print 2020).

The most exceptional state was Kerala. At the early stage of the Covidian crisis, the state government was successful in managing COVID-19 by reducing its spread and achieving high recovery and low case fatality rates. This success was made possible due to the state government's prior investments in its public healthcare system and its high levels of community participation, volunteer engagement, and awareness generation through radio and in local languages. Local governments were actively involved in these pandemic mitigation efforts (Isaac and Sadanandan 2020). On the other hand, there is a huge gap between the creation and implementation of knowledge and understandings about COVID-19 in national policy, and knowledge uptake and negotiation at the village level. Most rural and older villagers gathered knowledge from literate neighbors who are also village council (*panchayat*) members; whereas younger people often relied for information on social media (via mobile phone, WhatsApp, Facebook, and others). The information obtained by both generations was often misleading at best and completely incorrect at worst, as also found by Vrega and Bode (2021) and by many of the chapter authors. In this context, and as suggested by Vijayan (2020), I argue for the need to develop strong, trustworthy and organic relationships among national and state governments and local people. *Negotiations cannot be effective when they are based on misinformation.*

Micro-Level Understandings with Special Reference to Indian Tribes

The pandemic crisis in India has significantly affected all communities, particularly members of vulnerable social groups, including those living below the poverty line, elders, persons with disabilities, children, and Indigenous peoples. Despite meticulous "rituals of containment" (Ali 2021a) at national and state levels to deal effectively with the COVID-19 crisis, local and micro-level communities have suffered the most, and have tried to negotiate this crisis among themselves. People in such communities have been negotiating with each other and with their local and regional governments around whether or not to follow safety measures such as wearing masks, handwashing, and physical distancing. Many have chosen and are choosing not to comply, in some cases due to their lack of accurate information about the severity of the disease resulting from ineffective governmental education measures, and in others due to outright misinformation. Other types of negotiations occurred between landless migratory laborers and their employers around their daily wages, yet the employers would not compromise, so these workers have had to compromise their physical and mental health to keep on working in order to feed themselves and their families. Also adversely affected have been those who experienced discharge from their previous jobs or salary cuts due to COVID-19.

In general, COVID-19 and the succeeding lockdown threatened the livelihoods of tribal members and forest dwellers, according to a joint preliminary assessment report, which had been submitted to the Ministry of Tribal Affairs during first week of May 2020 by the Community Forest Rights-Learning and Advocacy (CFR-LA), the All India Forum of Forest Movements (AIFFM), and other rights groups (Newsclick 2020). This threat was likely since most of the forest-dwelling Indigenous groups depended for approximately 60% of their incomes on annual collection of Minor Forest Produce (MFP) or Non-Timber Forest Produce (NTFP), including bamboo, brush wood, stumps, cane, cocoons, honey, wax, lac, *tendu* or *kendu* leaves, medicinal plants and herbs, roots, and tubers, which takes place annually between April and June. For two years now, these periods have coincided with lockdowns, meaning restrictions on the movements needed to do this sort of work, from collecting the products to selling them in nearby markets—primarily in the central and eastern parts of India. As a result, incomes from the selling of NTFPs declined, these tribal groups fell into food insecurity, and their remote geographical locations, poor infrastructure, malnutrition, and existing morbidities made them more susceptible to COVID-19 infection (Behera and Dassani 2021). Nevertheless, the infection rates among them have remained surprisingly low.

By August 2020, only 3% of tribal members had been infected nationwide. The Ministry of Tribal Affairs took on the challenges of ensuring the wellbeing of the tribal populations, in part by limiting viral spread among them. Ministry members tried to build awareness among these groups and to provide masks and essential supplies (ALEKH 2020), as their subsistence activities do not produce a surplus that can serve as a backup in financially challenging times. Some tribal women who had to travel to various villages to sell their products were stigmatized by being labeled as "coronavirus carriers" (Wakharde 2021). However, one study reported that some tribal members have successfully negotiated challenges to their livelihoods in various forms. For example, the women vendors from the Tribal Market Complex in Imphal, Manipur State, negotiated among themselves during COVID-19 to reduce participation in the market and also to minimize the selling of various goods to their customers (Haokip et al. 2020).

My primary data as collected from the Indigenous groups I have described above showed that they conceptualized and assimilated the uncertain disease conditions, negotiating them via their religious beliefs and their cultural constructions of disease. Initially, all of the studied groups had misinterpreted the emergence of the novel coronavirus by conceptualizing it as part of preexisting diseases such as the common cough and cold, and seasonal flu. And many of these groups, such as the Bodo tribes of north Bengal, have relied heavily on their religious beliefs to negotiate COVID, such as increasing their worship of the village deity, Lord Shiva, locally termed as *Shijou*. Lord Shiva is the primary God in Hindu mythology. Hindus believe that his powers of destruction and recreation are used even now to destroy the illusions and imperfections of this world, paving the way for beneficial change. In addition, every Bodo household performed rituals of the worship of the goddess *Khasuli* (the goddess of coughs and colds) and *Chakha* (the goddess of pneumonia), believing that pleasing these goddesses would overcome the crisis, and reflecting their general understanding of COVID-19 as akin to these diseases. Such rituals were generally performed both at the village and household levels. But during the pandemic, this use of ritual was intensified—as generally occurs during crises (see Davis-Floyd and Laughlin 2022). A group of villagers repeatedly performed these ceremonies on the bank of the river adjacent to the village. They offered eggs and pounded rice flour by floating them on the river. In addition, to treat the symptoms of what they saw as "pneumonia," tribal members have used their traditional medicines such as extract of ginger (*Zingiber moiga*) mixed with honey; the juice of the *vasaka* flower (*Justicia adhatoda*) mixed with honey or fried with onions; and the juice from the leaves of Asian pigeonwings (*Clitoria ternatea*), and have encouraged others to do the same.

Similar rituals have been performed by the Santal villagers of the Purulia District of West Bengal; all villages have their distinct community place of worship, called *Jaher Than*. As I collected data from various villages, I observed that *every* Santal village of Purulia District had begun performing the worship of the deities *Marang-buru and Jaher-era*[1] in the traditional *Jaher-than* (sacred grove), starting immediately after the lockdown. They prayed together to their traditional gods and goddess to save them from this unknown disease, and promised to perform a grand feast and worship in their *Jaher-than* once the situation was under control. After one year, when I visited them again, I noted that they had not as yet performed that grand feast because the pandemic situation was not yet under control.

Although religious beliefs vary among the Rabha people of North Bengal and the Khasi and Hmar people from northeast India, most of them are Christians; hence local churches have played significant roles in directing their behaviors around and perceptions of the COVID-19 crisis. Initially, group church prayers were performed to ask for God's blessing. Then, via a productive negotiation process, their community leader (the head man of the village), along with government officials and the priest of the local church, decided to postpone community prayers in the church for the next two months, specifically the Sunday prayers. In another example of fruitful negotiation, the *Arr-Rinam* ritual was performed by the members of the Galo tribe of Arunachal Pradesh, a state bordering northeast India and China. The Galo community member whom I interviewed explained that Arr-Rinam is the Galo equivalent of lockdown; the difference is that it is imposed by societal consensus rather than government mandate whenever an epidemic strikes (Karmakar 2020). In this way, the Galo have managed to syncretically assimilate their perceptions of this new disease into their cultural value and belief system.

In addition to the ritualistic behaviors of the communities under study, I noted the cooperation and sense of belongingness among the Hmar tribes of northeast India, where local NGOs (non-governmental organizations) and the Hmar Students' Association have been providing food to those who need it, as has the local church, due to the fact that the free rations from the national government were not enough for all in this rural and remote Hmar community in Dima Hasao District. However, I did not find these kinds of positive Covidian negotiating attitudes among the Shabar in Odisha state, where the rice and money distributed to the economically poor were not sufficient and were unequally distributed. These micro-level negotiations and actions, when successful, illustrate how tribal members build trust, promote community participation in COVID-19 control, and provide meaningful healthcare management via the use of existing, or the creation of new, local cultural models of negotiation, which will stand them in good stead should another epidemic or pandemic arrive (Ennis-McMillan and Hedges 2020).

Traditionally, stigma and so-called "othering" have not been common features among Indian tribal peoples. However, due to the influence of urbanization and close contact with other non-tribal peoples, they have by now developed some forms of stigmatization within their own communities, such as around HIV infection and tuberculosis (Vlassoff et al. 2012; Joseph et al. 2019). In contrast, they are often the victims of stigmatization and "otherization" from their non-tribal counterparts (Kharshiing 2020). In a previous study, Bhanot et al. (2020) observed racial and ethnic discrimination and stigmatization across the country. Yet in my current study, I did not see any COVID-19 related stigma against tribal groups, since there is rarely any evidence of COVID-19 infection among the studied communities.

Because the coronavirus originated in China, people who appeared to be Chinese suffered the deepest forms of discrimination, according to Suhas Chakma, Director of the Rights and Risks Analysis Group (RRAG)—an independent think-tank based in New Delhi, India. He stated that India's

Mongoloid-looking people were called "coronavirus," "Chinese," and *Chinki*. They were forced to leave restaurants to make others comfortable and to endure the fact that no one wanted to share transport with them; spat on; forcibly quarantined despite showing no COVID-19 symptoms; denied entry into their apartment complexes; and sometimes forced to leave their apartments or threatened with eviction (Chakma 2020). There was no negotiation here, just ill-informed resentment and stigmatization. The desire to blame someone for this global crisis is often strong: the Chinese, or even people who look like they might be Chinese, are held guilty by association—in India and elsewhere.

In order to minimize the spread of infectious diseases, it is of course essential that public health administrators clearly communicate the need for preventive measures—such as good hygiene behaviors like handwashing, physical distancing, and cleaning surfaces—to all citizens, including rural and remote tribal people, through mass media and other feasible ways. It is also important to honor efficacious local remedies. For example, tribal groups from the Kandhamal District of Odisha State in India were using *Sal* (*Shorea robusta*) leaf masks made of leaves from the Sal evergreen tree as protection from COVID-19, due to the shortage of cloth masks during the initial crisis (*Sambad* English Bureau 2020). During this crisis, social group belongingness, strong kinship cohesiveness, and belief in traditional healers seem to have put them in an advantageous position.

Negotiations between tribal peoples and their local governance appear vital for obtaining long term and sustainable preventive equipment against COVID-19. Due to the rural and remote locations of the Indian tribal communities, respective Village Councils (*Panchayat*) and local police stations can be seen to play a crucial role in generating civic awareness and monitoring lockdown within these communities, yet I found that this role was too limited. In the absence of official help from above, their reliance on religious activities to protect their community and prevent viral spread increased greatly, along with the use of their Indigenous methods of healing and maintaining health and negotiations through community participation. These measures undoubtedly helped them to cope with the multiple stresses induced by the pandemic far more than the Panchayat and the police.

An Overview of COVID-19 Vaccination in India: Differences and Shortages

Approximately 10 months after the imposition of its first lockdown, India began administering COVID-19 vaccines on January 16, 2021, in an effort to vaccinate 300 million high-risk people, such as the elderly and people with co-morbidities, by the end of July 2021. As of May 2, 2021, India had administered nearly 150 million doses of COVID-19 vaccines; 120 million people had received their first dose and 30 million had also received the second dose. Yet these seemingly high numbers account for only around 12% of the population. Most of those vaccinated (88%) have been 45 or older; men have slightly outnumbered women; and these numbers vary among Indian states (GI 2021). Two companies in India are producing COVID-19 vaccines. Serum Institute of India, based in Pune, was working with AstraZeneca to produce Covishield; Bharat Biotech, based in Hyderabad, was given a manufacturing license from the Indian Council of Medical Research (ICMR) to produce Covaxin (DTE 2021). More of those who have been vaccinated have received the Covishield vaccine than the Covaxin vaccine. Yet despite being one of the world's largest vaccine suppliers, India faced vaccine shortages during March 2021 and negotiated to halt exports temporarily (Padma 2021). At present, several Indian states have run out of vaccines against COVID-19, exacerbating a dire second wave of infections that left hospitals and morgues overflowing while families scrambled for increasingly scarce medicines and oxygen. Therefore, Indian governments (both central and state) have been in ongoing processes of negotiating vaccines in terms of availability, accessibility, and public acceptance (Brunson and Schoch-Spana 2021).

Public acceptance—or the lack thereof—is a major challenge to vaccine uptake in India due to large differences in knowledge and attitudes towards vaccination in general (Cvjetkovic, Jeremic, and Tirosavljevic 2017). When I inquired about acceptance of COVID-19 vaccination among the urban Indian population, my interlocutors often asked if they could even get the vaccine, given the national shortage. Some who had received their first dose worried that they might not receive the second dose should this shortage continue. Others, especially in rural areas, expressed vaccine hesitancy and often outright resistance, stemming in part from the spread of the news that by March 29, 2021, 180 people in India had died after vaccination against COVID-19, though no direct causal link has been found (Scroll 2021). Thus it is easy to see how, based on this accurate information, many rumors have been generated among villagers that COVID-19 vaccination can result in death. And I found that villagers from the Purulia District of West Bengal are very afraid that getting the vaccine will cause them to test positive for COVID-19. As a result, I observed that even after developing symptoms similar to those of COVID-19, these villagers refused to report those symptoms to the appropriate authorities, fearing that they might die in the still-underprepared healthcare system. Clearly, there is enormous mistrust of the government, especially among India's tribal and village populations. Therefore, collectively negotiating trust in healthcare personnel and in biomedical facilities remains a significant challenge to stopping the pandemic in India. In this context, Gupta and Baru (2020) rightly argued that transparency and full information will be required to ethically increase vaccine update in India and to negotiate effective future policymaking for the vast and diverse Indian population.

Conclusion: India's Culture of Negotiation

In this chapter, I have described the *culture of negotiation* in India among various governmental levels and their citizens. To illustrate this culture of negotiation, I discussed the issues and challenges of negotiated behaviors at both the macro and micro levels among the Indian population during the COVID-19 crisis, from the initiation of the pandemic to the administrations of vaccines. At the micro level, I gave special attention to varying Indigenous peoples and their internal and external negotiations around COVID-19, showing the efficacy of their cooperative methods and demonstrating their reliance on religion and on their traditional healers and healing methods, which likely do no harm, surely generate a sense of confidence, and may be efficacious in preventing viral contraction and/or treating symptoms. At the macro level, I described national, state, and local governmental negotiations around COVID-19 and how best to control its spread.

To recap, despite the existence of two COVID vaccines in India, the country is at this time of writing (May 2021) suffering a destructive second wave, this time of an even more dangerous mutated virus, B.1617. Thus, there is enormous uncertainty regarding how long this pandemic crisis will last and how much more damage it will do to the life and livelihoods of the Indian people. Reaching mutual understandings and agreements on actions to be taken will require strengthening the negotiation processes between central, state, and local governments, and among laypeople. The country's massive diversities can make these challenges seem overwhelming. Nevertheless, within India's culture of negotiation, stronger linkages among national, state, district, block, village *panchayat,* and village level administrations should be prioritized in every state. I suggest that these linkages should negotiate existing forms of disparities, poverty reduction for the marginalized migrant workers and for Indigenous groups, re-forming the health care infrastructure, and performing smooth and ethical vaccine administration by generating community participation and consensus on the importance of vaccine uptake.

Note

1 Marang-buru and Jaher-era are considered as God and Goddess of traditional Santal rituals. These are two *Sal* trees (*Shorea robusta*) planted in a row in the Santal Sacred Grove. These are the principal deities of Santal, worshipped in various community festivals and rituals.

References

ALEKH (A Learning Endeavour for Knowledge in Healthcare). 2020. *COVID-19 response in the tribal regions of India.* Ministry of Tribal Affairs, Government of India. Vol. 1. https://tribal.nic.in/downloads/Swasthya/ALEKH_Edition1_Aug%2020.pdf

Alfredson T., and A. Cungu. 2008. *Negotiation Theory and Practice. A Review of the Literature.* EASYPol Module 179. FAO. www.fao.org/easypol

Ali, I. 2021. Rituals of containment: Many pandemics, body politics, and social dramas during COVID-19 in Pakistan. *Frontiers in Sociology* 6: 648149. https://doi.org/10.3389/fsoc.2021.648149

Aneja, A. 2020. Coronavirus: India in negotiations with China on much-needed medical supplies. www.thehindu.com/news/national/coronavirus-india-in-negotiations-with-china-on-much-needed-medical-supplies/article31287923.ece

Bajpai, V. 2014. The Challenges Confronting Public Hospitals in India, Their Origins, and Possible Solutions. *Advances in Public Health* 898502. https://doi.org/10.1155/2014/898502

Behera M., and P. Dassani. 2021. Livelihood vulnerabilities of tribals during covid-19 challenges and policy measures. *Economic and Political Weekly* LVI(11): 19–22.

Bhagat, R.B., R.S. Reshmi, H. Sahoo, A.K. Roy, and D. Govil. 2020. The COVID-19, migration and livelihood in India: Challenges and policy issues. *Migration Letters* 17(5): 705–718.

Bhamoriya, A.V., P. Gupta, M. Kaushik, A. Kishore, R. Kumar, A. Sharma, et al. 2020. India's food system in the time of covid-19. *Economic and Political Weekly* LV(15): 12–14.

Bhanot, D., T. Singh, Sk. Verma, and S. Sharad. 2020. Stigma and discrimination during COVID-19 pandemic. *Frontiers in Public Health* 8: 577018. doi: 10.3389/fpubh.2020.577018

Biswas, S. 2021. Covid-19: How India failed to prevent a deadly second wave www.bbc.com/news/world-asia-india-56771766

Brunson, E., and M. Schoch-Spana. 2021. What makes vaccines social? *Sapiens.* www.sapiens.org/culture/vaccines-anthropology/

Chakma, S. 2020. Coronavirus pandemic: India's mongoloid looking people face upsurge of racism. www.rightsrisks.org/by-country/india/coronavirus-pandemic-indias-mongoloid-looking-people-face-upsurge-of-racism/

Chakrabarty, S. 2019a. "Socio-Economic Inequalities and Food Security among the Rabha Tribe Living in Fringe Forest Areas of North Bengal." In U.K. Dey and M. Pal (eds.), *Development and Deprivation in the Indian Subcontinent,* 369–385. Kolkata: Levant Books.

Chakrabarty, S. 2019b. Rehabilitation and Tribal Health Status: A Case Study among the Shabar tribe in Odisha, India. In R. Ray (ed.), *Tribal Health Care System: A Tribute to P.O. Bodding,* 263–278. Kolkata: The Asiatic Society.

Chandrasekhar, C.P. 2020. A faulty response to the covid-19-induced crisis. *Economic and Political Weekly* LV(37): 10–12.

Chinchwadkar, R., and V. Kathuria. 2020. Post-COVID-19 challenges in the Indian IT industry. *Economic and Political Weekly* LV(42): 17–20.

Cvjetkovic, S.J., V.L. Jeremic, and D.V. Tirosavljevic. 2017. Knowledge and attitudes toward vaccination: A survey of Serbian students. *Journal of Infection and Public Health* 10: 649–656.

Das Gupta, M., and M. Rani. 2004. India's Public Health System How Well Does It Function at the National Level? World Bank Policy Research Working Paper 3447. https://openknowledge.worldbank.org/bitstream/handle/10986/14215/WPS3447.pdf?sequence=1&isAllowed=y

Davis-Floyd, R., and C.F. Laughlin. 2022. *Ritual: What It Is, How It Works, and Why.* New York: Berghahn Books.

Dev, M. 2020. COVID-19 crisis: An opportunity for long-delayed agricultural reforms in India. IFPRI Blog, Guest Post. www.ifpri.org/blog/covid-19-crisis-opportunity-long-delayed-agricultural-reforms-india

Down To Earth (DTE). 2021. A dose of truth: The real story of India's COVID-19 vaccination programme. www.downtoearth.org.in/news/health/a-dose-of-truth-the-real-story-of-india-s-covid-19-vaccination-programme-76548

Drabble, L., F.T. Karen, S. Brenda, P.C. Walker, and R.A. Korcha. 2016. Conducting qualitative interviews by telephone: Lessons learned from a study of alcohol use among sexual minority and heterosexual women. *Quality Social Work* 15: 118–133. https://doi.org/10.1177/1473325015585613

Ennis-McMillan, M.C., and K. Hedges. 2020. Pandemic perspective: Response to COVID-19. *Open Anthropology* 8 www.americananthro.org/StayInformed/OAArticleDetail.aspx?ItemNumber=25631&utm_source=informz&utm_medium=email&utm_campaign=cta.

Geographic Insights (GI). 2021. *Harvard Center for Population and Development Studies. Center for Geographic Analysis.* Cambridge, MA. https://geographicinsights.iq.harvard.edu/

Gupta, I., and R. Baru. 2020. Economics and ethics of the covid-19 vaccine: How prepared are we? *Indian Journal of Medical Research* 152: 153–155.

Haokip, H., A. Haokip, and T. Gangte. 2020. Negotiating livelihood during Covid-19 urban tribal women vendors of Manipur. *Economic and Political Weekly* LV(46): 19–22.

Hardiman, D. 2012. The influenza epidemic of 1918 and the *Adivasis* of western India. *Social History of Medicine* 25(3): 644–664.

Hindu. 2020a. India lifts export ban on hydroxychloroquine. www.thehindu.com/news/national/india-lifts-export-ban-on-hydroxychloroquine/article31806635.ece

Hindu 2020b. Coronavirus: PM lights lamp as nation joins hands against virus. www.thehindu.com/news/national/coronavirus-pm-lights-lamp-as-nation-joins-hands-against-virus/article31264682.ece

Hindu. 2020c. Data: An Estimated 12.2 Crore Indians Lost Their Jobs during the Coronavirus Lockdown in April, CMIE, May 7, www.thehindu.com/data/dataover-12-crore-indians-lost-their-jobs-duringthe-coronavirus-lockdown-in-april/article31520715.ece

Isaac, T.T.M., and R. Sadanandan. 2020. COVID-19, public health system and local governance in Kerala. *Economic and Political Weekly* LV(21): 35–40.

Jha, A. 2020. COVID-19 relief package will central largesse help construction workers? *Economic and Political Weekly* LV(17): 20–22.

Joseph, A., A. Kumar, I. Krishnan, and A. Anilkumar. 2019. The tribal community's perception on tuberculosis: A community based qualitative study in Tamil Nadu, India. *Journal of Family Medicine and Primary Care* 8: 3236–3241. www.jfmpc.com/temp/JFamMedPrimaryCare8103236-4279506_115315.pdf

Joshua Project. 2018. How Many People Groups Are There? Colorado Springs, CO: Joshua Project. https://joshuaproject.net/ assets/media/articles/how-many-people-groupsare-there.pdf

Kanupriya. 2021. COVID-19 and the Indian textiles sector: Issues, challenges and prospects. *Vision* 25(1): 7–11.

Karmakar, R. 2020. Arunachal's tribes revive indigenous lockdown rituals – The Hindu. www.thehindu.com/news/national/other-states/arunachals-tribes-revive-indigenous-lockdown-rituals/article31186665.ece.

Kharshiing, K.D. 2020. Identity and otherisation in northeast India: Representations in media texts. *Psychology and Developing Society* 32: 65–93 https://journals.sagepub.com/doi/abs/10.1177/0971333619900046

Kocher, V.K. 1966. Village deities of the santal and associated rituals. *Anthropos* 61: 241–257.

Kumar, A.P. 2020. Lawless lawmaking in a COVID-19 World. *Economic and Political Weekly* LV(25): 10–12.

Levesques, A. 2020. India-China tensions: What next for India? IISS. www.iiss.org/blogs/analysis/2020/07/sasia-india-china-tensions

Newsclick. 2020. COVID-19 and lockdown threatening livelihoods of tribal communities and other forest dwellers: A report. www.newsclick.in/COVID-19-lockdown-threatening-livelihoods-tribal-communities-forest-dwellers-report

Padma, T.V. 2021. India's COVID vaccine woes: by the numbers. *Nature* 592: 500–501.

Pandey, R., Kukreja S., and K. Ravipriya. 2020. COVID-19 mental healthcare without social justice? *Economic and Political Weekly* LV(31): 16–20.

PIB. 2020. Finance Minister announces Rs 1.70 Lakh Crore relief package under Pradhan Mantri Garib Kalyan Yojana for the poor to help them fight the battle against Corona Virus. Ministry of Finance, Press Information Bureau, Press Release, March 26, https://pib.gov.in/ PressReleseDetailm.aspx?PRID=1608345

The Print. 2020. Health a state subject, but Covid proved how dependant India's states are on Centre. https://theprint.in/opinion/health-a-state-subject-but-covid-proved-how-dependant-indias-states-are-on-centre/442602/

Roberts, G.C. 2021. Indian coronavirus variant – What is it and what effect will it have? https://theprint.in/health/indian-coronavirus-variant-what-is-it-and-what-effect-will-it-have/645722/

Sambad English Bureau. 2020. Amid COVID-19 Outbreak, Odisha villagers use sal leaf mask as protection. https://sambadenglish.com/amid-covid-19-outbreak-odisha-villagers-use-sal-leaf-mask-as-protection/

Saya, G.K., Chinnakali, P., and Premarajan, K.C. Determinants of COVID-19 transmission in India: Issues and challenges. *Indian Journal of Community and Family Medicine* 6 (2): 88–92.

Scroll. 2021. Covid: 180 people died after vaccination in India till March 29, over 6 crore inoculated by then. https://scroll.in/latest/991807/coronavirus-180-people-have-died-after-vaccination-in-india-till-march-29

Sharma, P., and K. Veer. 2020. Action and problems related to the COVID-19 outbreak in India. *Infection Control and Hospital Epidemiology* 41: 1478–1479, https://doi.org/10.1017/ice.2020.18

Singh, A., P. Deedwania, K. Vinay, A.R. Chowdhury, and P. Khanna. 2020. Is India's health care infrastructure sufficient for handling COVID 19 pandemic? *International Archives of Public Health and Community Medicine* 4: 041. doi.org/10.23937/2643-4512/1710041

Singh, S.K., V. Patel, A. Chaudhary, and N. Mishra. 2020. Reverse migration of labourers amidst COVID-19. *Economic and Political Weekly* LV(32 & 33): 25–29.

Statista Research Department (SRD). 2020. Impact on household income due to the coronavirus (COVID-19) in India from February to April 2020. www.statista.com/statistics/1111510/india-coronavirus-impact-on-household-income/

Swaroop, K., and J. Lee. 2021. Caste and COVID-19 Notes on sanitation in a pandemic. *Economic and Political Weekly* LVI(13): 35–42.

Vijayan, P. 2020. Challenges in the midst of the COVID-19 pandemic. *Economic and Political Weekly* LV(24): 11–13.

Vlassoff, C., M.G. Weiss, S. Rao, F. Ali, and T. Prentice. 2012. HIV-related stigma in rural and tribal communities of Maharashtra, India. *Health Population and Nutrition* 30: 394–403.

Vraga, E.K., and L. Bode. 2021. Addressing covid-19 misinformation on social media preemptively and responsively. *Emerging Infectious Diseases* 27(2): 396–403. https://doi.org/10.3201/eid2702.203139

Wakharde, S.B. 2021. COVID-19 pandemic and tribal women in Nanded District of Maharashtra. *Economic and Political Weekly* LVI(11). www.epw.in/node/158119/pdf

15 Contesting COVID-19 in Bangladesh

Government Responses and Local Perceptions

Inayat Ali and Sudipta Das Gupta

Introduction: A Brief Overview of COVID-19 in Bangladesh

Bangladesh recorded its first case of COVID-19 on March 7, 2020, but many believed that the then-novel coronavirus had already entered the country long before its first official identification (Anwar, Nasrullah, and Hosen 2020). Between January 3, 2020, and June 2, 2021, the WHO reported 802,305 confirmed cases of COVID-19 in Bangladesh, with 12,660 deaths (WHO 2021). As in almost all other countries, the coronavirus pandemic has adversely impacted every sector of Bangladesh, particularly its healthcare facilities and its economy, which has suffered due to coronaviral spread and the measures taken against it. The nationwide shutdown has halted almost all economic activities except agriculture; thus many people have lost their jobs, and others live in fear of the same thing happening to them. As we write (June 2021), international trade orders are being canceled in large numbers, particularly in the ready-made garments industry.

The syndemics of structured disparities (Ali and Ali 2020; Ali, Sadique, and Ali 2020; Singer and Rylko-Bauer 2021) remain as the leading causes of the severe effects of the disease in this country, given that Bangladesh has a dense population and limited resources, including health facilities and healthcare providers. Considering the importance of local knowledge, attitudes, perceptions, and practices, this chapter deals with local perceptions and practices concerning various aspects of the pandemic. The central questions we ask and answer include: How do laypeople in Bangladesh perceive COVID-19? How do they perceive the preventive measures and other government responses to the pandemic? What home remedies or other medical systems, if any, have they relied on? What are their first-hand experiences of contracting COVID-19, if any? What are their perceptions of COVID-19 vaccination, and what do they think about when and how the pandemic might end? In brief, we ask, how have laypeople negotiated the pandemic? In answering these multiple questions, we show both dissonance and resonance in local perceptions and practices surrounding COVID-19 in Bangladesh.

DOI: 10.4324/9781003187462-19

Bangladesh: An Overview of Its Sociocultural, Economic, and Healthcare Systems

Bangladesh is a Southeast Asian lower-to middle-income country of approximately 147,570 square kilometers (56,980 sq mi). Although some claim that it has a "rapidly" expanding economy, it has a low per capita Gross Domestic Product (GDP), and around 20% of the population is impoverished (Islam et al. 2020). Approximately 163 million people of different religions and ethnicities live in Bangladesh—one of the most densely populated countries in the world. Over the past decade, Muslims have accounted for 90.4% of Bangladesh's total population, while Hindus, Buddhists, and Christians have accounted for 8.5%, 0.6%, and 0.3%, respectively (Moinuddin Haider et al. 2019).

Bangladesh currently has 5.3 doctors for every 10,000 people; 0.3 nurses for every 1,000 people; 0.87 hospital beds for every 1,000 people; and 0.72 ICU beds and 1 ventilator for every 100,000 people (Islam et al.2020). The pandemic has revealed numerous flaws in the healthcare system that can be summarized under three themes: (1) poor governance and increasing corruption; (2) inadequate healthcare facilities; and (3) poor public health communications (Al-Zaman 2020). Furthermore, during this crisis, many hospitals, doctors, nurses, and other health officials have been unwilling to treat COVID-19 patients because they fear becoming infected due to a lack of protective equipment. Thus, Bangladesh's Health Ministry appointed 2,000 doctors and 6,000 nurses to attend to people with COVID-19, giving them no choice and leaving many other citizens without needed medical care (Dhaka Tribune 2020).

The Politics of COVID-19 in Bangladesh: An "Extremely Irresponsible" and "Suicidal" Lockdown Lifting

As a low-to-middle-resource country with limited healthcare resources, Bangladesh has not responded well enough to minimize the spread of COVID-19 in the country by, for example, identifying cases and tracing the contacts of potentially infected people. As with many other countries, the Bangladeshi government has employed what Inayat Ali (2021) calls "rituals of containment" to deal with the pandemic by following WHO guidelines and taking preventive measures, such as prohibiting all public gatherings, placing restrictions on travel, promoting physical distancing, fighting misinformation, shutting down educational institutions, keeping traffic off the streets, and implementing lockdowns on significantly impacted cities (Islam et al. 2020). However, these did not happen all at once, so cases surged in specific areas, and the initial lockdown was not in place for long enough. There was a large gap, from March 8, 2020 (when the first case in the country was identified) to March 26, 2020, when, after the deaths of four COVID-19 patients, the Bangladesh government finally decided to impose a nationwide lockdown in terms of suspending water, rail, air travel, and public transport; this lockdown was later extended to May 30, 2020. After 65 days, on May 31, 2020, the government lifted the nationwide lockdown, but partial and complete lockdowns were re-imposed in different periods and places as the COVID-19 situation worsened (Kamruzzaman and Sakib 2020).

These measures were politically contested at the national level when the government decided to lift the first lockdown, as the opposition party leaders named this decision "suicidal," while, in unusual agreement, the leftist alliance called it "extremely irresponsible." The leftist parties' alliance alleged that, in lifting the first lockdown, thereby allowing a large increase in viral spread, the government had opted for "herd immunity"—which refers to resistance to infectious disease spread within a population that is based on the pre-existing immunity of a high proportion of individuals as a result of previous infection or vaccination. In this case, the leftist parties were alleging that the government wanted a high degree of viral spread to gain herd immunity, not by mass vaccination but by mass infection. In response to this severe criticism, the government has argued that all of its decisions have been taken to save lives and livelihoods. There was tremendous social and economic pressure on the government to release the first and subsequent lockdowns (see below), even though opening things up would likely increase the spread of COVID-19, which it did (Choudhury 2020).

The World Health Organization (WHO) has reported that when the number of people testing positive for COVID-19 drops below 5%, then the first wave of COVID-19 is over. At the end of January 2021, the infection rate in Bangladesh remained below 5% for seven days (Dhaka Tribune 2021d; Khan 2020); thus, the government concluded that the first wave had passed. Then in mid-March 2021, the number of daily recorded cases and deaths again rose dramatically, and the second wave began. According to the ICDDRB (International Centre for Diarrheal Disease Research, Bangladesh), the Beta variant of the coronavirus, first discovered in South Africa, was detected in more than 80% of sampled individuals in Bangladesh between March 18–24, 2021.

In Bangladesh, the Beta variant was first discovered on January 24, 2021 (Faiaz 2021). On April 14, 2021, the government imposed a new week-long nationwide lockdown—later extended until June 6, 2021—to address the deteriorating COVID-19 situation. However, despite the lockdown and considering the country's severely affected economy, the government approved reopening shops and malls across the nation on April 25, 2021, and relaxed restrictions on long-distance public transportation on May 25, 2021 (Dhaka Tribune 2021b; The Business Standard 2021). As of that date, infection rates in the bordering districts of Chapainawabganj, Satkhira, and Rajshahi had increased to 55%, 42%, and 33%, respectively. Some of these border districts have been placed on strict lockdown to disrupt the transmission of the Kapa (B.1.617.1) and Delta (B.1.617.2) variants first found in India (Faiaz 2021).

The government urged the country's people to maintain mandatory physical distancing to limit viral spread, yet many did not comply, and thus community transmission continued (Choudhury 2020). Starting on July 21, 2020—very late in the game—the government also urged its citizens to wear masks properly, and mandated mask-wearing in public places (UNB 2020b). In addition, the government deployed the military to assist the local governance in controlling the pandemic in all districts (The Business Standard 2020).

COVID-19-related treatments have been available in some government and private healthcare centers, which, as in other countries, were all initially unprepared to deal with the crisis (Faiaz 2021). To ensure proper medical treatment for COVID-19 for its officials, the government inaugurated a telemedicine service available only to those officials (UNB 2020a). On March 17, 2020, the government closed all educational institutions until June 12, 2021, later extending the closure until June 30, 2021 (Dhaka Tribune 2021c). In addition to its prevention programs, the government began to provide real help to those who needed it most. One of the ten directives of the Prime Minister of Bangladesh to prevent coronaviral spread was the *Ghor a Fera Kormosuchi* (Back to Home Program); in this program, low-income urban people affected by the outbreak have been provided assistance such as food supplies and economic support (Daily Bangladesh 2020).

Once vaccines were available, the Bangladesh government asked people to register for the COVID-19 vaccine on a website. Starting on February 7, 2021, around 8,700,000 doses of the vaccine Oxford-AstraZeneca, produced by the Serum Institute in India, had been administered by June 2, 2021 free of charge—but these were "just a drop in the bucket" for the total population of around 165 million. And after India cut back on the export of its vaccine to Bangladesh, the first dose administration was stopped, and there were no shipments in April and May 2021 as India prioritized its own domestic needs (Dhaka Tribune 2021a).

Methods and Materials

Participants and Procedures

For this chapter, we conducted an online survey of middle-class, English-speaking Bangladeshis during January 2021. The survey contained 34 qualitative and quantitative questions concerning: (1) socio-economic and demographic data; (2) perceptions of COVID-19 and of vaccination against it; and (3) thoughts about when the pandemic might end, and how. Inayat Ali formulated the interview guide and Sudipta Das Gupta distributed our questionnaire on social media, for example, WhatsApp and Facebook, and emailed it to friends and acquaintances in Bangladesh. A total of 45 respondents participated. We ceased data collection when we reached saturation—that is, when respondents' answers became repetitive. We received written consent from all respondents.

Data Analysis

Since all data were already in English, as all respondents were educated and proficient in this language, there was no need for translation nor transcription, as we received all data in written form. Inayat Ali developed an initial codebook and then refined it according to the themes we identify below.

Our Respondents' Compositions

28 of our respondents were around 18–25 years of age; 15 respondents were 26–35; 2 were over 36. 24 participants were women and 20 were men. Reflecting the composition of the population as a whole, Muslims constituted the majority of respondents (30), followed by Hindus (8), Buddhists (4), and atheists (2). 26 were in the process of obtaining their Bachelor's degrees; another 26 were working on their Master's degrees; and the remaining respondents had some form of advanced schooling, a college education, or had obtained their Master's of Philosophy degrees. 33 of them were students; 2 were working for the government; 7 for an international non-governmental organization; and 4 were self-employed. 41 were living in a nuclear family, and 4 in a joint family. 35 were living in urban areas and the remaining 10 were from rural areas. Most were from the Chittagong Division, followed by those from the Dhaka Division. 16 had a monthly family income of more than US$600–700; 6 of $500–$600; 11 of $250–350; and the remaining had a monthly income of between $100–$200US.

Results and Discussion

Trout and Kleinman (2020) rightly called COVID-19 a "social disease" that demonstrates an interplay among sociocultural, economic, and political factors. Our research resulted in deep understandings of this interplay in Bangladesh. During our analysis, four themes emerged as primary: (1) perceptions of COVID-19, including testing and preventive measures; (2) first-hand experiences of COVID-19; (3) COVID-19 vaccination; and (4) thoughts about when and how the pandemic might end in Bangladesh. In what follows, we will discuss these themes and their assigned sub-themes in that order.

Perceptions of COVID-19: Testing and Preventive Measures

Clearly, experiencing a given phenomenon greatly affects one's perceptions of it. At the beginning of the pandemic in Bangladesh, many people were greatly suspicious of the existence of the coronavirus, though most of them also felt anxiety and even panic due to multiple factors, including the shutting down of economic activities and/or facing quarantines. In our data collection during January 2021, we found that of our 45 respondents, 91% (41) considered COVID-19 to be a dangerous and potentially fatal disease; all of these had either contracted the disease themselves or their loved ones had. Around 9% believed that it is a non-dangerous disease; these respondents had no first-hand experience of COVID-19. 55% (25) of them thought that the virus is not a conspiracy but a phenomenon that has naturally evolved. In contrast, around 37% (17) of our respondents stated, "Maybe it is a conspiracy," while 7% (3) thought that COVID-19 most certainly is a conspiracy—most likely of some influential countries who want to fulfill their vested interests. For instance, the conspiracy theory circulated that China wanted to use people from Bangladesh as "guinea pigs" for vaccine trials (Islam et al. 2021).

Perceptions of COVID-19: Rumors and Conspiracy Theories

As indicated just above, many rumors and conspiracy theories around COVID-19 are circulating in Bangladesh concerning health, politics, religion, crime, entertainment, and other topics. Although the examples provided below are not from our own dataset, we provide them nonetheless as a concrete means of illustrating what our numerous respondents who mention "conspiracy theories" are likely referring to. Here we draw from the work of Al-Zaman (2021) who has listed the following rumors and conspiracy theories currently circulating in Bangladesh by topic:

Health

"Kalazira (fennel flower) prevents coronavirus."
"Hot water mixed with salt-vinegar can cure corona infection."
"A medical team of 37 Chinese has arrived in Bangladesh."
"Coronavirus is a myth mainly to control people."
"Drink boiling water to prevent corona infection."

Politics

"Italy's PM says: 'The only solution of the pandemic is in the sky.' "
"Putin deploys 800 tigers and lions in the streets of Russia to force people to stay at home."
"86 countries will file a case against China for spreading coronavirus."
"Rizvi [the spokesperson of the Bangladesh Nationalist Party] dreamt that the coronavirus will vanish from Bangladesh if Khaleda Zia [the former Prime Minister of Bangladesh] is released."

Religion

"Quarantine was first invented by [the Holy Prophet] Mohammad: US researcher."

"The Saudi government canceled the Hajj this year due to the pandemic."[1]

"Two million Chinese people accepted Islam in six months because of coronavirus."

"*Allahu Akbar* is written on the roads of Europe to avoid corona."

"Coronavirus is a curse of Allah for the infidels and real Muslims will be exempted from it."

"Life and death, both are in the hands of Allah, coronavirus can do nothing about it."

Crime

"More than 20 million people are missing in China during the pandemic."

"COVID-19 positive dead bodies are found in the streets of Italy."

"Local public vandalized a Saudi immigrant's house suspecting corona positive."

Entertainment

"Due to COVID-19, Netflix will give out three months free subscription."

"COVID-19 positive vs COVID-19 negative football match in Mymensingh."

According to our observations, some COVID-19 related rumors are popular in the social media and among the local people. These include: "COVID-19 affects the rich people, not the poor people"; "COVID-19 vaccines imported from India are not trustable, these are not real vaccines"; and "those who work in a hot environment and are involved in rigorous physical labor (cook, rickshaw puller) won't be affected by COVID-19." These rumors and conspiracy theories need to be studied within historical and present sociocultural, economic and (geo-)political contexts (Ali 2020a). These narratives have added fuel to the fire of local Bangladeshis' fears and anxieties surrounding the coronavirus pandemic, as will be illustrated in some of our respondents' statements below.

Preventive Measures: Local Remedies Against COVID-19

While in Bangladesh, as elsewhere, biomedicine is hegemonic, medical pluralism abounds. Ancient healing systems such as Ayurveda and Unani-Tib co-exist with biomedicine and are widely employed, as are folk home remedies that have often been passed down over generations. Thus, in response to COVID-19, many people started using home remedies to strengthen their immune systems, including 54% of our respondents. The following are some of the remedies they used:

- *Masala* [spices] tea containing bay leaf, cardamom, and cinnamon (without milk or sugar).
- Tea mixed with ginger, basil, lemon, mint leaves, cinnamon, cardamom.
- Water boiled with cinnamon, ginger, lemon, and black pepper.
- Water boiled with cinnamon, clove, bay leaves, black pepper, ginger, and lemon juice.
- Water boiled with cinnamon bark, cardamom, and clove.
- Lukewarm water with lemon, honey, and ginger.
- Fruits and foods that contain Vitamin C.
- Vitamins C and A, garlic, cumin seed, black seed.
- Lemon juice.
- Breathing hot steam will kill germs and remove any blockages.
- Gargling with water mixed with lemon and salt.

These home remedies should be contextualized within existing contentions between biomedicine and Indigenous medicines. Unsurprisingly, from biomedical perspectives these remedies have been called "non-scientific" and the results of "misinformation," thereby highlighting the conceptual hegemony of biomedicine in Bangladesh and elsewhere. Yet these home remedies are grounded within Bangladeshi economic, political, and sociocultural patterns and the country's pluralistic healthcare systems. A large percentage of people live below the poverty line and cannot afford biomedical care; the biomedical healthcare system is quite limited, as shown above; and many biomedical practitioners refuse to treat people who contract COVID-19. Thus, like many people around the world, Bangladeshis often deem home remedies as essential to their wellbeing, along with the larger "alternative" healing systems often used (see Chapters 10 and 14 for detailed descriptions of these "alternative" and "complementary" medicinal systems in China and India).

COVID-19 (Non)Testing

A look at COVID-19 testing reveals various forms of disparities; for example, it has been a great challenge in low-resource countries to conduct large-scale testing (Ali and Ali 2021). Bangladesh, with its low per capita GDP of around $3 billion, which accounts for only 0.25% of the global economy (Rahman 2015), could not afford massive testing; such is also the case with our respondents. Those who have limited economic resources cannot afford to be tested, while the wealthier ones can. Nevertheless, out of our 45 respondents, the majority, 91% (41), including those who could afford it, did not choose to get tested for COVID-19. Only 9% (4) of respondents did choose to do so.

Taking or Ignoring COVID-19 Preventive Measures: Underlying Reasons

Our interlocutors' perceptions of preventive measures resonate with each other, and at the same time show dissonance. 20% of respondents stated that they have neither performed any preventive measures nor have they seen anyone using these measures. For instance, one respondent stated, "I have not observed any physical distancing or masks usage in my surrounding. Everybody is roaming freely." Another respondent shared, "Most people do not care about the virus and those who are maintaining the preventive initiatives are not doing it properly. Most of them do not know how to use face masks. They are just wearing it [wrongly] or carrying it!" Another respondent stated:

> some people are maintaining social distance, wearing a mask, and not going anywhere if it is not too necessary. But most people are traveling without a mask and there is no social distance. When I have to go out, I notice that most people are not maintaining these. I think the reason behind this is their unawareness of COVID. Some people, especially illiterate people, do not even know what COVID-19 is. On the other hand, some people question the existence of COVID-19.

Another respondent answered, "No! as in my region people use a mask or any other protective equipment only as a formality in different situations. On the other hand, some people (a very small portion) use this equipment as a safety measure. Finally, physical distance is not seen around here in any public area."

A few respondents said that people do not follow preventive measures because they either believe in superstitions or in a supernatural being. One respondent stated, "I have been experiencing a few people [taking] preventive measures. As people in Bangladesh are not so much educated and [are] superstitious as well...they fail to comprehend its severity and do not intend to be much concerned about it." Similarly, another respondent replied, "People of rural areas, they think that it's a normal issue. 'If Allah is with us, COVID-19 cannot attack us.' For this reason, they don't [keep] physical distance or wear a mask."

Revealing the influence of group pressure, some respondents did not follow preventive measures because no one around them was doing so. As one of them admitted, "It is very tough for me to wear things when others don't use them." In contrast, the views of 80% (36) of our respondents resonate with each other; they stated that they have taken preventive measures and have also seen other people doing so. One respondent, who had high health literacy, noted:

> Yes, I wear a mask and am doing physical distancing to avoid getting COVID-19, because we all know that this virus spreads primarily

through droplets generated when an infected person coughs, sneezes, or speaks. So, I can also become infected by touching a contaminated surface and then touching your eyes, nose, or mouth before washing your hands. To protect me, keep at least 1-meter distance from others and disinfect frequently touched surfaces. Clean my hands thoroughly and often, and avoid touching your eyes, mouth, and nose.

This respondent's words "as we all know" were clearly misguided: our survey results show that in fact, many of those with low health literacy do not know how COVID-19 is spread. This respondent was assuming that "we all" have the same level of health literacy that he enjoys, which "we" do not.

One respondent emphasized some measures over others, saying, "Mask and sanitizers are the two most important things which I follow, as these are the primary steps which help to limit the risk factors." In comparison, some respondents noted the *partial* practice of preventive measures. For instance, one respondent said, "I am observing that around 20% of people in my area are wearing masks. But nobody is maintaining physical distances."

Reasons Given for Not Following Preventive Measures

Our respondents mentioned different reasons behind people's decisions not to follow preventive measures. One respondent stated four reasons: "(1) the government has lost its control and the proper initiatives were not taken tightly enough; (2) low test rate; (3) [stopping] the daily TV press briefing on the affected and the deaths; (4) opening up the tourist spots." Another respondent stated:

First of all, the lack of proper knowledge about the pandemic or the virus is responsible for such carelessness of people. Most of them do not care about the virus. As for Bangladesh, religion (not any specific one) plays an unavoidable role here. People are defining this virus as a punishment from the creator. And some issues are influencing mass people to follow the preventive measures such as health consciousness, fear of being fined or charged by the [police] force etc.

One respondent said, "Many people are conscious about COVID-19 to protect themselves. On the contrary, a few people [think that] this virus has no presence [does not exist]. Therefore, they are moving around as usual, and don't even wear a mask." One respondent described "Not enough publicity or awareness. There are also many conspiracy theories going around, which some people tend to subscribe to. Many are frustrated because of the measures and at the same time social distancing is actually affecting many families as they don't get to see each other…" Another respondent said, "Maintaining physical distance is not possible in my area as [it] is densely populated."

Governmental Responses: Public Mistrust and Suggestions for Improving Them

Around 64% (29) of respondents were not satisfied with the government's efforts to deal with COVID-19; 36% were satisfied. These views showing mistrust in the government need to be historically and politically contextualized, as a relationship of mistrust has long been prevalent between the people and the government. Starting from Bangladesh's independence from Pakistan in 1971, a civilian government, a military government, or a civilian—but not an elected—government has ruled the country. Most of these governments were characterized by violence, instability, and mistrust among the main political parties, providing the means for developing the current military-backed civil government, which intentionally avoids public participation and transparency (Sobhan 2004; Rahman 2015). When people do not elect governments, their members do not feel accountable to their citizens. A patron-client relationship prevails, as large political parties tend to favor people with money and muscle to win local and national elections, which has allowed corruption and mistrust to become entrenched in Bangladeshi society. Affecting all government departments at all levels, corruption prevails in education, healthcare, the judiciary, police, government procurement, social protection, and in banking and financial services (Rahman 2015). This systemic corruption has ultimately affected poverty alleviation, leading to Bangladesh's low per capita GDP, and creating a vicious circle.

Many of our respondents provided specific suggestions for the government to deal with the effects of COVID-19. One respondent suggested, "The government should provide economic security to the lowest status holders in the economic hierarchy because they are the most vulnerable people. They have to go out daily for winning the bread, therefore physical distancing is an impossible task." One respondent stated, "There should be proper distribution of knowledge. All of a sudden mass people heard some totally unfamiliar terms like 'isolation,' 'quarantine.' They do not know what this means and [are] making wrong meaning out of these or perceiving these as something terrifying or harmful." Another respondent stated:

> [First the] government has to prove its legitimacy in every sector for its political initiative to deal with this pandemic...as we [have] much corruption in the regulatory system. Secondly, this pandemic shows us literally how many social disparities have existed in our living world and it's now time to re-organize our education system and make it more useful for getting a better social life. And finally, I have to say in economic regard that we aren't as insufficient as we were before. Our BD government works fruitfully in solving the economic insufficiency so that Bangladesh starts to grow as an economically potential [country].

Some respondents pointed towards issues in the healthcare system that need to be fixed. For instance, one respondent stated, "'Hospital Management' should be improved. Government should maintain discipline there. 'Middlemen' are creating nuisance in government hospitals in every activity (i.e., in diagnosis, purchasing medicine)." Another respondent affirmed, "Government should apply punishment policy [for those who do not follow preventive measures in the ways that] other countries are maintaining." A few respondents strongly suggested the implementation of a strict lockdown; as one respondent stated, "[There should be] lockdown for 14 days everywhere in Bangladesh [so that] no one can move from [their] house." Some respondents also suggested mass testing across the country.

Contracting COVID-19: The Resonance of First-Hand Experiences

One can easily see a resonance of perceptions and effects of COVID-19 in our respondents who had first-hand experiences of this disease. Their experiences clearly illustrate what Inayat Ali (2021) has called the "emotional/psychological pandemic," which, worldwide, has taken a heavy toll on people's emotional and psychological wellbeing. 62% of respondents told us that either they were infected by the virus themselves, or that the virus had infected one or more of their family members and friends, and that it was a "terrible" experience. For example, one 25-year-old female student, who lives in a rural part of Bangladesh, stated:

> My father contracted COVID-19 because of the forced travel (by his office) to Dhaka. It was troublesome since he has a history of cardiovascular disease, high bp, and diabetes. He had a moderate fever, a slight breathing problem, and acute coughing. The whole experience was energy draining because of the stress and anxiety we had as a family.

A 25-year-old Muslim student from the Chittagong Division described that her relatives who had contracted the virus "were in a terrible state. They had a severe fever, headache, and most importantly, they had difficulties in breathing. They took one or in some cases two months to cure completely. Their body became too weak. They said this was one of the most painful experiences [that they had ever had to live through]."

Some respondents had lost loved ones due to COVID-19. One respondent stated, "My friend's father has died due to COVID-19. Their family is completely broken." Another said, "Until now I'm safe. But some people in my area were infected. And their experience was horrible. Some of them died." Another described, "My cousins' husband has died on December 26 [2020] suffering from COVID-19. He was also a kidney transplant patient. So he didn't survive." In resonance, another respondent stated, "My family was infected. Although most of them had mild symptoms, my father had to go through a lot. He was in the hospital for 20 days. We do not take this virus lightly at all." Another respondent stated, "My uncle was infected. He died at the age of 58 though he was strong...he had so many difficulties in breathing. Covid-19 is indeed a serious concern for all." In contrast, some of our respondents stated that, even though either they or their loved ones contracted the virus, they perceived this disease as "normal." For instance, one respondent practicing Buddhism and working on his Master's degree, living in the urban area of the Chittagong division, shared that, "one of my relatives...was admitted to the hospital. I talked to him and told him not to fear at all. It's just a disease like other diseases. He did not fear at all."

Perceptions of Vaccination: Effective Yet Unsought

Like other themes we have addressed, local perceptions and practices of vaccination simultaneously resonate and differ. Regarding their perceptions of vaccines and vaccination, 56% of respondents perceived that "It is safe and good as it protects against diseases." 42% "don't know" about it, and one respondent thinks, "It is unsafe and bad since it does not protect against diseases." Although most of our respondents perceive vaccines in general as "effective," nevertheless, most of them have not gotten vaccinations for themselves nor for their children (see Figure 15.1).

Around 96% of our respondents stated that no vaccination teams visit them for routine vaccinations against diseases such as polio and measles. Only two of them said that mobile vaccination teams visit their homes. In contrast, in response to the question about whether or not they take a child/sibling/cousin to a healthcare facility for vaccination, 35% of respondents stated "yes," and 35% said "no," while 31% have "sometimes" done so. We also asked if they or their children or family members had ever received any vaccines thus far? And if so, which ones? Around 47% of respondents replied "no," while 6% of them said they "don't remember." In contrast,

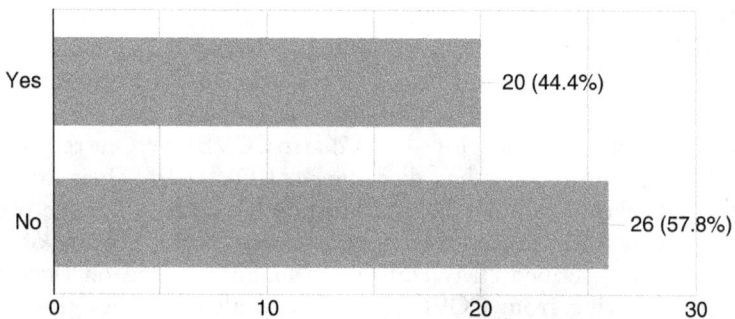

Figure 15.1 Vaccinating Their Children.

47% stated they or their family's children had received vaccines for diseases such as measles, polio, hepatitis A, and chickenpox.

COVID-19 Vaccination: Local Knowledges and Attitudes

During our data collection in January 2021, only 9% of respondents were unaware of the COVID-19 vaccine, while the remaining 91% of respondents knew of it (see Figure 15.2). Most respondents (78%) believe that the COVID-19 vaccine is safe, and said they would like to receive it. However, the remaining 12% have a reason not to receive the vaccine (see Table 15.1).

To recap from above, 78% of our respondents felt that the vaccine was safe and would like to receive it. Most respondents (53%) even wanted to pay money to receive the COVID-19 vaccine; 11% did not want to pay; and 36% stated "maybe." However, they shared different views on how people in

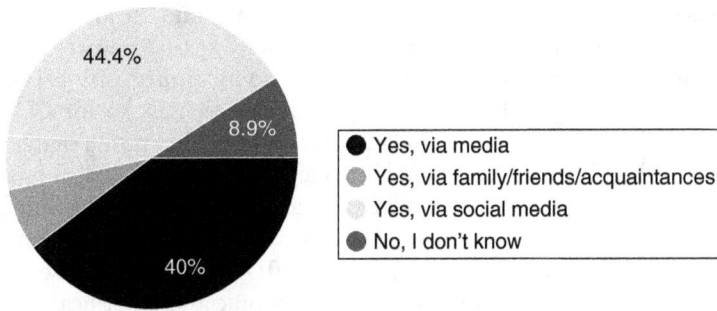

Figure 15.2 Knowledge about the COVID-19 Vaccine.

Table 15.1 Attitudes towards the COVID-19 Vaccine

Yes, vaccines are safe, and this vaccine will protect me against COVID-19.	78% (35)
No, I believe in natural immunity and the vaccine is unsafe and may disturb the body's mechanism.	9% (4)
I still can't decide.	2.2% (1)
I know that this virus is having a mutation every time, so I don't know if the vaccine will work properly or not, but I want to be vaccinated.	2.2% (1)
Vaccines are safe and create immunity to certain viruses or bacteria but in the case of the COVID-19 vaccine, I am not satisfied as it has some negative impact in humans. So, I will not go for the vaccine right now. I think it needs more trial and time.	2.2% (1)
I am confused.	2.2% (1)
I am not sure about it.	2.2% (1)
I don't know.	2.2% (1)

their communities perceive the COVID-19 vaccine and whether or not they will receive it. 35% of respondents said that people in their communities are eager to receive this vaccine because, as one respondent ironically put it, "people want to get rid of the fear of COVID-19 and most surprisingly they want to get rid of the mask!" Nine respondents were skeptical: "maybe" or "maybe not." Around 44% said that people in their community would not receive this vaccine mainly due to "lack of education and knowledge," and "Most of them are against taking this vaccine because they have doubts about its effects." Regarding whether or not the government would be successful in vaccinating the entire population of the country, 49% thought that the government "may or may not be successful"; 38% stated, "No, the government would not succeed; and only 13% said "Yes."

On the subject of whether or not a vaccine would be a good solution to end this pandemic, our respondents were divided again. 40% think that a vaccine is not a solution. As one respondent stated, "No! It is not a permanent solution. The vaccine may lose its power. So, people should continuously follow the safety guidelines." Another respondent noted that "ensuring proper vaccinations to everyone will take some time and, in the meantime, the virus may spread further or just be mutated again." However, 26% believe that a vaccine is a solution. As one respondent argued, "[since] earlier vaccines have saved people from many deadliest diseases, so for COVID-19, a vaccine is the best solution. The vaccine should be more reliable and safer for people." 34% were skeptical. As one respondent argued, "I have no accurate answer about that. But maybe this vaccine can stop spreading from one person to others, and no one will die. This vaccine creates immunity in the human body which will fight against COVID-19." Another respondent stated, "If the vaccines have no side effects for people and other health issues and problems then it will obviously be the solution, but people also should maintain some preventing steps, so that they can assure a better, safe and healthy life." Another respondent answered, "Yes for now. I don't have any evidence except for the studies. I know some elderly relatives who took the vaccine and are doing well. I think this will provide some protection if not complete protection from the virus." Some respondents emphasized that a vaccine can be a solution if taken in tandem with other preventive measures, such as observing cleanliness and wearing a mask.

When Will the Pandemic End?

Although much regarding the pandemic has been discussed within scientific, media, and political circles, how local people interpret and view the end of this pandemic is less documented. Thus, we asked our respondents: "When do you think the pandemic will end? And how do you think it will end?" At this time of writing (June 2021), the pandemic continues and is likely to do so for quite some time, especially in low-resource countries like Bangladesh. Holding different views and logics about the end of the pandemic, most of our respondents just "wonder" when it will end. Although mass vaccination has opened up several old and new debates concerning its acceptance, affordability, and acceptability (Ali, Ali, and Iqbal 2021), many people, including ourselves, see vaccination as the "game-changer" that can bring this pandemic to an end (provided that enough people take it to achieve herd immunity). In resonance, some of our respondents think the pandemic will be over, "As soon as every individual gets vaccinated," or "after obtaining herd immunity [through vaccination]."

As in Pakistan, where people have associated this pandemic with supernatural causes (Ali 2021; Chapters 16 and 17, this volume), a few of our respondents believe that only supernatural authority will bring the pandemic to an end. As one such respondent stated, "*InshaAllah* [if Allah wills it]! The pandemic will be over as only Allah makes possible." Some respondents were concerned that the pandemic may not end soon—or maybe ever—due to the new mutations of the coronavirus, which are proving more dangerous than the original virus. For instance, one respondent stated: "I don't think that this pandemic will easily end because recently we see that corona again creates its new mutant like B117, which is more dangerous and spreads more than 70% easier than the current corona …and it happens especially in young people."

In contrast, some respondents said that they were unable to predict the pandemic's endpoint. For example, one respondent stated, "I don't know [when this pandemic will be over]. We need to improve our immunity naturally and should wear masks and maintain social distances to avoid getting infected before getting a more reliable vaccine." This statement illustrates medical pluralism at work in Bangladesh. On the one hand, this respondent believes in natural immunity, in which vaccination may been seen as disturbing the "natural mechanisms" of the body (Ali 2020b). This perception can be situated within Bangladesh's millennia-old healthcare systems such as Unani Tib and Ayurveda (see Chapters 10 and 14), which holistically focus on gaining and maintaining good health. On the other hand, this respondent also emphasizes the importance of adopting biomedically recommended preventive measures. Thus, this respondent demonstrates how different medical systems can work together and complement each other, especially during a health crisis. Just as medical systems like Ayurveda and Unani-Tib can be "alternative" or "complementary" to biomedicine, so biomedicine can be "alternative" or "complementary" to other medical systems.

Conclusion: Dissonance and Resonance of Perceptions around COVID-19

In this chapter, we have presented the results of a survey taken by 45 Bangladeshi respondents from a diverse variety of backgrounds, and have addressed the primary themes that emerged from their responses—their perceptions, beliefs, and behaviors around preventive measures; vaccination and the COVID-19 vaccine; their personal experiences of COVID-19; and their thoughts about when and how this pandemic might end. We have shown that the Bangladesh government has taken numerous measures to deal with the coronavirus pandemic, including implementing lockdowns and then lifting them to shore up the economy. Revealing the government's stratagem, we have also shown that these measures have been politicized at the national level, as some political groups have labeled them "extremely irresponsible" and even "suicidal"—most especially regarding the lifting of the first lockdown on May 31, 2020.

According to local perspectives, the government's initiatives seem insufficient. Around 64% of our respondents were not satisfied with the government's efforts to deal with this pandemic. Our respondents suggest that the government should ensure economic security to people belonging to low-income families and provide much-needed awareness of the virus and its dangers. The majority of our respondents view COVID-19 as a dangerous disease, which often is due to their first-hand experiences of either contracting the virus themselves or knowing someone who had. Such experiences have led them to follow the preventive measures; 80% of our respondents, including the people around them, do observe these measures. In contrast, 20% avoid following them and see the same behaviors in their surroundings, which is a major reason for their own avoidance that illustrates the strong effects of group pressure. Our respondents explained that the reasons that lead people not to follow preventive measures include lack of appropriate awareness of the dangers of the coronavirus and lack of awareness that the virus actually exists. As in many other countries, the conspiracy theories around COVID-19 that circulate in Bangladesh, many of which are listed above, make laypeople suspicious. Some people also believe that certain influential countries are behind COVID-19; here we recall the conspiracy theory mentioned above that the Chinese want to use Bangladeshis as guinea pigs for vaccine trials.

A great majority of our respondents (78%) consider the COVID-19 vaccine to be safe and even want to pay money to receive it. 35% of respondents said that people in their communities are eager to have this vaccine as "people want to get rid of the fear of COVID-19." In contrast, around 44% think that people in their community would not accept this vaccine, mainly due to a "lack of education and knowledge" and doubts about its effectiveness. 40% of respondents judiciously suggest that a vaccine is not the only solution to this pandemic and that people should also take preventive measures. However, as previously noted, 26% think that a vaccine *is* a solution. Nonetheless, some respondents believe that only supernatural authority would bring the pandemic to an end, and so put their faith and trust in Allah.

In sum, our study has shown both dissonance and resonance between government policies and local perceptions and practices by revealing their similarities and contestations. With this research, we hope to provoke further anthropological studies, both on- and off-line, of local people's perceptions of and reactions to the coronavirus pandemic and to the preventive measures utilized in various countries, with the goal of highlighting local perspectives in ways that can help researchers and governments to better define and refine those measures in accordance with local people's perceptions, needs, and levels of health literacy.

Note

1 In fact, the Saudi government did not cancel the 2020 Hajj, but they did limit attendance to Saudi Arabian residents only.

References

Ali, I. 2020a. Impacts of rumors and conspiracy theories surrounding COVID-19 on preparedness programs. *Disaster Medicine and Public Health Preparedness* 1–6. doi:10.1017/dmp.2020.149

Ali, I. 2020b. *Constructing and Negotiating Measles: The Case of Sindh Province of Pakistan*. (PhD Thesis). Vienna: University of Vienna.

Ali, I. 2021. Rituals of containment: Many pandemics, body politics, and social dramas during covid-19 in Pakistan. *Frontiers in Sociology* 6(83). doi:10.3389/fsoc.2021.648149

Ali, I., and Ali, S. 2020. Why may Covid-19 overwhelm low-income countries like Pakistan? *Disaster Medicine and Public Health Preparedness*. doi:10.1017/dmp.2020.149

Ali, I., and Ali, S. 2021. Covid-19 in Pakistan and Papua New Guinea: Reflections on massive testing and challenges. *Primary Health Care Research & Development* 22(e71): 1–4. doi.org/10.1017/S1463423621000724

Ali, I., Ali, S., and Iqbal, S. 2021. Covid-19 vaccination: Concerns about its accessibility, affordability, and acceptability. *Frontiers in Medicine* doi:10.3389/fmed.2021.647294

Ali, I., Sadique, S., and Ali, S. 2020. Covid-19 significantly affects maternal health: A rapid-response investigation from Pakistan. *Frontiers in Global Women's Health* 1. doi:10.3389/fgwh.2020.591809

Ali, I., Sadique, S., and Ali, S. 2021. Covid-19 and vaccination campaigns as "Western plots" in Pakistan: Government policies, (geo-) politics, local perceptions, and beliefs. *Frontiers in Sociology* 6(82). doi.org/10.3389/fsoc.2021.608979

Al-Zaman, M.S. 2020. Healthcare crisis in Bangladesh during the COVID-19 pandemic.
The American Journal of Tropical Medicine and Hygiene 103(4): 1357–1359. https://doi.org/10.4269/ajtmh.20-0826

Al-Zaman, M.S. 2021. Covid-19-related online misinformation in Bangladesh. *Journal of Health Research* 35(4): 364–368.

Anwar, S., Nasrullah, M., and Hosen, M.J. 2020. Covid-19 and Bangladesh: Challenges and how to address them. *Frontiers in Public Health* 8(154). https://doi.org/10.3389/fpubh.2020.00154

The Business Standard. 2020. March 24. Armed forces deployed in all districts to control the coronavirus. *The Business Standard* Retrieved from https://tbsnews.net/coronavirus-chronicle/coronavirus-bangladesh/armed-forces-deployed-all- districts-control-coronavirus

The Business Standard. 2021. May 31. Bangladesh govt extends coronavirus lockdown restrictions till June 6. *The Business Standard* Retrieved from www.business-standard.com

Chowdhury, M.H. 2020. May 29. Bangladesh set to step into coronavirus new normal with a lot at stake. *bdnews24* Retrieved from https://bdnews24.com/bangladesh/2020/05/29/

Daily Bangladesh. 2020. March 23. PM's 10 directives to prevent corona. *Daily Bangladesh* Retrieved from www.daily-bangladesh.com

Dhaka Tribune. 2020. April 27. Coronavirus: Govt to recruit 2,000 doctors, 6,000 nurses within a week. *Dhaka Tribune*. Retrieved from www.dhakatribune.com

Dhaka Tribune. 2021a. April 29. 8.6 million doses of Covid-19 vaccine administered in Bangladesh. *Dhaka Tribune* Retrieved from www.dhakatribune.com

Dhaka Tribune. 2021b. May 2. Covid surge in Bangladesh: Experts say lockdown likely to pay off. *Dhaka Tribune* Retrieved from www.dhakatribune.com

Dhaka Tribune. 2021c. May 26. Bangladesh pushes back plan to reopen educational institutions to June 13. *Dhaka Tribune* Retrieved from www.dhakatribune.com

Dhaka Tribune. 2021d. January 25. Covid-19: Daily test positivity rate stays below 5% for last 7 days. *Dhaka Tribune*. Retrieved from www.dhakatribune.com

Faiaz, Z. 2021. June 3. Bangladesh's 'reactionary' COVID-19 response is working, but for how long? *The Diplomat* Retrieved from https://thediplomat.com

Islam, K., Ali, S., Akanda, S.Z.R., Rahman, S., Kamruzzaman, A.H.M., Pavel, S.A.K., et al. 2020. COVID -19 pandemic and level of responses in Bangladesh. *International Journal of Rare Diseases & Disorders* 3: 019. doi.org/10.23937/2643-4571/1710019

Islam, M.S., Kamal, A.H.M., Kabir, A., Southern, D.L., Khan, S.H., Hasan, S.M., et al. 2021. COVID-19 vaccine rumors and conspiracy theories: The need for cognitive inoculation against misinformation to improve vaccine adherence. *PloS ONE* 16(5): e0251605.

Islam, M., Talukder, A., Badruzzaman, M., and Khan, M. 2020. Health service facilities are positively linked with outcome of COVID-19 patients in majority of the countries: The global situation. *Journal of Advanced Biotechnology and Experimental Therapeutics* 3(3): 36. https://doi.org/10.5455/jabet.2020.d154

Kamruzzaman, M., and Sakib, S.M.N. 2020. March 25. Bangladesh imposes total lockdown over COVID-19. *Anadolu Agency*. Retrieved from www.aa.com.tr/en/asia-pacific/bangladesh-imposes-total-lockdown-over-covid-19/1778272#

Khan, K.M. 2020, December 5. Second wave of COVID-19 in Bangladesh and concerns. *The Daily Star*. Retrieved from www.thedailystar.net

Lescure, F.X., Bouadma, L., Nguyen, D., Parisey, M., Wicky, P-H., Behillil, S., et al. 2020. Clinical and virological data of the first cases of COVID-19 in Europe: A case series. *The Lancet Infectious Diseases* 20: 697–706.

Moinuddin, H.M., Rahman, M., and Kamal, N. 2019. Hindu population growth in Bangladesh: A demographic puzzle. *Journal of Religion and Demography* 6(1): 123–148. https://doi.org/10.1163/2589742x-00601003

Rahman, M.A. 2015. *Governance Matters: Power, Corruption, Social Exclusion, and Climate Change in Bangladesh*. Tuscon, AZ: University of Arizona.

Singer, M., and Rylko-Bauer, B. 2021. The syndemics and structural violence of the covid pandemic: Anthropological insights on a crisis. *Open Anthropological Research* 1(1): 7–32. doi.org/10.1515/opan-2020-0100

Sobhan, R. 2004. Structural dimensions of malgovernance in Bangladesh. *Economic and Political Weekly* 39(36): 4101–4108.

Trout, L.J., and Kleinman, A. (2020). Covid-19 requires a social medicine response. *Frontiers in Sociology* 5. https://doi.org/10.3389/fsoc.2020.579991

United News of Bangladesh (UNB). 2020a. June 28. Covid-19: Telemedicine service launched for govt officials. Retrieved from https://unb.com.bd/category/Bangladesh/covid-19-telemedicine-service-launched-for-govt-officials/53811

United News of Bangladesh (UNB). 2020b. July 21. Coronavirus: Bangladesh makes wearing masks mandatory. Retrieved from https://unb.com.bd/category/bangladesh/coronavirus-bangladesh-makes-wearing-masks-mandatory/54963

World Health Organization (WHO). 2021. June 2. Bangladesh: WHO Coronavirus disease (COVID-19) dashboard with vaccination data. Retrieved from https://covid19.who.int/region/searo/country/bd/

Part IV

Negotiating COVID-19 in Pakistan

Cultural Conceptions and Pandemic Responses

16 Social Constructions of the Concept of COVID-19 in Pakistan

An Anthropological Investigation

Sara Akram and Rao Nadeem Alam

Introduction

Pakistan, as a low-income country, faces severe economic and political challenges that have resulted in a lack of funds for its healthcare budget allotment, which put the country at a higher risk of being overwhelmed by the pandemic (Ali and Ali 2020). Economically, insufficient funds have created a gap between high demands for equipment such as ventilators, medicines, hospital gowns, and protective kits, and lack of sufficient supply during this still-ongoing pandemic (Hamid 2020; Ladiwala et al. 2021). Even with firm measures imposed by the government authorities, as of April 2021, the country had reported over 24,954 cases, with the addition of 1300 cases in a single day (Abrar 2020).

Public responsiveness to preventive measures helps to lessen the intensity of viral dispersion frequency and diminishes the death rate from COVID-19 (Ali and Bhatti 2020), yet such responsiveness has been sorely lacking in Pakistan, especially in its rural areas. Sociocultural and religious patterns have significantly influenced the uptake of the government preparedness programs to effectively deal with COVID-19 (Ali and Ali 2020; Ali 2020a, b). Some religious leaders rejected the government-enforced complete lockdown from March to May 2020 and counseled people to continue their congregational prayers at mosques (Ali, Sadique, and Ali 2020). Many people continued—and continue—to congregate, arrange marriages, and perform religious festivals (Ali and Ali 2020). Even as the pandemic progressed, numerous national, political, and religious gatherings and crowds were witnessed (Latif 2020), demonstrating both a lack of the necessary knowledge about viral spread and the existing mistrust between the government and the people (Ali 2020; Munawar 2021).

Although much anthropological literature has been produced to explore various aspects of COVID-19 in Pakistan,[1] the widespread refusals to follow the government-recommended preventive standard operating procedures (SOPs) beg anthropological investigation of the reasons behind these refusals, which involve popular perceptions of COVID-19. Therefore, this study aimed to explore the knowledge, perceptions, and attitudes of Pakistanis

DOI: 10.4324/9781003187462-21

towards COVID-19, and to identify key misperceptions that affect Pakistan's healthcare system and SOP up/downtake. The cultural constructions of this disease can be best understood by identifying the characteristics and attributes that people attach to the concept of "coronavirus." Beliefs about the origin of the virus, its presence in Pakistan, its means of transmission, and its prevalence are the themes we will investigate, in order to uncover the sociocultural rationales Pakistanis use to negotiate COVID-19 and the SOPs in their daily lives. Viral spread cannot be stopped until local perceptions and levels of awareness are fully understood and taken into account.

Methods and Materials

During this pandemic, many ethnographers have had to change their research methods to cyber resource utilization (Johnson and Abramson 2020; Senior and Chenhall, this volume). Accordingly, we conducted cyber-ethnography using in-depth interviews and online focus group discussions (FGDs) from May to August 2020. But first, we conducted a preliminary survey and observations of online dialogues relevant to our topic. We then carried out two FGDs, in which 7 to 9 persons participated via online resources, and conducted 321 online interviews. We found our interlocutors via convenience and snowball sampling: co-authors Rao and Sara simply contacted family members and friends, who led us to others. All those who showed interest were invited for interviews. We collected our data primarily in the local languages—Urdu and Punjabi—and then both authors worked equally on transcribing these data into English.

We organized our qualitative data into specific themes for analysis; and ran our quantitative data through Excel to obtain frequency distributions (see Table 16.1). In this chapter, we provide brief dialogic narrative vignettes that help to understand how our interlocutors construct COVID-19. As we will show, rumors, conspiracy theories, controversies, religion, and varying types of logic, beliefs, and evidence are in play in these Covidian vignettes. We ground our analyses in the relevant literature, in these vignettes, and in the information presented in our five Tables.

Data Presentation and Analysis

In Table 16.1, we present some important demographic information about our interlocutors, describing their age ranges; genders; monthly household incomes; family structures—nuclear or joint; household locations—city, town, or village; and levels of education.

General Awareness of Coronavirus Existence

During the most critical phase of the pandemic in Pakistan—from March to May 2020—we asked various questions to determine our interlocutors'

Table 16.1 Socio-economic Characteristics of Respondents

	Characteristics	Percentage based on (N=321)
Age	15–25	46%
	25–35	37%
	35–45	10%
	Above 45	7%
Gender	Male	51%
	Female	49%
Household monthly income	Less than 20,000 PKR/120US$	32%
	20000–40000 PKR/120-240US$	21%
	40000–60000 PKR/240-360US$	13%
	Above 60000 PKR/360US$	34%
Family Structure	Nuclear	49%
	Joint	51%
Household location	City	66%
	Town	6%
	Village	28%
Education	Above 16 years education	18%
	16 years education	57%
	14 years	13%
	12 yeas	7%
	10 years	3%
	Less than 10 years	2%

levels of information about COVID-19. Our first questions involved people's opinions about this novel coronavirus, as shown in Table 16.2.

When talking about the dangers of COVID-19, 80% of respondents agreed that it is caused by a deadly virus. They were of the view that this awareness was being spread through the media by the government, which had launched an info-campaign on March 28, 2020. Specifically, this campaign was launched by the Pakistan's National Command and Operation Center (NCOC), with the cooperation of the health secretaries of each province. Moreover, social media were filled with pictures of dying people and the lack of needed hospital beds; these created fears of death among our interlocutors. In contrast, 20% of respondents believed that no such virus exists, saying things like, "If someone has a cough or a temperature due to effects of changing weather, doctors declare them COVID patients."[2] This statement resonates with the title of Chapter 4 on Kenya: "As soon as people see you cough, they say you have the disease."

The origin of the virus remained very controversial among our interlocutors. Some expressed conspiracy theories such as, "It is the start of a biowar among power states." A male PhD professor, who is a 42-year-old

Table 16.2 Opinions about the Coronavirus

Summary of Survey responses

Questions	Answer Options	Percentage based on (N=321) (out of 100%)
1. Do you think that the coronavirus is deadly?	Yes No	80% 20%
2. Is the coronavirus human-made?	Yes No	42% 58%
3. Are there treatments available for the coronavirus?	Yes No	45% 55%
4. Can medicines used to treat other diseases be used to alleviate the symptoms of the coronavirus?	Yes No	64% 36%
5. Is the coronavirus equally dangerous for infants/children?	Yes No	79% 21%
6. Is the coronavirus equally as dangerous for women as for men?	Yes No	83% 17%

well-known statistician currently working at a well-respected university, stated, "The third world war will happen via the Internet and this spread of disease is part of that." It was generally believed that "the virus was produced through laboratories intentionally to destroy the economies of countries." Some further added that viral videos on social media showed the intentional spread of the virus by some Chinese people in their own country. They were clearly seen in the video coughing on grocery store items, touching "infected" hands on elevator surfaces and operating buttons, and also distributing "infected" masks among ordinary citizens. The Chinese people in the video were quite likely unaware of their viral status, but the video made it appear that they were intentionally attempting to spread the virus, thereby reinforcing this geopolitical conspiracy theory (see Ali 2020b).

About possible treatments, respondents were fairly evenly divided: 45% believed that COVID-19 treatment was available and the rest did not. Participants expressed varying views: "It is the combination of medicines that effectively helps to cure the illness"; "Since the death ratio of this disease is very low, then why is it labeled 'incurable'?" 55% of respondents believed that "There is no specific treatment yet invented." These were of the view that the medications currently in use are parts of clinical trials, and that sometimes they work effectively and sometimes not. Some also believed that the intensity of viral spread and human response differ among communities and countries. They felt that the type of virus identified in Pakistan is the "weak type" that does not badly affect the masses and could be treated with light medications. Some also believed that more deadly forms of the virus exist in Europe and the United States, and that if these come to Pakistan, there would be complete destruction. It was generally believed that the existing kind of virus in Pakistan could be treated, while the other forms found only abroad could not.

A full 83% of our respondents believed that COVID is equally dangerous for both men and women, and including children. Nevertheless, 17% of our respondents believed that men are more vulnerable to catching COVID-19 than women, as men have to leave home to earn money and buy food to meet their families' needs, and thus have a high probability of contagion. An elderly, poor, and uneducated woman, who was the head of her rural household, clarified:

> My son goes out every day to earn our bread and butter. If he catches the disease, we may not be able to survive. There would be nothing to eat at home. But if the daughter-in-law catches the virus, other females like the mother-in-law and the daughters can replace her work. There is no substitute for male earning. That is the main reason to support and provide him with better safety.

This statement can best be understood against the backdrop of existing structural disparities in Pakistan, where many male members are dominant due to holding economic resources; thus the illness of the male is taken more seriously than that of the female (see Ali 2020d).

Physical Distancing, Handshaking, and Cultural Activities

Since the term "social distancing" has been highly criticized by anthropologists due to its denial of the primary human characteristic of sociability (Ali and Davis-Floyd 2020), we here employ the term "physical distancing," which does not mean "don't socialize" but rather means "stay at a physical distance of around six feet from those who do not belong to your family and household both indoors and outdoors." Physical distancing is a major part of the government SOPs, in combination with various other preventive actions like cleaning hands, avoiding surface touching, and wearing masks (Maclellan 2020). People are advised to stay at home and avoid face-to-face interactions. Current research illustrates the consequences of negligence in following the SOPs: according to Gregory Poland, infectious disease expert at the Mayo Clinic (one of the largest and most respected medical research institutions in the USA), "When you extend your hand, you are extending a bioweapon" (quoted in Lufkin 2020: 2). Poland calls handshaking an "outmoded custom" that should cease to exist (ibid).

In our research (see Table 16.3), around 97% of respondents stated that they currently avoid handshaking and hugging. Echoing Poland's words above, one of our interlocutors, who worked as a lecturer in a university, stated that, "In my opinion, we may never be able to shake hands ever

Table 16.3 Cultural Activities

Summary of survey responses	Question Options	Answers Percentage based on (N=321) (out of 100%)
7. Do you avoid cultural activities like shaking hands/embracing/hugging?	Yes No	97% 3%
8. Do you attended funerals to offer your condolences?	Yes No	58% 42%
9. Do you visit relatives/friends/family homes?	Yes No	42% 58%
10. Do you offer prayers in the mosque during the Ramzan in pandemic?	Yes No	51% 49%
11. Do you welcome guests on Eid al-Adha at your home? (Eid al-Adha is an Islamic religious festival that commemorates Ibrahim's willingness to sacrifice his son to God.)	Yes No	55% 45%

again in the future." A respondent who is a government official added that: "Extending a hand is equal to having a bomb in the other hand that would explode if you shake hands, and the person would die."

During an FGD, one of the discussants, who works as a primary school teacher in a city, expressed his irritation by saying, "Although everybody knows that shaking hands can be harmful, various people still extend a hand for greetings. Such ignorant behavior is beyond understanding." Only 3% of our interlocutors still tried to shake hands when greeting others. They were of the view that handshaking is a social ritual that cannot be ignored so easily. One of these participants, a 35-year-old security guard, said, "Tightly holding hands shows the warming welcome of meeting others. If we don't shake hands, how will others know that we are happy to see them?" A participant who works as a shopkeeper turned out to be another conspiracy theorist; he responded that "There is no such virus that actually exists; it is only a drama by the government to restrict the [economically] poor and kill them to reduce the population." Clearly, his statement is oxymoronic—if the virus does not exist, then how can it kill the poor? The oxymoronic nature of this statement reflects the lack of health literacy and scientific understanding that was shared by a substantial number of our participants, as we will further show below.

Returning here to the topic of physical distancing, we note that a full 58% of our interlocutors chose to attend funerals despite the danger of viral spread. The general opinion was that "When you are a member of a society, funerals and condolences can never be ignored due to social pressure to attend." One well-educated housewife interlocutor had attended the funeral of a COVID-19-infected person. When we inquired why, she responded, "It was the death of a close relative. When I participated in the funeral, I felt like I was at the frontline of a war border. Anyway, I could not ignore the sympathy visit; otherwise, I would have had to face the criticisms of my relatives, which would have been quite stressful for me." In contrast, 42% of our participants said that they avoided funerals, replacing condolence visits with either a phone or a video call. During our conversation, one of our male interlocutors, who ran a textile business, stated that "We pray for the departed souls online." The pre-COVID cultural way of offering condolences was to pray for the eternal peace of the departed soul during a visit to the mourning family's home (see Ali 2021a). This practice has been converted by many into sending online wishes or updating prayer status on social media.

Even at the peak of viral spread, 42% of our respondents ignored the SOP of physical distancing and continued to visit their relatives and friends; 58% said that they avoided such activities. One respondent working as a government bureaucrat complained that "The government closed everything to maintain social distance, while people considered it as a public holiday and started to visit relatives for the sake of enjoyment." A middle-aged lawyer who was trying to follow the SOPs stated, "I had pasted a written note outside of the gate to our home saying that we had a COVID-positive patient inside to keep people from coming in, but people came in anyway for the sake of wishing a healthy recovery!"

Regarding religious activities, 51% of our interlocutors said that they had gone to mosques to pray. The government closed the mosques during its initial lockdown, yet many were reluctant to accept this restriction. Later in May 2020, during Ramazan (the Pakistani name for the Islamic holy month in which Muslims observe fasting), it was made compulsory to maintain 6 feet of distance between those praying (see Abi-Habib and ur-Rehman 2020). These respondents, both male and female (as during Ramazan, in this patriarchal society even women voluntarily participate in *Juma* [Friday] communal prayers), never missed a Friday congregational prayer. One of them, a female factory worker with 10 years of education, insisted that "A virus cannot enter sacred places; a mosque is a clean, pious place. It is the symptom of weak religious belief to skip the mosque prayer." Her statement both reveals a lack of scientific awareness of the means of viral transmission and shows how contagion deniers can stigmatize and blame the contagion-conscious for not following religious norms.

A young female student expressed the Pakistani cultural belief in *Qismat* (destiny or fate) when she stated, "Our time of death is pre-written; if it comes due to congregational prayer, it would be equal to martyrdom." One male teacher stated, "I have never seen such a huge crowd for prayer at mosques ever before, not even during Ramazan. People are anxious with the horror of death with COVID-19." We note here the power of ritual to comfort and calm (Davis-Floyd and Laughlin 2022): so reassuring is a formal prayer to these people that they will risk contagion in order to practice this ritual for the psychological (and perhaps supernatural) benefits it brings. In contrast, 49% of respondents stated that either they don't pray, or do so at home individually.

Another important Muslim ritual practice is the performance of sacrifices, including animal sacrifices, to overcome or deal with a difficult situation, especially during certain religious ceremonies and festivals (Nougairede 2013). Animal sacrifices and Muslim rituals in general have become even more important during COVID-19 as people pray to Allah to protect them and their loved ones from this disease and to end the pandemic. Yet 45% of our interlocutors said that they avoid community gatherings, particularly religious ones. In contrast, almost 55% of participants said that they invited people to gatherings—religious or otherwise—where food was served. One respondent, a 41-year-old man running his own frozen food business, shared his experience, "We have a cultural custom to bring salty meat and rice from homes and eat together. I felt that I had to participate, as not doing so would symbolize me as a coward who fears death. But after this *Eid* [a Pakistani religious festival] lunch, I became very sick and caught the virus." During pandemic times, clearly, many cultural customs can be downright dangerous, causing every Pakistani who believes that COVID-19 is real to have to choose between two dangers: that of not following custom and perhaps getting sick, and that of breaking custom to avoid contagion and suffering negative sociocultural consequences.

Rational and Irrational Approaches to Mask Wearing and Physical Distancing

With the outbreak of COVID-19, the use of masks became essential to prevent viral spread. Initially, masks—especially medical masks—were in short supply in many countries, revealing how unprepared the world was for a pandemic. To tackle the situation, WHO issued a call for the increased production of masks, and also set distribution priorities to provide healthcare workers and the most vulnerable communities first. In the case of Pakistan, the NCOC had declared in early March 2020 that people must wear masks in public places.

Regarding Table 16.4, the first and foremost response from our participants was the positive use of a mask. Almost 76% responded that they do not care what others think, as they consider masking to be the only source of protection to avoid viral contagion. The rest of the respondents were negatively affected by the opinions and comments of others regarding mask wearing, as we further discuss below.

Here we highlight a few interview responses that represent people's general attitudes. One young graduate stated, "One of my relatives, while visiting my home, asked me why I wear a mask at home, even though it is

Table 16.4 Mask Wearing and Physical Distancing

Summary of survey responses	Question Options	Answers Percentage based on (N=321) (out of 100%)
12. I do not cover my face with a mask/cloth because people would make fun of me.	Never Concerned Occasionally Sometimes Always	76% 6% 10% 8%
13. I avoid distancing because my environment does not support it.	Never Occasionally Sometimes Always	42% 12% 26% 20%
14. I do not wear a mask because (I cannot breathe, feel hot, have shortness of breath)	Never Occasionally Sometimes Always	52% 8% 26% 14%
15. The coronavirus is not as dangerous as presented by the media.	Never Occasionally Often Sometimes Always	34% 11% 13% 29% 13%
16. I avoid distancing because people would tag me as a coward.	Never Occasionally Sometimes Always	71% 3% 14% 12%

possible to avoid close interaction with guests." Another person working in a hospital as a helper said, "I was *living* with a COVID positive patient. Still, people would ask me the reason for wearing a mask all the time although they were well aware of my work." For many Pakistanis, mask wearing symbolizes certain personal characteristics: that the people wearing the masks do not trust in Qismat—that everything is predetermined, including the timing of one's death (Ali 2020c)—and/or that they are cowards. One female respondent working as a housemaid stated, "Covering the face is thought to make you look like a clown." One educated Muslim homemaker expressed her religious belief that "In the beginning, modern fashionable ladies—though Muslims—used to make fun of those women who wore a *Burqa* [a long cloth veil used by many women in Pakistan to cover their entire body, either including the entire face with slits for seeing, or just the mouth and nose, leaving the eyes uncovered]. Now, the fact that everyone is compelled to hide one's face is the result of a minor act of God." In this way, she manages to productively use her religious faith to justify the resemblance of mask usage to wearing a burqa and as a fulfillment of God's will. Considering the socio-cultural conceptions of covering the face, we note the contrast between facemask use as a hygienic practice and as a practice that modern, urban Pakistani women stigmatize. And we note that one positive effect of universal mask usage is that it prevents discrimination against sick individuals, for whom mask wearing has long been mandatory in Pakistan.

In regard to physical distancing, around 60% of respondents said that they face some form of difficulty in their efforts to distance themselves from others. Either they were living in an environment that did not support such distancing, or were working in a crowded place (see Ali and Ali 2020). A woman living in a hostel said, "Living alone is tough while you are supposed to live with three other roommates and share a common room as well." A Food Panda (a food delivery service) delivery boy insisted, "It's better to stay in a congested living place rather than to be homeless and on the street." A housemaid said, "Working as a maid at various homes and trying to sustain space are two parallel things that cannot be accomplished at the same time." In contrast, 40% of respondents said that they had been keeping physical distance. A 62-year-old farmer elaborated, "We can maintain physical distance only if we stop receiving guests, ignore friends, and minimize our social life."

Here we turn to the exploration of three key themes that emerged from our data: (1) viral awareness—or its lack; (2) the protective measures adopted by our interlocutors—or not; and (3) the religious interpretations of COVID-19 that greatly affected people's behaviors in potentially harmful ways.

Regarding the stigma of being a "coward," many respondents ignored that stigma and said that they keep physical distance despite it. In contrast, 29% of respondents had been negatively affected by being labeled a coward. One 26-year-old student stated, "[Because I wear a mask in public], my community members say that I am afraid of death, while I am just trying to avoid sickness." A 52-year-old businessman said, "Meeting a sick person is the same as exposing yourself to an atomic bomb. People do not understand that death is the ultimate truth but committing suicide is something different." His words reflect his scientific understanding of COVID-19 transmission routes and his concern for people who lack or deny this understanding.

The Negatively Perceived Role of the Media

About the dangers of the virus, the media worked to spread awareness and the need to follow the SOPs. Yet one interlocutor, who was working as a freelancer, insisted that "The media created more fear than awareness." A government official said, "The media did not play a positive role and exaggerated the degree of viral spread." During our FGDs, several negative opinions about the roles played by the media were expressed, such as:

- The media presented COVID-19 as incurable and reported an incorrect number of deaths that compelled people to hide their sickness instead of going for treatment.

- The image created by the media was unsupportive of patients. People started to avoid going for tests and tried to hide their sickness.
- No campaign was launched for immunity boost-up.
- The media did not show any single positive perspective. The media never interviewed people who had recovered from COVID.

These points are well taken; indeed the media, in Pakistan as elsewhere, should have done a much better job that took such perspectives into account.

Religious Interpretations of COVID-19: Anxiety, Qismat, and Ignoring the Virus

Two primary factors involved in perceptions of COVID-19 are "anxiety" and "religious healing," both of which we sought to identify during our conversations with our interlocutors. Anxiety is traced in words such as "My hands get numb when I hear about death due to virus attack." One interlocutor spoke for many when he said, "I lie awake at night with the fear that I might get the virus." During our discussions with university students, the following responses emerged:

- My hands get clammy and my heartbeat gets disturbed when I imagine myself as a patient of COVID.
- Every single night I sleep with the fear that I might have caught the virus. In contrast, every following day after having a good sleep, I find myself refreshed—which reveals that on that past night it was only tiredness, not disease symptoms.
- I am afraid if I catch the infection, no one from my family would take me to the doctor for treatment.

Regarding religious healing, our interlocutors emphasized that religion does provide them with emotional support. For instance, "[I recited] verses [from the Quran] to help to gain the emotional strength to fight COVID." A respondent who was working as a sales officer at a shopping mall, whose father had died due to COVID, strongly believed in Qismat—predefined destiny—and stated, "Death is predetermined by God. The virus attack was just an excuse for his death."

Yet at the societal level, personal beliefs and behaviors are contradictory. Those who are religious consistently defied the SOPs, such as the prohibitions on handshaking, sharing food, and large gatherings. One large congregation of around 80,000 people gathered in early March 2020 in Lahore, Punjab and became a major source of viral spread; 539 confirmed cases were reported as a result of this gathering. Government Minister Fawad Chaudhary railed against the "stubbornness of the clergy" who had insisted on holding this gathering (Chaudhry 2020). This religious congregation became the epicenter of initial viral spread across the country. To justify such behaviors, religious practitioners generated conspiracy theories about the virus and its scientific identification, such as those presented above (Bentzen 2020). The closing of religious gathering places was viewed by many as a "sign of anger" from the government against certain religious leaders and local *Mulas* (heads of mosques).

Infectious diseases possess a well-established history of carrying stigma resulting from their social constructions, which can contribute to discrimination and social disharmony (Das 2020). In Pakistan, coronavirus spread was stigmatized by religious leaders as "punishment for prevalent illegal sexual dishonesty." The illicit sexual relations referred to here are secret affairs between men and women, or girlfriends and boyfriends, without *nikah*—the Islamic marriage contract.

Conclusion

Our study has shown that the level of awareness among our interlocutors about COVID-19 and its dangers and the need to follow the SOPS is relatively high. Yet a substantial number of our participants showed low levels of knowledge about COVID-19 that often led to a nonchalant attitude, making it harder to control the disease. In the absence of sufficient knowledge, people may fail to assess the potential harms that could result from their non-compliant actions (Wagner 2003). Pakistan, with its insufficient infrastructure, deficiency of medical emergency preparedness, and low testing rates, struggles to combat COVID-19. The number of cases grew exponentially, especially after the lifting of lockdown, which was established on March 15, 2020 and removed on May 8, 2020 to allow festive religious activities. Both Ramazan and the religious festival of *Eid al-fitar* were celebrated enthusiastically all over the country. For these events, and due to pressure from religious leaders and the people's wishes, the government relaxed its lockdown and opened the markets for fixed hours, five days a week. Highly placed government officials gave permission to prepare for these occasions, asked people to observe the SOPs, and sought to ensure the implementation of these SOPs via police vigilance.

On the one hand, many of our interlocutors were truly frightened of dying from COVID-19; on the other, many believed that God predetermines their time of death (see Ali 2020b); thus for them, COVID-19 is irrelevant. Many were personally willing to practice physical distancing, but when their social environments did not support this practice, ultimately either they dropped the idea or accepted being stigmatized as cowards. Some chose not to engage in physical distancing, often due to their religious beliefs, as we have shown. Although viral dispersion peaked during the religious festivities, many ignored the SOPs in favor of the emotional and psychological comfort that the performance of religious rituals can provide. Our results have shown that religious faith can serve both as a source of comfort and courage and as a source of viral spreading behaviors. To believe that one's death is predetermined can translate to doing nothing to prevent contagion. Why bother? Hence, our study results clearly show the influence of both religion and culture on COVID-related beliefs and behaviors in Pakistan.

Yet COVID-19 can also constitute an agent of social change. Most Pakistanis have changed their social behaviors to follow the SOPs, yet such changes are often only slowly accepted. Over time, we believe that Pakistanis will learn to better cope with this situational stress and will more universally adopt changed interaction patterns. This kind of Covidian adaptation will most likely need to continue for many months or even years to come. Even the expected arrival of a vaccine is not likely to keep COVID-19 at bay in Pakistan, as we can expect that vaccine uptake will be insufficient to create herd immunity, for some of the same reasons that many refuse to follow the SOPs, and because many Pakistanis, especially in rural areas, oppose or are suspicious of vaccination in general (see Ali 2020b, c, d; Ali and Ali 2020; Ali 2021b; Ali, Sadique and Ali 2021).

In conclusion, we reiterate that, although their responses to our questions show a high level of COVID-19 knowledge among our interlocutors, some expressed misperceptions and engaged in behaviors that enhanced viral dispersion. Inappropriate understandings and behaviors keep people at high risk of acquiring the virus, highlighting the need to increase local understandings. Most especially, we argue that the Pakistani media must not promote precautionary measures in ways that instill the kinds of fears that our interlocutors expressed, which resulted in many people not getting tested and trying to hide their illness, in what Mayarí Hengstermann (this volume), calls the "prevention paradox." Instead of showing and telling the kinds of horror stories that generate such fears, the media should focus more on telling the stories of people who have recovered, as an interlocutor suggested, or who, despite direct exposure, have successfully staved off contagion by effectively following the SOPs. In other words, the media should not promote the SOPs via negative fear-mongering, but rather as positive ways to fulfill people's desires to protect themselves and others from viral contagion.

Notes

1 See Ali 2020a, b, c; Ali and Ali 2020; Ali and Davis-Floyd 2020, 2021; Ali, Sadique, and Ali 2020; Ali 2021a, 2021b; Ali et al. 2021.
2 These findings are similar to those of other studies—see Ali, 2020a, b; Ali and Ali 2020; Ali, Sadique, and Ali 2020; Ali et al. 2021.

References

Abi-Habib, M., and ur-Rehman, Z. 2020. Imams Overrule Pakistan's Coronavirus Lockdown as Ramadan Nears. *New York Times*. Retrieved from www.nytimes.com/2020/04/23/world/asia/pakistan-coronavirus-ramadan.html

Abrar, M. 2020. Pakistan eases lockdown as Covid-19 kills 46 in single-day spike. *Pakistan Today*.

Ali, I. 2020a. The COVID-19 pandemic: Making sense of rumor and fear. *Medical Anthropology* 39(5): 376–379. doi:10.1080/01459740.2020.1745481

Ali, I. 2020b. Impacts of rumors and conspiracy theories surrounding COVID-19 on preparedness programs. *Disaster Medicine and Public Health Preparedness*, 1–6. https://doi.org/10.1017/dmp.2020.325

Ali, I. 2020c. *Constructing and Negotiating Measles: The Case of Sindh Province of Pakistan*. PhD dissertation. Vienna, Austria: University of Vienna.

Ali, I. 2020d. Impact of COVID-19 on vaccination programs: Adverse or positive? *Human Vaccines and Immunotherapeutics* 16(11): 2594–2600. doi:10.1080/21645515.2020.1787065

Ali, I. 2021a. From Normal to Viral Body: Death rituals during ordinary and extraordinary Covidian times in Pakistan. *Frontiers in Sociology* 5: 133.

Ali, I. 2021b. Rituals of containment: Many pandemics, body politics, and social dramas during COVID-19 in Pakistan. *Frontiers in Sociology* 6, 83.

Ali, I., and Ali, S. 2020. Why may COVID-19 overwhelm low-income countries like Pakistan? *Disaster Medicine and Public Health Preparedness* 1–5. doi:10.1017/dmp.2020.329

Ali, I., and Davis-Floyd, R. 2020. The interplay of words and politics during COVID-19: Contextualizing the universal pandemic vocabulary. *Practicing Anthropology* 42(4): 20–24.

Ali, I., Sadique, S., and Ali, S. 2020. COVID-19 Significantly affects maternal health: A rapid-response investigation from Pakistan. *Frontiers in Global Women's Health* 1. doi:10.3389/fgwh.2020.591809.

Ali, I., Sadique, S., and Ali, S. 2021. COVID-19 and vaccination campaigns as "Western plots" in Pakistan: Government policies, (geo-) politics and local perceptions and beliefs. *Frontiers in Sociology* 6: 82.

Ali, I., Sadique, S., Ali, S., and Davis-Floyd, R.E. 2021. Birthing between the "traditional" and the "modern": Dāi practices and childbearing women's choices during COVID-19 in Pakistan. *Frontiers in Sociology* 6: 49.

Ali, M. Y., and Bhatti, R. 2020. COVID-19 (Coronavirus) pandemic: Information sources channels for the public health awareness. *Asia Pacific Journal of Public Health* 32(4): 168–169.

Chaudhry, A. 2020 *Tableeghi Jamaat in hot water in Pakistan too for Covid-19 spread*. DAWN. Retrieved April 8, 2021.

Das, M. 2020. Social construction of stigma and its implications: Observations from COVID-19. *Social Science and Humanities Open* 27. Retrieved from: https://papers.ssrn.com/sol3/papers.cfm?abstract_id=3599764

Davis-Floyd, R., and Laughlin, C.D. 2022. *Ritual: What It Is, How It Works, and Why*. New York: Berghahn Books.

Davis-Floyd, R., and Laughlin, C.D. Forthcoming. *Ritual: What It Is, How It Works, and Why*. New York: Berghahn Books.

Hamid, N. 2020. Govt warns stern actions against traders who raise face mask price: Pakistan. *Daily Times*. Retrieved from https://dailytimes.com.pk/567976/govt-warns-stern-actions-against-traders-who-raise-face-mask-price-nausheen-hamid/

Johnson, J.E., and Abramson, C.M. 2020. Ethnography in the time of COVID-19. *American Sociological Association* 48(3). Retrieved from www.asanet.org/news-events/footnotes/may-jun-2020/professional-challenges-facing-sociologists/ethnography-time-covid-19

Ladiwala, Z.F.R., Dhillon, R.A., Zahid, I., Irfan, O., Khan, M.S., Awan, S., et al. 2021. Knowledge, attitude and perception of Pakistanis towards COVID-19; a large cross-sectional survey. *BMC Public Health* 21(1): 21. doi:10.1186/s12889-020-10083-y

Latif, A. 2020. Pakistan: "Politicization" of COVID-19 leads to confusion. *Politics Asia-Pacific*. Retrieved from www.aa.com.tr/en/asia-pacific/pakistan-politicization-of-covid-19-leads-to-confusion/2080214

Lufkin, B. 2020. Will COVID-19 end the handshake? *BBC*. Retrieved from www.bbc.com/worklife/article/20200413-coronavirus-will-covid-19-end-the-handshake

Maclellan, L. 2020. Coronavirus: Here's how to avoid handshakes without offending anyone. *World Economic Forum*. Retrieved from www.weforum.org/agenda/2020/03/handshake-coronavirus-work-hygiene/

Munawar, K., and Choudhry, F.R. 2021. Exploring stress coping strategies of frontline emergency health workers dealing Covid-19 in Pakistan: A qualitative inquiry. *American Journal of Infection Control* 49(3): 286–292.

Nougairede, A., Fossati, C., Salez, N., Cohen-Bacrie, S., Ninove, L., Michel, F., et al. 2013. Sheep-to-human transmission of Orf virus during Eid al-Adha religious practices, France. *Emerging infectious diseases* 19(1): 102.

Siddiqui, N. 2020, October 28. Wearing face mask made mandatory as second wave of Covid-19 sweeps across Pakistan: www.dawn.com/news/1587447

Wagner, W.E. 2003. Commons ignorance: The failure of environmental law to produce needed information on health and the environment. *Duke LJ* 53: 1619.

17 Local Perceptions of COVID-19 in Pakistan's Sindh Province

Political Game, Supernatural Test, or Western Conspiracy?

Inayat Ali, Salma Sadique, and Shahbaz Ali

Introduction

In Pakistan, the Ministry of Health confirmed the first two COVID-19 infections on February 26, 2020: one person in Karachi and another in Islamabad.[1] Within the next 15 days, the virus "officially" infected around 20 people, while the suspected number of infected people was around 470. The highest number of infections was in Sindh province, followed by Gilgit Baltistan (Imtaiz Ali et al. 2020). All those confirmed to be infected had traveled from Iran, Syria, or London. Infections rapidly escalated, and by the end of August 2020, the virus had infected around 30,000 people, of whom over 6,000 died. This spread led the Pakistani government to impose lockdown, and thereafter what the government called "smart" lockdown, which is the same as the "targeted" lockdowns imposed in the USA (Ali and Davis-Floyd 2020). Nevertheless, by the end of April 2021, the virus had infected around 826,000 Pakistanis, of whom approximately 18,000 had died (WHO 2021). Owing to a rapid escalation of infection, the government re-imposed smart lockdown in 20 cities across the country, including the capital, Islamabad. By April 2021, as anticipated, the third wave of the pandemic caused a critical situation in Pakistan, despite the apparent efforts of the government to control the situation.

The novelty and scale of this disease, along with its uncertainties and ambiguities, have made it critical for health authorities to plan appropriate strategies for effective preparedness. The government's efforts to contain the virus have included: early case detection and tracing and tracking contacts; efforts to communicate the risks of the virus to the public; and mandating physical distancing, quarantine, and isolation—including from one's family—for COVID+ people. The government opened specific quarantine centers, which were heavily criticized for being like "jails" that kept COVID sufferers imprisoned, and for not having the necessary facilities.

People's continuous worries and fears have created a fertile environment for local perspectives and narratives in the forms of rumors and conspiracy theories to emerge; thus the local perspectives of laypeople from villages and

DOI: 10.4324/9781003187462-22

from a small town of Pakistan's Sindh province constitute the subject matter of this chapter. We will analyze these perspectives after situating them within global as well as sociocultural, economic, and political perspectives.

Methods and Materials

During May and June 2020, we carried out the study we report on here in a small town of the *Matiari* District in Sindh province of Pakistan. Located in the southeastern portion of the country, Sindh is geographically one of the largest of the four provinces of Pakistan. We collected our data using well-established anthropological research methods. To conduct anthropological research, one needs ample time to build rapport, mingle with interlocutors, develop tools, and gather data methodically as well as through observation. Although the research for this chapter did not encompass long-term ethnographic fieldwork on COVID-19, it does draw on our earlier long-term ethnographic fieldwork projects in Pakistan, mainly in Sindh province, which we have been conducting since 2005: Inayat Ali (2005 to the present), Salma Sadique (from 2013 on), and Shabazz Ali (from 2012 on). The fieldwork projects of Inayat Ali (2008–2011 and 2013–2020), and Shabazz Ali (2014–2020) on health and illness provide background and context for this present chapter.

For the primary data collection in the selected village, we drew on Salma's long-term fieldwork (2013–2020); for this particular project, Salma simply contacted her prior interlocutors. Given the constraints of the pandemic, and using convenience sampling, we conducted ten online group discussions, seven one-on-one interviews, and 30 cellphone discussions. We made every effort to make our sampling inclusive in terms of decisive sociocultural factors: gender, religion, level of formal education, and occupation/job. We obtained data from women, men, Muslims and non-Muslims, the formally educated and non-educated, government employees, and daily wage laborers. The purpose of this diverse sampling was to incorporate multiple and differing perspectives, as all these identities play pivotal roles in shaping the ideas and practices of the people in the selected locale. To perform content analysis, we used social media such as WhatsApp and Facebook.

This study forms part of a project that was approved by Pakistan's National Bioethics Committee (reference No.4-87/NBC-471-COVID-19-09/20/). It included an informal interview guide that encompassed 14 central themes related to COVID-19, including the necessary socio-economic information about our interlocutors on which this chapter draws. The intention behind using an informal interview guide was to avoid affecting the views of interlocutors, as well as not making them feel uncomfortable with a "formal" interview. To maintain ethical considerations, we sought verbal consent from our interlocutors and have anonymized their names. Again, our analyses of our current data on COVID-19 build on our above-noted ethnographic fieldwork projects in Pakistan, including in Sindh province.

COVID-19 from a Local Perspective in Sindh

While globally, (mis)information about COVID-19 is circulating rapidly around the sociocultural landscape, Pakistanis have their own, unique, and socioculturally rooted (mis)information and (mis)conceptions about COVID-19 (Ali 2020c). As the number of affected people increased, people's perceptions of COVID-19 also gradually changed. Everyone is affected by the pandemic directly or indirectly, yet some people, including many Pakistanis, still consider it to be "propaganda." As in other countries, various local perspectives and narratives about COVID-19 have emerged in Pakistan (Ali 2020c, e, 2021; Ali et al. 2020). For a non-COVID-related example of how rumors and conspiracy theories can spread in local areas, Inayat Ali reports that he repeatedly heard varying narratives in Sindh province concerning an unfamiliar, aggressive and dangerous small animal that appeared and attacked. This story held that:

> the animal was an Indian conspiracy to cause havoc in Pakistan— someone imported them from an Indian zoo to deliberately set them free in Pakistan. The other held that the animal had emerged from an unknown area. As fear grew larger and stronger, villages started assigning duties to various individuals to provide 24-hour security. People, especially children, were afraid to sleep. The male members stopped sleeping at an Otāq (a male guest house) or walking outside the house after sunset. Frequent announcements broke out about seeing the animal, which caused villagers to gather with their dogs and their weapons—rifles, pistols, axes, and sticks. These gatherings attracted the local media. A few deaths occurred, in which the bodies were said to contain "paw"-like marks, which added further fear into an already chaotic situation. Despite the fact that such an animal was never captured, the rumor continued unabated for over a month.
>
> (Ali 2020b: 260)

Similarly, multiple competing narratives have been surrounding vaccination campaigns—that these campaigns contain "hidden interests" and are a "Western plot to sterilize Muslim women," leading to vaccine resentments and refusals (Ali 2020b). The "Western plot" and "hidden interest" narratives became a reality in 2011 when the media reported a fake vaccination drive that the American Central Intelligence Agency (CIA) organized in Abbottabad city to locate Osama bin Ladin. This critical event was termed "vaccination suicide" for Pakistan, as it negatively affected the Expanded Programme on Immunization (EPI); many vaccinators were attacked, and more than 100 were killed (ibid.).

Likewise, various narratives have surrounded COVID-19 about the "hidden agent" behind it. Some believe that either the USA or Big Pharma has "bioengineered" COVID-19. People also started circulating information about home remedies, for example, drinking garlic water or "blowing hot air from a hair dryer through your nostrils"; or keeping one's throat moist on the recommendation of the country's Health Ministry (Dawn 2020). Two highly prevalent narratives in Sindh province were about prevention:

(1) A widespread rumor broke out in Sindh province, from its district *Hyderabad* to district *Ddaharki*, that shaving one's head protects against the virus. As soon as this rumor traveled, many men (the shaving of a woman's head is considered shameful) immediately shaved their heads—a very affordable preventive measure that costs only US5-10 cents. In one village of Sindh, over 50 men had their heads shaved.

(Ali 2020e, 2021: 677)

This rumor is a good example of how a society can come up with an easily accessible "cure" in the absence of a practical and effective healthcare system, and in the presence of a disease that to date has no actual proven biomedical cure. The second narrative that emerged concerned an infant in the northern part of Sindh Province; it quickly spread in many districts with multiple forms but with the same idea as given below:

(2) After this baby's miraculous birth, he started talking: "I will not survive. I am here to tell you something important about the current coronavirus, that the disease is deadly. I will die at noon and will bring the coronavirus with me," said the child. It could kill everyone if a recommended measure was not taken. The measure was brewing green tea, and every person should drink five sips. The one who would drink these five sips would survive; the rest would die. "As long as my heart beats, I ask you to please drink tea." After conveying this message, the child died.

(Ali 2020e, 2021: 677)

Following the wide dissemination of this narrative, many laypeople got on their mobile phones to make calls and send messages to their family, friends, and acquaintances. Some even paid in-person visits to their neighbors to bring the great news of this miraculous treatment, showing the locals' strong belief in the supernatural. In contrast, some local people feel that COVID-19 does not exist but is just a "political game" being played because the Pakistani government wants funds from high-income countries and from the International Monetary Fund (IMF). Inayat Ali (2020e, 2021) discovered that many people in Sindh and Punjab provinces believe that "the government is only imposing lockdowns to receive global attention for potential foreign aid and that there is no danger." Therefore, many believe that the government is "fabricating" the statistics, which is why the number of infected people is escalating. Some interlocutors believe that COVID-19 is a *Yahudi Sazish*

(Jewish conspiracy) to stop Muslims from going to mosques. Those who do not believe that this pandemic exists freely go to markets and roam around. They believe that there is no reality in the coronavirus as presented in the media; they reason, "If COVID-19 exists, why have we not been affected?"

In contrast, some Pakistanis who do believe that it is real fear contracting it; hence, they have been maintaining self-quarantine. Sorath—a 35-year-old woman from Sindh Province working in a nongovernmental organization (NGO) in Matiari District —stated that:

> Our life is totally at risk. We are fearful of contracting the virus, as the pandemic has affected millions of people worldwide. Owing to that fear, there are people who even have a simple cough; they think they have contracted the virus. My uncle died due to heart failure. Since he had symptoms of COVID-19, he was brought for a test for this virus to a nearby hospital. On his way, he got heart failure because he was significantly under stress and fearful of contracting COVID-19. Consequently, he died when he was on the way to a hospital. He was worried, like many people in Sindh, to be tested for the coronavirus due to the attached fear that he will be put in quarantine.

Moreover, some interlocutors perceive that the coronavirus is only dangerous when one does not follow the required measures such as physical distancing, wearing masks, and using a sanitizer. If a person follows precautions, eats a healthy diet, and does not go outside, then s/he is safe from this virus. As Qudarat, who is in her late 40s and a gynecologist at a government hospital of Matiari District, explained:

> COVID-19 has created an alarming situation for us. We must take precautions because we will also be dealing with it soon. It is better to make our body prepared and strong while eating a healthy diet and practicing physical distancing. The most important thing is to make our minds strong enough to deal with this critical disease.

Most interlocutors argued that they have not in actuality met any COVID-infected person; however, they have constantly been reading and watching about them on social and print media. Thinking about COVID-19 has resulted in psychological depression in some people, as they fear that the government might enforce quarantine and isolate them from their families. And being diagnosed with COVID-19 may stigmatize them in the eyes of others. Habiba, aged 29, from the Matiari District, who also works in the private sector, shared that:

> One of our colleagues has been tested COVID positive, therefore, our organization has decided to conduct COVID tests of all employees and communities who remained in physical contact with the employee

in the last week. Nonetheless, due to fear, people are refusing to get the coronavirus tests. The underlying reason is that if they are tested positive, it will mean shame for the community and the government will not allow them to live with the family members, and we will be put in an isolation center. Yet some people consider it an opportunity: if tested positive, then they will be spared from work.

As Habiba notes, for some people, COVID-19 has emerged as an opportunity to get some free time to spend with their families. For example, a colleague of Habiba, named Halima—in her late 30s from Matiari District—stated, "We want our COVID test to be positive because after declaring as positive, we will take a rest for a few days, as our organization will give us leave without pay. And this way we will have time to spend time with family."

One year after we obtained our original data for this chapter, the situation of COVID-19 became more critical in Pakistan as people got used to the presence of the virus and became less or non-serious about protecting themselves from it—as described by our interlocutor Sakeena, who is around 40 years old and works as a nurse at a private hospital in a town of Matiari District:

> When the coronavirus infection was first confirmed in Pakistan, most people were following precautionary measures, such as wearing masks and gloves, observing physical distance during going outside from home. However, the current condition is critical because many people are not taking COVID-19 seriously anymore. People have become habituated to it by now.

As shown in the preceding chapter, some people have attributed the etiology of the pandemic to a supernatural act. Inayat Ali (2020e, 2021) found interpretations of COVID-19 as a supernatural act in Punjab province, where laypeople considered the virus as the punishment of Allah, which occurred due to "the opening of cinemas in Saudi Arabia and general disbelief in God in the Global North, where everything is 'too open,' especially romance." People believed that "Allah has shown us how powerful He is in that science is unable to deal with the pandemic." Many Pakistanis hold the idea that their strong belief in Allah is the reason why viral infections are significantly less in Pakistan than in the US and Europe (ibid.). For example, Asad Ali, age 45, who is a college teacher from Matiari District, argues:

> COVID-19 is a punishment for unbelievers. As we are followers of Ali (the son-in-law and cousin of the prophet Muhammad), we would not be infected by the virus under any circumstances. [In Urdu] *Jis Ka Ali Waris, Usay Kiya Kre Ga Coronavirus* [literally meaning: If Ali is our protector, then we won't be affected by the coronavirus].

Similar are the views of Kamalan, who is around 60 years old, from Matiari District with no formal education, and a house worker; she stated:

> None of us has a fear of coronavirus; instead, we are afraid of God. The occurrence of a disease and its cure is the will of Allah. Nobody except Allah would ever cause any disease to anyone. Despite that, we are living in the scientific world and cannot make or unmake an illness because it occurs by the decision of Allah. Presently, the coronavirus has been described by a religious leader and many people as a disease from Allah to test individuals and put them on the right track. Many people are stating that the coronavirus spread because people are not performing *Namāz* (praying) and [reading the] *Qurān*. Once Allah is pleased with us, then the disease will soon end, as we are not able to prevent ourselves from the disease—only Allah can do so.

Interestingly, the Bāgarrī—a nomadic Hindu hunting and gathering community of Sindh—have adopted a distinct set of preventive measures. They have performed various rituals and have used cow urine for prevention, because they consider cows to represent a goddess—which particular goddess depends on the specific Bāgarrī cultural group, as each group worships a different goddess. As Jariya, a 50-year-old Bāgarrī woman with no formal education who works as a wage laborer, shared:

> We wash our bodies with cow urine as the cow Mātta is our goddess. Firstly, we make sweet bread and distribute it to children, and then children offer the bread to a cow. After an hour, when the cow urinates, then we keep that urine in a metal jug and recite some *Bhajjan* (sacred songs of Hinduism). After that, every family member, irrespective of age and gender, washes their body with that urine. Furthermore, we also sprinkle urine on every space of our house. Our deliberation is that the virus will not affect us, with the blessing of our cow Mātta.

Other cultural groups have also used cow urine as a sacred measure for negotiating COVID-19. In accordance with this belief, members of All India Hindu Mahasabha (All India Hindu Union) organized a *Gāūmūtrā* (cow urine worship) program, hosted by *Akhil Bharat Hindu Mahasabha*—a right-wing Hindu nationalist group. Hundreds of people attended this event and drank the urine, believing that this would immunize them against the virus. (A specific type of cow urine is used in Ayurvedic medicine, in which it is believed to have antioxidant and anti-microbial properties.)

Discussion

People's beliefs and perspectives are real, influence behavior, and help them to make sense of their lifeworlds (Ali 2020 a, c, d, e). These beliefs and perspectives are encoded in various narratives—for examples, rumors and conspiracy theories, which are social phenomena that reflect people's anxieties and fears (Ali 2020e). Believing that there is no coronavirus demonstrates the mistrustful relationship between the government and the people, which, again, created negative effects as people became more careless in taking preventive measures against a disease they do not believe even exists—or if it does, then both its cause and its cure are in the hands of Allah and/or of *Qismat*—fate. The deeper meanings of such perceptions can only be fully understood when they are placed within the historical contexts of colonization, poverty, corrupt or ineffective governance, and aid dependency (see Ali 2020b).

Some narratives can be downright dangerous. For example, based on a rumor that consuming highly concentrated alcohol disinfects the body and kills COVID-19 (WHO 2020), people started drinking alcohol excessively, and as a result, around 800 people died in Pakistan, and around 5,900 in Iran (Aljazeera 2020; Islam et al. 2020). Some Americans died from drinking bleach because then-President Trump actually recommended it, and Asian Americans across the United States are being vilified, attacked, and even killed because to some, they incarnate the belief that the virus was deliberately imported to the USA from China. Former President Trump repeatedly referred to COVID-19 as the "China virus," which apparently strengthened the association of Asians in general with the coronavirus in the minds of his followers, expressed through social media hate speech and actual attacks in various countries on people who "looked Chinese" (Jilani 2021).

Rumors, conspiracy theories, and infection-associated stigmas have also negatively affected people's willingness to comply with government measures to contain the virus (Ali 2020e). Yet such narratives may also exert positive effects. For example, linking the pandemic to the supernatural likely gives people great hope that pleasing and worshiping Allah will help to prevent and cure the disease. For another example, Inayat Ali (2020c, e) found that at the beginning of the pandemic, rumors circulated in Pakistan that the government shot or set fire to COVID-19 infected people. These narratives made family members, particularly parents, want the younger generations in their families to stay at home (ibid.). On the upside, these rumors might have caused people to intensify their efforts to avoid contagion by self-quarantining. Yet on the downside, such rumors caused many to avoid getting tested even if they were symptomatic.

Thus, paradoxically, such local perspectives may both increase and decrease panic and fear. Local narratives such as rumors and conspiracy theories often increase fear, whereas, for example, believing that health and illness—including COVID-19—are determined by God allows people to release their anxieties and fears through prayers. Similarly, listening to the sacred songs of *Bhajjan* (Hindu religious songs) also gives people hope that the virus will not infect them. According to Davis-Floyd and Laughlin (2022), "ritual stands as a buffer between cognition and chaos"—between people's ability and inability to cope with a stressful situation—because the performance of rituals can be calming and stabilizing. Thus it is no wonder that people everywhere use rituals to stabilize themselves in times of crisis (ibid.). Even the small daily rituals of handwashing, mask-wearing, and physical distancing give people a sense of confidence, while deeper rituals, such as performing prayers and engaging in large-scale ceremonies, greatly enhance that sense of confidence. Local knowledges, perceptions, and attitudes toward any disease, especially when they generate anxieties and fears, play integral roles in shaping a society's readiness to accept— or to reject—behavioral changes, and may further complicate measures to contain disease spread (Person et al. 2004).

Local perceptions and practices are shaped by wider sociocultural, economic, and political factors. When facing new and challenging diseases that may cause epidemics and pandemics, we should consider these different perceptions and practices because they will certainly affect people's responses and practices. We call attention to fear of stigmatization, which can result in refusals of testing, and to how that can be remedied by clear and effective information provided by health and governmental authorities—as occurred in Bhutan (see Chapter 13), but not in most of the other countries addressed in this volume. Public health interventions should consider cultural beliefs and assumptions to ensure that the interventions are culturally appropriate for the community (Napier et al. 2014; Shaikh and Hatcher 2005). It is crucial to avoid correlating the disease with questionable cultural causations, as this may lead to blaming specific populations for their high prevalence rate or to the stigmatizing of those infected (Sovran 2013).

We note that it is essential to conduct in-depth studies to generate thorough understandings of these numerous perspectives: what do such narratives reveal and why do they emerge? To document and analyze these narratives and to answer such questions are undoubtedly vital. Such documentation and analysis will lead us to those historical, sociocultural, economic, and political factors that significantly shape these seemingly irrational perspectives, which, in Pakistan and many other countries, develop in the presence of multiple and syndemic disparities, including lack of effective educational and healthcare systems and an inefficient and corrupt governmental regime (see Ali 2020e, 2021; Singer et al. 2017).

Conclusion

Analogous to other countries, Pakistan has been overwhelmed by the pandemic. Since COVID-19 is still unfolding and there are as yet (June 2021) no or not enough vaccines available in many countries, including Pakistan, distinct perceptions, attitudes, and practices surrounding COVID-19 have emerged there, as elsewhere. We have described these in this chapter, showing that the practices around COVID-19 in Pakistan range from harmless home remedies like drinking green tea to extremely harmful "preventive measures" like drinking oneself to death. We have also shown how local beliefs and attitudes about COVID-19 have strongly influenced behaviors in both positive and negative, rational and irrational, ways.

Understanding local attitudes, beliefs, and practices and their underlying rationales could greatly help health officials to present science-based strategies for preventing infection in culturally appropriate and acceptable ways. For example, government protocols could recommend drinking green tea and performing rituals and prayers—harmless practices that carry great psychological benefits—while also noting that the beneficial effects of such home remedies or large-scale ceremonies would be greatly enhanced by also wearing masks, hand-sanitizing, and physical distancing. In such ways, government SOPs could be presented as a package that includes local remedies and honors local beliefs. We hope that this present research on Sindhis' perceptions of COVID-19 may aid in such efforts.

Acknowledgments

Although we received no specific funding for this article, Inayat Ali acknowledges the Higher Education Commission (HEC) of Pakistan's grant (PD/OSS-II/Batch-IV/Austria/2012/9903), which supported the PhD research that has significantly informed this article. We also thank the National Bioethics Committee, Pakistan (reference No.4-87/NBC-471-COVID-19-09/20/) for its ethical approval of this study.

Note

1 This chapter is another version of an article that has been published under open access agreement: Ali, I., Saddique, S., & Ali, S. (2021). Local Perceptions of COVID-19 in Pakistan's Sindh Province: "Political Game", Supernatural Test, or Western Conspiracy?. *Disaster Medicine and Public Health Preparedness*, 1–6. https://doi.org/10.1017/dmp.2021.220.

References

Ali, I. 2020a. Anthropology in emergencies: The roles of anthropologists during the COVID-19 pandemic. *Practicing Anthropology*, 42 (3), 16–22. https://doi.org/10.17730/0888-4552.42.3.4
Ali, I. 2020b. *Construction and Negotiation of Measles: The Case of Sindh Province of Pakistan*. Vienna: University of Vienna.
Ali, I. 2020c. The COVID-19 pandemic: Making sense of rumor and fear. *Medical Anthropology* 39(5): 376–379. https://doi.org/10.1080/0145 9740.2020.1745481
Ali, I. 2020d. COVID-19: Are we ready for the second wave? *Disaster Medicine and Public Health Preparedness* 14(5): e16–e18. https://doi.org/10.1017/dmp.2020.149
Ali, I. 2020e. Impacts of rumors and conspiracy theories surrounding COVID-19 on preparedness programs. *Disaster Medicine and Public Health Preparedness*, 1–6. https://doi.org/10.1017/dmp.2020.149

Ali, I. 2021. COVID-19 amid rumours and conspiracy theories: The interplay between local and global worlds. In N. Rezaei (ed.), *Coronavirus Disease (COVID-19)*. New York: Springer, pp. 673–686.

Ali, I., and Davis-Floyd, R. 2020. The interplay of words and politics during COVID-19: Contextualizing the universal pandemic vocabulary. *Practicing Anthropology* 42(4): 20–24. https://doi.org/10.17730/0888-4552.42.4.20

Ali, I., Sadique, S., and Ali, S. 2020. COVID-19 significantly affects maternal health: A rapid-response investigation from Pakistan. *Frontiers in Global Women's Health* 1. https://doi.org/10.3389/fgwh.2020.591809

Ali, I., Shah, S.A., and Siddiqui, N. 2020, Feburary 27. Pakistan confirms first two cases of coronavirus, govt says "no need to panic." *Dawn*. www.dawn.com/news/1536792

Aljazeera. 2020. Iran: Over 700 dead after drinking alcohol to cure coronavirus www.aljazeera.com/news/2020/04/iran-700-dead-drinking-alcohol-cure-coronavirus200427163529629.html

Davis-Floyd, R., and Laughlin, C.D. 2022. *Ritual: What It Is, How It Works, and Why*. New York: Berghahn Books.

Dawn. 2020, 31 March. Covid-19 misinformation. *Dawn*, 06. https://epaper.dawn.com/DetailNews.php?StoryText=31_03_2020_006_003

Islam, M.S., Sarkar, T., Khan, S.H., et al. 2020. COVID-19-related infodemic and its impact on public health: A global social media analysis. *The American Journal of Tropical Medicine and Hygiene* 103(4): 1621–1629. https://doi.org/10.4269/ajtmh.20-0812

Jilani, Z. 2021. Why are Asian Americans being attacked and what can you do about it? *The Greater Good Science Center*, 1–6. https://greatergood.berkeley.edu/article/item/why_are_asian_americans_being_attacked_and_what_can_you_do_about_it

Napier, A.D., Ancarno, C., Butler, B., et al. 2014. Culture and health. *The Lancet* 384(9954): 1607–1639. https://doi.org/10.1016/S0140-6736(14)61603-2

Person, B., Sy, F., Holton, K., et al. 2004. Fear and stigma: The epidemic within the SARS outbreak. *Emerging Infectious Diseases* 10(2): 358.

Shaikh, B. T., and Hatcher, J. 2005. Health seeking behaviour and health service utilization in Pakistan: Challenging the policy makers. *Journal of Public Health* 27(1): 49–54.

Singer, M., Bulled, N., Ostrach, B., and Mendenhall, E. 2017. Syndemics and the biosocial conception of health. The Lancet 389(10072): 941–950.

Sovran, S. 2013. Understanding culture and HIV/AIDS in Sub-Saharan Africa. *Sahara-J: Journal of Social Aspects of HIV/AIDS* 10(1): 32–41.

World Health Organization (WHO). 2020. *Alcohol does not protect against COVID-19 and its access should be restricted during lock down* World Health Organization. Retrieved August 31 from www.emro.who.int/mnh/news/alcohol-does-not-protect-against-covid-19-and-its-access-should-be-restricted-during-lock-down.html

World Health Organization (WHO). 2021, April 25. *Coronavirus disease 2019 (COVID-19) dashboard*. World Health Organisation. Retrieved April 26 from https://covid19.who.int/

18 Negotiating Online Shopping Behaviors after the COVID-19 Outbreak in Pakistan

Tayyaba Rafique Makhdoom, Sanaullah Jamali, and Maria Tufail Memon

Introduction

E-commerce has revolutionized the old trade patterns; its invention dates back to 1979. Afterwards, the development of the first worldwide web (www) server and browser in 1990 gave impetus to large stores to launch online businesses, which resulted in a rapid shift towards online shopping and the global flourishing of the e-commerce sector. Pakistan had a slower pace in e-commerce development as compared to higher-resource countries, though by now, online shopping has penetrated Pakistan's culture as well. Nowadays in Pakistan, metropolitans, people from the suburbs, and dwellers of small towns (with sufficient Internet connectivity) shop online.

Pakistan recorded its first case of COVID-19 on February 26, 2020, started observing lockdown from March 24, 2020, and ended the official lockdown in August 2020 (Ali et al. 2020). Since then, it has been implementing "smart" (targeted) lockdowns in various sensitive cities, and stressing compliance with standard operating procedures (SOPs) (Ali and Davis-Floyd 2020; Chapters 16 and 17, this volume). Pakistan is rich in cultural diversity, and a variety of festivals and traditions are celebrated with zeal and devotion. During the lockdown in 2020, the nation nevertheless celebrated the two most significant religious festivals—*Eid ul Fitr*[1] and *Eid al Adha*[2]—along with fasting during the Islamic holy month of Ramazan (its spelling in Pakistan). As usual, these festivals and the month of Ramazan, along with matrimonial rituals and ceremonies, tempted people to spend on food, clothing, gifts, and other accessories.

Just as the spread of COVID-19 has had adverse effects on human lives, it also has hampered world economic markets (Javed 2020). Many business operations were halted, with ensuing detrimental effects on workers—especially daily wage laborers, many of whom lost their jobs. In Pakistan, multiple economic activities were suspended during lockdown, and a large number of Pakistanis lost their jobs or experienced income reductions. According to the Planning Commission of Pakistan, nearly 20.8 million people—forming nearly 37.2% of the country's total labor force (consisting of 55.7 million workers)—suffered livelihood losses due to the shutdown

DOI: 10.4324/9781003187462-23

of businesses and the mobility restrictions enforced between April and June 2020 to halt coronaviral spread (Pakistan Bureau of Statistics 2021).

This study aimed to probe into buying behaviors among the people of Pakistan after the advent of COVID-19 and during lockdown to provide insight into buyers' attitudes, preferences, and their propensities for future shopping. Evaluating the buying behaviors of consumers in regard to demographic factors, we have studied online shopping behaviors in terms of platforms used for buying online, payment methods, influencing factors, returning to physical stores instead of shopping online, the products shopped for the most, and tendencies toward e-browsing and impulse buying. We hope that our results will help in understanding national and individual shopping behaviors, and will assist in negotiating this pandemic and any future ones that may arise.

A Situational Analysis of COVID-19 and Consumers' Purchasing Behaviors

Given that the pandemic has drastically affected national and global economies and individual lifestyles, businesses have had to formulate new policies and to alter the prevailing and conventional patterns of offers and sales. A boost has been observed in digital commerce; essential and cleaning products' sales are rising, while the sales of non-essential products have fallen rapidly (Accenture 2020). During lockdowns, consumers have adopted new technologies and have sought innovative ways of shopping that facilitate work, education, and consumption at home. Furthermore, consumer behavior and all consumption are time and location bound, as existing habits and necessities are abandoned or sacrificed and consumers adopt new habits and activities (Sheth 2020). The buying behaviors of consumers during the COVID-19 pandemic seem to greatly depend on fear: the greater the fear, the greater the change in shopping behaviors (Eger et al. 2021). Due to the coronavirus pandemic, changes have been observed in food-related products as people have shown less interest in restaurants and increased interest in recipes for preparing food at home. Shopping for non-perishable and ready meals has decreased, while consumers have become more likely to purchase more fresh vegetables to enhance their health. Google's (2020) COVID-19 community mobility report highlighted that changes in consumer behavior negatively affected cafeterias, restaurants, and grocery and convenience stores, as well as their suppliers. Moreover, Ali, Khalid and colleagues (2020) investigated the situational influences of COVID-19 that affected online behavior in Pakistan. Optimism and innovation showed positive effects on the adoption of technology for online food delivery ordering services, and demographic factors were found to be significant in influencing consumers' intentions towards the adoption of new technology for the online delivery services.

Findings from the Relevant Literature

As the COVID-19 pandemic has drastically affected consumers' buying behaviors, their COVID-related demands have affected economies and societies globally. Li, Hallsworth, and Stefaniak (2020) collected data via an online survey, which revealed that local independent small retailers enjoyed the highest degree of stability with regards to customer retention. In contrast, farmers' markets suffered, as people were afraid to shop in them. For India, Kulkarni and Barge (2020) also collected data via an online questionnaire: out of 340 respondents, 283 preferred online shopping, especially when the number of positive cases was high in that country. Similarly, for the USA, Grashuis, Skevas, and Segovia (2020) reported that US consumers have been preferring home delivery methods during the pandemic.

Online shopping has long been predicted to become dominant. In 2013, Wainewright predicted that the future of retail is going to be "click-and-collect" rather than the traditional brick-and-mortar stores; hence traditional retailers have to learn how to survive the transition into the digital age. Qureshi, Fatima, and Sarwar (2014) investigated consumer behaviors regarding online shopping in Pakistan. They identified the factors that influence online shopping as perceived risk, product varieties, website design, and social norms. They concluded that online shopping is difficult for women and for consumers who have low income and education. However, in his investigation of the factors affecting the online purchasing behavior of people in Pakistan, Adnan (2014) found that website design was an insignificant variable, along with hedonistic motivation. Moreover, Adnan identified both the positive impacts of perceived advantages and psychological factors, and the negative impacts of perceived risks (fear of losing money, the risk of receiving malfunctioning goods, or non-delivery of the items ordered) of consumer buying behavior. In addition to its many other global impacts, the COVID-19 pandemic has significantly influenced e-commerce, which has grown rapidly worldwide due to the pandemic-related self-quarantines and the resultant social isolation. The coronavirus has constrained many buyers to using the Internet to fulfill their needs (Abiad, Arao, and Dagli 2020).

People often spend their leisure time on "window shopping" at brick-and-mortar stores, but usually end up buying nothing (Shy 2014). Due to the pandemic, window shopping has largely been replaced by e-browsing—the process of spending much time in online marketplaces but not purchasing anything or even without any intention to buy (Kukar-Kinney and Close 2010). Several authors have argued that the Internet favors e-browsing and "impulse buying" (Jeffrey and Hodge 2007; Verhagen and van Dolen 2011). Impulse buying occurs when a consumer experiences a sudden, often powerful and persistent urge to buy something immediately (Rook

1987: 191). The ease of choosing a product and clicking on it may create temptation and thus increase the likelihood of impulse buying (Greenfield 1999). Lowe (2020) anticipated an increase in e-browsing and impulse buying due to the pandemic.

Mehta, Saxena, and Purohit (2020) compared consumer behaviors in normal and pandemic times through the critical analysis of literature, and inferred that, during pandemics, the public will be financially burdened due to healthcare costs and loss of income, and will therefore tend to be more economical in the future. Shafi and colleagues (2020) used an exploratory approach and also collected data via an online questionnaire using snowball sampling, and concluded that businesses are facing problems of fall in demand, loss in sales, and reduction in profits. They also found that many companies adopted different strategies, such as applying for loans, terminating employees or reducing their wages, and downsizing their businesses (see Chapter 11, this volume).

Collecting questionnaire data on Spain, Laguna and colleagues (2020) evaluated people's changed behaviors regarding food using various search engines and viewing ads on YouTube and messages on Twitter. Their results showed no significant changes in shopping location for that country. Conversely, they noted that shopping frequency was minimized during the initial period of COVID-19 in Spain. Prasetyo and colleagues (2021) indicated that hedonistic motivation has the highest effect on customer satisfaction, followed by price, information quality, and promotion, since people in low-resource countries have been extensively utilizing online food delivery services during the new normal of COVID-19. Examining the effects of the pandemic on the buying behaviors of consumers of the department stores of Rivers State in Nigeria, Acee-Eke and Ogonu (2020) demonstrated that the COVID-19 pandemic forced a market shutdown and changed the patterns of consumption, including the buying behaviors around particular essential products. Nguyen and colleagues (2020) investigated the influence of COVID-19 on book purchasing, using an online survey method on a sample of 275 Vietnamese consumers. Results showed that the COVID-19 pandemic had significant positive effects on the intentions of consumers regarding online book shopping, whereas the nexus between hedonistic motivation and online purchase intention showed insignificant positive results.

For India, Chauhan and Shah (2020) noted that due to lockdown, more consumers are buying essentials, while many brick-and-mortar stores have shut down, sometimes temporarily. Likewise, for the USA, Mason, Narcum, and Mason (2020) showed that consumers' satisfaction levels have decreased, that consumers have increased their online purchasing behaviors, and that some marketers will face difficulty in regaining customer loyalty in the future. Similarly, Koch, Frommeyer, and Schewe (2020) found that trends established during this crisis may remain stable into the future, inflicting serious consequences on physical stores due to the rapid increase in e-commerce. As we will demonstrate later on, this will likely not be the case in Pakistan. Yet due to nationwide and targeted lockdowns, Pakistani consumers have also been compelled to renegotiate their shopping habits to buy online rather than in physical stores.

Methods and Materials

We developed an online questionnaire for our survey in the English language, which most of the users of social media understand to some degree. Our questionnaire contained 16 items: 4 concerned demographic factors; 3 addressed employment and earning; and 9 items inquired about participants' online shopping behaviors. Responses were measured on a nominal scale for 12 items, and rating scales were used for measuring the responses to 4 of the items. Eight of the 16 items were adapted from an article by Etzioni (2020) about online shopping during the pandemic on the website of Namogoo—a Digital Journey Continuity platform that enables online brands to drive their customer journeys forward and clear the path to purchase. The platform autonomously adapts to each customer visit in real time, which helps to improve online customer journeys and business results for global retail brands. The remaining eight items were developed from articles by Wold (2020) and Lowe (2020) about online shopping during COVID-19.

We posted the survey questionnaire on various social media groups and sent it to personal contacts through email, Facebook, and WhatsApp. The sample is convenient because it reached the people who were in contact (directly or indirectly) with the researchers. A total of 334 respondents participated in the survey from July 7, 2020 to October 17, 2020. We analyzed the data via bar charts, double-doughnut diagrams, frequency and percentages, and crosstabs, using SPSS 20 and Microsoft Excel. Items about demographic factors, the effects of COVID-19 on online shopping, earning situations, and intentions to shop online in the future were analyzed with cross-tabulations. Items about the platforms used for online shopping, payment methods, influencing factors, and using the physical store as a substitute are presented in double-doughnut diagrams, while items about products shopped the most and e-browsing and impulse buying are presented in bar charts. All monies detailed throughout are in US dollars.

Findings

Demographics and Their Effects on Online Shopping

Our demographic data show that 53% of our survey respondents are female and 47% are male. 15% were 20 years of age or under; 55% were 21–40; 23% were 41–60; only 7% were above 60. 48% of our participants were married and 52% were unmarried (single, separated, divorced, widowed).

The majority of the respondents are well-educated; 40% have post graduated (completed their 16/18 years of education; any year of study over 14 is considered postgraduate in Pakistan); and 31% have graduated (completed 14 years of education); 6% have a doctorate. 15% of participants have an intermediate education level (passed the exam after the end of 12th grade), and 6% have matriculated (passed the exam after the end of 10th grade). Only 2% have education below matriculation. 19% are full-time government employees; 23% are full-time private job holders. People with part-time jobs constitute 9% of our survey respondents; 16% are homemakers; and 21% are students. 8% are unemployed and 4% are retired. 42% have a monthly family income of $400–$800; 29% percent have an income less than $400. 15% and 7% belong to income groups of $900–$1,200 and $1,300–$1,600 respectively; 7% have a family income above $1,600.

35% of participants stated that they increased online shopping after the advent of the pandemic; 27% stated that they shopped online for the first time after the lockdown imposition. 25% reported no effect on their shopping behaviors, and 13% stopped or decreased online shopping after the outbreak of COVID-19. In accordance with our Pakistan results, for India, Kulkarni and Barge (2020) and for the USA, Grashuis and Colleagues (2020) also reported that a large number of their study participants preferred online shopping after the outbreak of COVID-19. Table 18.1 exhibits these results.

Table 18.1 shows the cross-tabulations for demographics and their effects on online shopping. It is interesting to see how demographic factors affected the shopping behaviors of consumers in Pakistan. Our female respondents increased their online shopping due to lockdown, whereas most of the men shopped online for the first time, and others (31%) reported no effect on their shopping behaviors. From the age group of under 20 to 20 years, 40% increased their online shopping. Similarly, from the age group of 21 to 40 years, 36%, and from the age group of 41 to 60, 35%, also increased shopping online. On the other hand, from the age group of above 60, 46% shopped online for the first time during the lockdown. Married and unmarried responses were not significantly different in terms of changes in online shopping due to COVID-19, as both reported an increase in their online shopping.

Education was found to influence shopping behavior. 71% of our PhD participants increased their online shopping. 34% of post-graduate participants did so as well, while 31% of post-graduate participants shopped online for the first time during the lockdown. The responses of participants having education less than postgraduation were not significantly different in terms of effects on online shopping. Regarding employment status, 55% of full-time government jobholders increased their online shopping, as did 40% of homemakers and 42% of students. 61% of the retired people in our sample did their first-time online shopping during lockdown. On the other hand, there was no effect on the online shopping behaviors of 48% of

Table 18.1 Demographic Factors and Their Effects on Online Shopping

Demographics		Effects on online shopping				Total
		Decreased/stopped online shopping	Increased online shopping	No effect	Shopped online for the first time	
Total		42(13%)	118(35%)	84(25%)	90(27%)	334
Gender	Female	23	78	36	41	178(53%)
	Male	19	40	48	49	156(47%)
Age	Under 20–20	4	20	12	13	49(15%)
	21–40	29	66	46	43	184(55%)
	41–60	8	27	19	23	77(23%)
	Above 60	1	5	7	11	24(7%)
Marital status	Married	20	55	36	49	160(48%)
	Unmarried	22	63	48	41	174(52%)
Education level	Less than Matriculation	0	4	2	1	7(2%)
	Matriculation	0	5	9	4	18(6%)
	Intermediate	7	19	14	11	51(15%)
	Graduate	18	29	27	29	103(31%)
	Post graduate	17	46	29	42	134(40%)
	Doctorate	0	15	3	3	21(6%)
Employment status	Full - Time (Government job)	0	35	11	18	64(19%)
	Full - Time (Private job)	17	19	20	21	77(23%)
	Part - Time	7	7	10	7	31(9%)
	Homemaker	5	21	10	17	53(16%)
	Retired	0	0	5	8	13(4%)
	Student	11	29	15	14	69(21%)
	Unemployed	2	7	13	5	27(8%)
Family income (monthly)	Less than $400	22	19	35	22	98(29%)
	$400 to $800	18	45	30	46	139(42%)
	$900 to $1,200	2	32	7	11	52(15%)
	$1,300 to $1,600	0	9	9	5	23(7%)
	Above $1,600	0	13	3	6	22(7%)

unemployed people, and no noticeable change in the shopping behaviors of full-time private jobholders nor among part-time jobholders.

Regarding income, for 36% of our respondents with a monthly family income of less than US$400, lockdown did not affect their online shopping behaviors. 33% of those with a family income of $400–$800 shopped online for the first time due to COVID-19, and a significant number—32%—from the same income bracket also increased their online shopping. 61% of our respondents with a monthly family income of $800–$1,200 also stated an increase in their online shopping. Among people with a family income of $1,200–$1,600, 39% increased their online shopping, while 39% reported no effect. 59% of those with a family income above $1,600 also increased their online shopping.

Earning Situations and Online Shopping

After the outbreak of COVID-19 and the imposition of lockdown, as previously mentioned, Pakistanis experienced various changes in their earning situations. Table 18.2 (vertically) provides the list of earning situations experienced by our respondents. 33% were not earning when they participated in the survey. 18% of respondents were receiving their usual pay with reduced hours, and 14% were working regular hours with usual pay. In contrast, 13% of self-employed respondents also mentioned a reduction in their incomes. 9% of the participants stated that their working hours and pay had been reduced, while 6% were laid off due to COVID-19. 4% of participants were still working without pay, whereas 3% of participants reported an increase in their incomes due to COVID-19. (See Table 18.2.)

Table 18.2 exhibits the cross-tabulation showing how earning situations have affected the online shopping behaviors of our survey respondents. 36% of the respondents who reported that they increased their online shopping were those who were not earning; this group might be the most dependent group, as it includes young adults and homemakers. 32% of these non-earners replied that they shopped online for the first time during the lockdown. 51% of those who also increased online shopping are employees whose working hours had been reduced yet were still receiving their usual pay. On the other hand, 25% of the participants who are not earning reported no effects on their shopping behaviors. 26% of self-employed respondents whose incomes had been reduced decreased their online shopping, while 26% of them reported no effects on their buying behaviors. 43% of respondents who were laid off during the lockdown decreased their shopping after the outbreak of COVID-19.

We asked the participants whether or not their online spending would be likely to change post-COVID. 34% responded that it would decrease slightly, whereas 32% said that it would stay the same. 19% of the participants anticipated that their online spending would decrease greatly, 12% thought

Table 18.2 Earning Situations and Their Effects on Online Shopping

Earning situations		Effect on online shopping				Total
		Decreased/ stopped online shopping	Increased online shopping	No effect	Shopped online for the first time	
	Total	42(13%)	118(35%)	84(25%)	90(27%)	334
Change in earning situation	Enhanced income(self-employed)	1	5	3	2	11(3%)
	Experienced lay-off (terminated)	9	4	5	3	21(6%)
	Not earning	7	40	28	36	111(33%)
	Reduced hours, reduced pay	4	9	8	10	31(9%)
	Reduced income(self-employed)	11	10	11	10	42(13%)
	Still employed, without pay	2	3	5	2	12(4%)
	Still working regular hours with usual pay	6	17	13	11	47(14%)
	Usual pay, reduced hours	2	30	11	16	59(18%)

that it would increase slightly, while 3% expected it to increase considerably. These results are shown in Table 18.3.

Table 18.3 presents the cross-tabulation of whether or not earning situations have affected people's propensities to shop online in the future. 36% of those whose incomes increased after the outbreak responded that their online shopping would decrease after the lockdown, likely meaning that they will return to physical stores. The majority of respondents who experienced layoffs and who are not earning, 38% and 41% respectively, said that there would be no effect on their shopping patterns post-lockdown. In contrast, the people with reduced hours and reduced pay, people who were still employed without pay, people who were still working regular hours with usual pay, and people who were working with usual pay but reduced hours—39%, 33%, 34%, and 46% respectively—also expected that their online shopping would slightly decrease. 36% of those whose income was reduced thought that there would be no effect on their shopping behaviors after the lockdown ended.

Online Shoppers' Buying Behaviors

There have been different modes used for shopping after the outbreak of the pandemic, and online shopping as the safest option has been a common consumer practice. We investigated the buying behaviors of our online shopper respondents and present our results in Figures 18.1–18.6.

As Figure 18.1 shows, there are various platforms used to shop online, on which a buyer can view the product and its categories, filter, sort out, purchase, negotiate, and pose queries about the product. We asked the participants which platform(s) they were using to purchase products online. 41% of respondents were using websites on their mobile phones. 18% replied "none," meaning that they did not shop online. 17% used Apps on mobile phones. Social media groups were used by 14%, while 8% used websites as their platforms for online shopping. 2% replied that they used other platforms for shopping online. Figure 18.2 presents the payment methods used.

Online payments and digital money have made payment faster and more convenient, though our respondents still preferred to pay cash—69% chose cash on delivery as a payment method for online shopping. 18% answered "none" as they did not shop online. The significance of electronic payments is also undeniable, as 69% paid by card, whereas 5% opted for Internet banking. These results are indicated in Figure 18.2, whereas Figure 18.3 shows the factors that influenced purchasing decisions.

While purchasing a product online, a customer is influenced by different factors; knowing about them can be very important for sellers, as they can add or improve such factors and thereby attract more customers. Price was the most influential factor for buying decisions, as indicated by 25% of our respondents. Fast and convenient delivery was the second most influential

Table 18.3 Earning Situations and Propensity to Shop Online in Future

Earning situations		Propensity to shop online in future					Total
		Will decrease greatly	*Will decrease slightly*	*Will stay the same*	*Will increase slightly*	*Will increase greatly*	
	Total	63(19%)	113(34%)	106(32%)	41(12%)	11(3%)	334
Change in earning situation	Enhanced income(self-employed)	2	4	3	1	1	11(3%)
	Experienced lay-off (terminated)	3	2	8	7	1	21(6%)
	Not earning	18	36	46	10	0	111(33%)
	Reduced hours, reduced pay	8	12	6	5	2	31(9%)
	Reduced income(self-employed)	8	12	15	5	2	42(13%)
	Still employed, without pay	2	4	2	1	3	12(4%)
	Still working regular hours with usual pay	6	16	13	10	2	47(14%)
	Usual pay, reduced hours	16	27	13	2	1	59(18%)

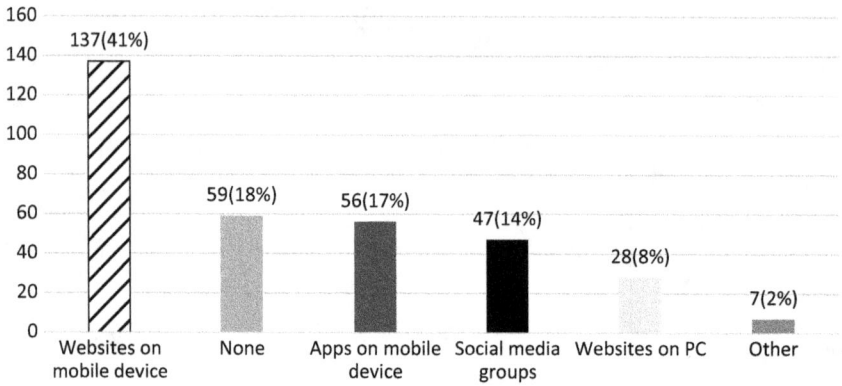

Figure 18.1 Platforms Used for Online Shopping.

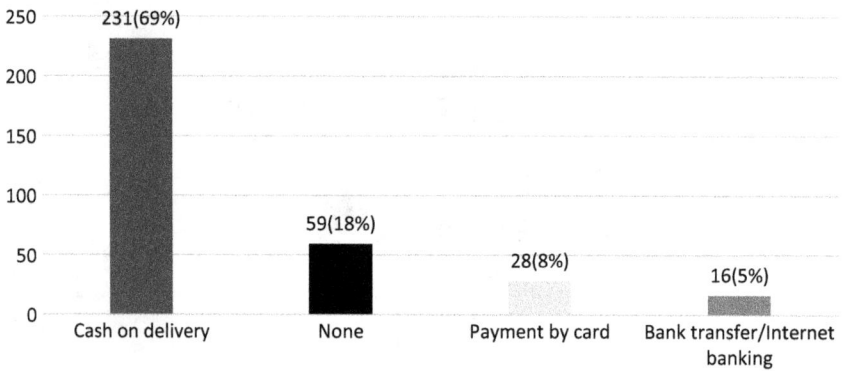

Figure 18.2 Payment Methods.

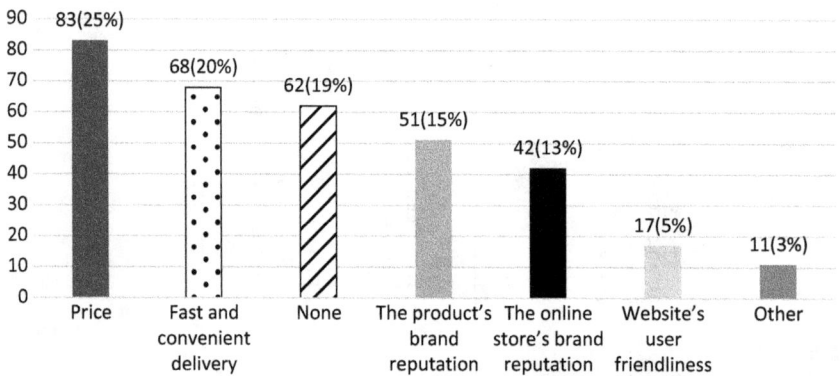

Figure 18.3 Influencing Factors in Purchasing Decisions.

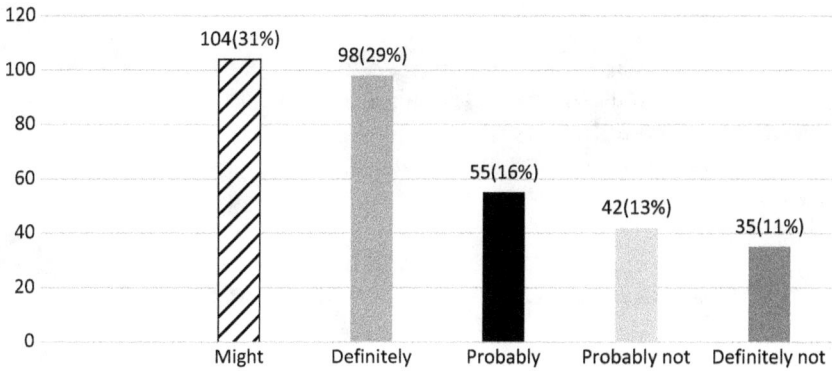

Figure 18.4 Preferring Physical Stores Over Online Shopping.

factor, as 20% indicated. 19% replied "none," while 15% were found to be influenced by the product's brand reputation and 13% by the online store's brand reputation. On the other hand, only 5% reported being influenced by the website's user-friendliness; this finding is very similar to the results of Adnan (2014), who found that website design is an insignificant factor. The remaining 3% were influenced by other factors. Figure 18.3 depicts these results, while Figure 18.4 indicates preferences for physical stores over online shopping.

Due to the COVID-19 lockdown, Pakistani citizens, especially those who were living in the large cities, were bound to their homes and had to rely on online shopping instead of shopping in brick-and-mortar stores. We asked participants, if they were given the option, would they opt for physical stores for shopping rather than shopping online, or not? 31% responded that they might have opted for a physical store, while 29% replied "definitely." 16% of the participants responded that they would probably opt for a physical store, and 13% responded they would probably not, whereas 11% responded they would definitely not opt for a physical store over online shopping. These results are shown in Figure 18.5.

We asked the participants about the type of products they shopped for the most online after the outbreak of COVID-19. As shown in Figure 18.5, clothing and accessories were the most shopped for items; 54% selected this option. Food items were also shopped for by a considerable number: 32%. Toys and games were bought by 7% of respondents; household items by 12%; electronic items by 12%; cosmetics and personal care products by 16%; books and magazines by 15%; and other items by 5% of our respondents. 18% did not shop for anything. Figure 18.6 illustrates our respondents' e-browsing and impulse buying behaviors.

The bar charts in Figure 18.6 highlight e-browsing and impulse buying. We asked the participants about their e-browsing tendencies; 28% reported

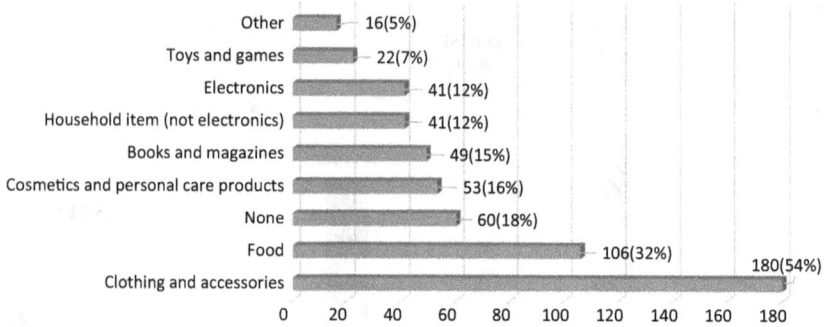

Figure 18.5 Products Shopped for the Most Online.

Note: This question was based on multiple item selection. Respondents were allowed to choose multiple options. Hence sum of the responses is not equal to the sample size or the sum of percentage is not 100.

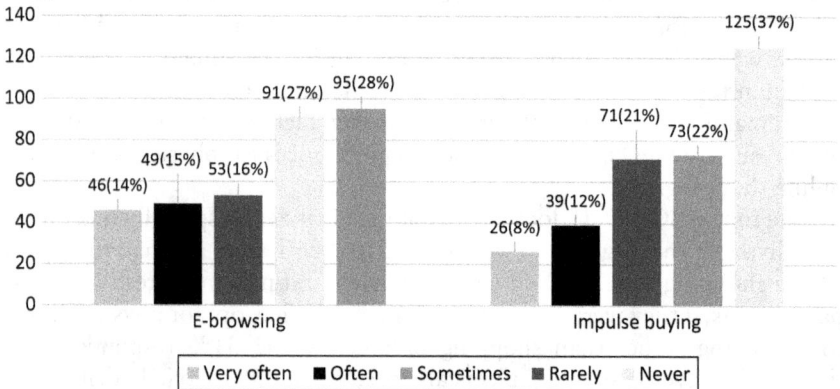

Figure 18.6 E-browsing and Impulse Buying.

having such tendencies sometimes, while 27% replied "never"; 16% "rarely"; 15% "often"; and 14% "very often" engaged in online "window shopping"/e-browsing.

Regarding our participants' impulse buying tendencies during the lockdown, 37% reported never shopping by impulse; 22% sometimes shopped by impulse; and 21% rarely engaged in impulse buying. On the other hand, 12% and 8% replied that they did so often and very often, respectively.

Discussion

Our results have shown that, among our respondents, women were more active online shoppers than men. Age has an inverse effect on online shopping;

most of the youngsters increased their online shopping, while most elders did not. Marital status has not affected our respondents' online shopping behaviors, whereas education level has affected them. Employment status has a significant impact: most of the full-time jobholders have increased their online shopping—yet most homemakers and students also increased online shopping. The effect of family income is pronounced: as common sense would dictate and as our data affirm, the higher the family income, the greater the increase in online shopping. A significant number of respondents were non-earners, had been laid off, or were working without pay; surprisingly, respondents' earning situations did not turn out to constitute an influencing factor, as a significant proportion of those who increased their online shopping were non-earners. In addition, a large number of people who were earning usual pay with reduced hours also increased their online shopping; hence, we could find no meaningful patterns in earning situations and their effects on online shopping. Regardless of their earning situations, most respondents expected that their online shopping will decrease slightly or greatly after COVID-19. Yet the majority of those who were laid off or not earning stated that there will be no post-COVID effect on their shopping patterns.

Websites on mobile phones were found to be the platforms most utilized by buyers. Cash on delivery was the most common payment method, whereas price was found to be the most influential factor in purchasing decisions. Physical stores are still deemed to be a priority, as the majority agreed that they would have opted for shopping in such stores had they been given this option during the lockdown. The products that were shopped for the most were found to be clothing and accessories, followed by food. This is somewhat consistent with the findings of Prasetyo and colleagues (2021), who found that food was the most shopped-for item in low-resource countries and particularly in Indonesia. In contrast, our results contradict those of Acee-Eke and Ogonu (2020) about Nigeria, and those of Chauhan and Shah (2020) about India, who found that the highest rates of shopping in those countries were for essential items such as food—yet our study found that in Pakistan, the most shopped-for items were clothing and accessories. We speculate that the reason for these differences in findings could be that in Pakistan during lockdown, essential items were also offered by physical stores but clothing and accessories were not, and Pakistanis, being relatively unwilling to follow SOPs, prefer to go to physical stores; hence they only shop online for items not available in physical stores.

Notwithstanding the anticipations of Lowe (2020) about a rise in e-browsing and impulse buying noted in our literature section, the results of this study show that our respondents were not eagerly involved in e-browsing or impulse buying. Most respondents replied that they sometimes went "window shopping" online, whereas a large number stated that they never did. And many reported that they never engaged in impulse buying during the lockdown, while others replied that they sometimes or rarely did.

Conclusion: Suggestions and Future Implications

This study provides valuable insights into consumers' shopping behaviors in Pakistan after the outbreak of the pandemic during the ensuing country-wide lockdown in 2020; this lockdown has been lifted and reinstated, especially in large cities, and is ongoing at this time of writing (May 2021) (see Chapter 17). We have shown that demographic factors have affected buying behaviors during the lockdown, yet varying earning situations have not significantly influenced online shopping behavior. Our results imply that Pakistanis tend to think economically, as price was the deciding factor in whether to purchase an item or not. Despite the fact that websites' user friendliness was not found to be an influencing factor in purchasing decisions, we nevertheless suggest that online stores should emphasize their websites, as the majority of consumers use them, and increased website attractiveness and user friendliness are likely to increase sales. Brick-and-mortar stores should also consider launching websites if they have not already done so, given that these can help them to generate large profits during a pandemic (see also Chapter 11, this volume). Clothing, accessories, and food have been widely shopped for online, suggesting that businesses should invest more in these products, especially during pandemics. Our study results have shown that although the COVID-19 pandemic did shift consumers to online shopping, in Pakistan this may well not be a long-term practice; it appears that physical stores will remain the primary sites for consumer shopping in Pakistan after the pandemic passes.

References

Abiad, A., Arao, R.M., Dagli, S., Ferrarini, B., Noy, I., Osewe, P., et al. 2020. The economic impact of the COVID-19 outbreak on developing Asia. *Asian Development Bank Briefs. No.128.* Retrieved October 20, 2020, from www.adb.org/publications/economic-impact-covid19-developing-asia

Accenture. 2020. COVID-19 will permanently change consumer behaviour. Retrieved April 15, 2021 from www.accenture.com/us-en/insights/consumer-goods-services/coronavirus-consumer-behavior-research.

Acee-Eke, B.C., and Ogonu, G.C. 2020. COVID-19 effects on consumer buying behaviour of departmental stores in rivers state, Nigeria. *International Journal of Scientific and Engineering Research* 11(6): 272–285.

Adnan, H. 2014. An analysis of the factors affecting online purchasing behavior of Pakistani consumers. *International Journal of Marketing Studies* 6(5): 133–148.

Ali, I., and Davis-Floyd, R. 2020. The interplay of words and politics during COVID-19: Contextualizing the Universal Pandemic Vocabulary. *Practicing Anthropology* 42(4): 20–24.

Ali, S., Khalid, N., Javed, H.M.U., and Islam, D.M.Z. 2020. Consumer adoption of Online Food Delivery Ordering (OFDO) services in Pakistan: The impact of the COVID-19 pandemic situation. *Journal of Open Innovation: Technology, Market, and Complexity* 7(1): 1–23.

Ali, I., Sadique S., and Ali, S. 2020. COVID-19 significantly affects maternal health: A rapid-response investigation from Pakistan. *Frontiers in Global Women's Health* 1(59): 1809.

Chauhan, V., and Shah, M.H. 2020. An empirical analysis into sentiments, media consumption habits, and consumer behaviour during the Coronavirus (COVID-19) outbreak. *Purakala Journal* 31(20): 353–378.

Eger, L., Komárková, L., Egerová D., and Mičík, M. 2021. The effect of COVID-19 on consumer shopping behaviour: Generational cohort perspective. *Journal of Retailing and Consumer Services* 61: 102542.

Etzioni, E. 2020. Consumer Survey: How COVID-19 Online shopping habits are shaping the customer journey, Namogoo. Retrieved July 5, 2020, from www.namogoo.com/ebooks/how-covid-19-online-shopping-habits-are-shaping-the-customer-journey/

Grashuis, J., Skevas, T., and Segovia, M.S. 2020. Grocery shopping preferences during the COVID-19 pandemic. *Sustainability* 12(13): 5369.

Greenfield, D.N. 1999. Psychological characteristics of compulsive Internet use: A preliminary analysis. *Cyberpsychology and Behavior* 2(5): 403–412.

Javed, A. 2020. Economic impact of coronavirus and revival measures: Way forward for Pakistan. *Policy Review, Sustainable Development Policy Institute (SDPI)*.

Jeffrey, S.A., and Hodge, R. 2007. Factors influencing impulse buying during an online purchase. *Electronic Commerce Research* 7(3/4): 367–379.

Koch, J., Frommeyer, B., and Schewe, G. 2020. Online shopping motives during the COVID-19 pandemic—Lessons from the crisis. *Sustainability* 12(24): 10247.

Kukar-Kinney, M., and Close, A.G. 2010. The determinants of consumers' online shopping cart abandonment. *Journal of the Academy of Marketing Science* 38(2): 240–250.

Kulkarni, S.R., and Barge, P. 2020. Effect of COVID-19 on the shift in consumer preferences with respect to shopping modes (offline/online) for groceries: An exploratory study. *International Journal of Management* 11(10): 581–590.

Laguna, L., Fiszman, S., Puerta, P., Chaya, C., and Tárrega, A. 2020. The impact of COVID-19 lockdown on food priorities. Results from a preliminary study using social media and an online survey with Spanish consumers. *Food Quality and Preference* 8(1): 104028.

Li, J., Hallsworth, A.G., and Coca-Stefaniak, J.A. 2020. Changing grocery shopping behaviours among Chinese consumers at the outset of the COVID-19 outbreak. Tijdschrift voor economische en sociale *geografie* 111(3): 574–583.

Lowe, S. 2020. How Covid-19 will change our shopping habits. *Worklife*, Retrieved July 6, 2020, from www.bbc.com/worklife/article/20200630-how-covid-19-will-change-our-shopping-habits

Mason, A., Narcum, J., and Mason, K. 2020. Changes in consumer decision-making resulting from the COVID-19 pandemic. *Journal of Customer Behaviour* 19(3). https://doi.org/10.1362/147539220X16003502334181

Mehta, S., Saxena, T., and Purohit, N. 2020. The New Consumer Behaviour Paradigm amid COVID-19: Permanent or transient? *Journal of Health Management* 22(2): 291–301.

Nguyen, H.V., Tran, H.X., Van Huy, L., Nguyen, X.N., Do, M.T., and Nguyen, N. 2020. Online book shopping in Vietnam: The impact of the COVID-19 pandemic situation. *Publishing Research Quarterly* 36(1): 437–445.

Pakistan Bureau of Statistics. 2021. Losses of Livelihoods. *Dawn*. Retrieved January 18, 2021, from www.dawn.com/news/1600525/loss-of-livelihoods

Prasetyo, Y.T., Tanto, H., Mariyanto, M., Hanjaya, C., Young, M.N., Persada, S.F., et al. 2021. Factors affecting customer satisfaction and loyalty in Online Food Delivery Service during the COVID-19 pandemic: Its relation with open innovation. *Journal of Open Innovation: Technology, Market, and Complexity* 7(1): 76.

Qureshi, H.A., Fatima, R., and Sarwar, A. 2014. Barriers to adoption of online shopping in Pakistan. *Science International* 26(3): 1277–1282.

Rook, D.W. 1987. The buying impulse. *Journal of Consumer Research* 14(2): 189–199.

Shafi, M., Liu, J., and Ren, W. 2020. Impact of COVID-19 pandemic on micro, small, and medium-sized enterprises operating in Pakistan. *Research in Globalization* 2(1): 100018.

Sheth, J. 2020. Impact of Covid-19 on consumer behavior: Will the old habits return or die? *Journal of Business Research* 117: 280–283.

Shy, O. 2014. Window shopping. *SSRN*. Retrieved June 15, 2020, from https://ssrn.com/abstract=2374720 or http://dx.doi.org/10.2139/ssrn.2374720.

Verhagen, T., and van-Dolen, W. 2011. The influence of online store beliefs on consumer online impulse buying: A model and empirical application. *Information and Management* 48(8): 320–327.

Wainewright, P. 2013. Clicks and bricks: The future of retail. *Diginomic*, Retrieved June 15, 2020, from https://diginomica.com/clicks-and-bricks-the-future-of-retail

Wold, S. 2020. How Covid-19 has changed shopper behaviour. *Marketingweek*. Retrieved July 2, 2020, from www.marketingweek.com/how-covid-19-has-changed-shopper-behaviour/

19 How Students Negotiated a University Closure

The Impacts of "Covistress" on Undergraduate Students of the University of Sindh During Online Education

Abdul Razaque Channa and Umbreen Soomro

Introduction: The Aims of This Study

In Pakistan, COVID-19 first appeared on February 25, 2020, in Karachi, the most populated city in the country. The news spread like wildfire through television, Facebook, Twitter, Instagram, and newspapers. Fear and questions grew around how Pakistan—a low-resource and struggling country—would manage and respond to the virus if the virus wreaked havoc there as it was doing in Europe and the USA. To contain a viral outbreak, the Government of Pakistan declared COVID a pandemic and enforced a national lockdown in March 2020. For a few months, a strict lockdown was imposed, then curtailed into "smart lockdown"—the equivalent of "targeted lockdown" in the United States and other countries. The recommended preventive measures—Standard Operating Procedures (SOPs)—included mass movement restriction, closure of academic institutions, maintaining social/physical distance, and practicing personal hygiene (especially regular and strict handwashing). Accordingly, the University of Sindh, Jamshoro and its associated sub-campuses closed down and moved to online education via Zoom. This shift led teachers and students to face many challenges, which we will discuss in the following sections. Our study aimed to investigate the influence of the COVID-19 pandemic on stress—which we term "Covistress"—and how Covistress has impacted students' mental health at the University of Sindh during online education as a result of unexpected lockdown.

Online Education and Its Effects on Students' Mental Health During COVID-19 pandemic

COVID-19 has highlighted Pakistani society's many nuances and profound vulnerabilities. Many of us took for granted the comfort zones we did not

DOI: 10.4324/9781003187462-24

realize we had until the coronavirus wrought havoc in our country. Many people considered online education to be a possible alternative for physical education with easy access for everyone. Although online education has benefited many users, it has also created tensions and difficulties. It has constituted a barrier for many who could not afford it or whose distant location prevented them from accessing the Internet. Our research examined online education and its impacts on mental wellbeing, touching on a variety of essential topics—both positive and negative—to understand further the complexities of Covistress and its relation to the sudden introduction of online education.

Prior to beginning online teaching, the University of Sindh, Jamshoro organized online Zoom meetings with academic staff to familiarize teachers with distance learning through the Zoom virtual network as a platform for teaching online classes. As online classes began, so did the challenges: only a few students had the needed devices and Internet connectivity, while the rest lacked both. The University of Sindh is Pakistan's public university, where most students come from very humble backgrounds. They attend the university from very far-flung areas where there are no basic facilities like electricity, gas, telephone, or potable water. Additionally, since most rural Pakistanis live in large and loud extended families, many students lacked a separate and quiet space for attending classes. Moreover, the unstable financial conditions resulting from the pandemic and knowing someone who had contracted COVID-19 increased the risks of severe anxiety and depression (Husky, Kovess-Masfety, and Swendsen 2020).

The students faced many difficulties, including unscheduled load-shedding (the power supply being cut off for several hours without notice), a lack of essential services, and unstable or no Internet access (Mishra, Gupta, and Shree 2020). Due to these and other factors described below, many students often felt that education was more about tension than learning. Numerous students had to walk for a mile or more in extreme heat to reach a location with Internet coverage—often only to find that accessibility was frequently disrupted and they were disconnected from Zoom during online lectures. Students sometimes cracked jokes about the situation in private Zoom talks. Occasionally, teachers inquired about them online by name, and became unreasonable and unable to fully comprehend the students' actual situation. And for socially and economically disadvantaged students, buying a compatible smartphone and finding a location that would appear attractive to their classmates when the video was turned on, the Internet bundle was often unaffordable and became a major source of stress. Many students simply lost interest in online education or just gave up. Certain students who excelled during physical classes often complained that they were falling behind due to weak Internet connectivity.

As a result of these conditions, students at the University of Sindh repeatedly appealed to Pakistan's Higher Education Commission (HEC), protesting against online education (see below). Thus, we argue that this pandemic has not only exposed Pakistani society's complex structural divisions, differences and inequalities, but has also resulted in many students experiencing critical mental health issues such as frustration, resentment, outrage, emotional pain, distress, and depression.

Materials and Methods

Conducting ethnographic fieldwork and following anthropological research protocols is challenging in pandemic times when there is a high risk of contracting the virus from the participants and vice-versa. Yet despite its multiple challenges, COVID-19 has also provided new opportunities for learning and new perspectives to researchers for conducting their research technologically. Due to the impossibility of conventional fieldwork, we collected data for this chapter via virtual meetings with students of the University of Sindh, Jamshoro, using Zoom conferencing tools and via email and WhatsApp messenger.

The University of Sindh, Jamshoro is the oldest public university in Sindh province and the second largest and oldest university in Pakistan after Punjab University, Lahore. Currently, there are around 32,000 students enrolled in numerous departments of various faculties. Due to the support of our colleagues and the students' enthusiastic reaction to participation in this research, we limited our research to students in the natural and social sciences and the Art and Design department. The office of Research, Innovation and Commercialization (ORIC) approved our study through the Institutional Bioethics Committee (IBC). We sought verbal and written consent from all study participants; they were first briefed about the study and its objectives. All research participants were from pakistan's Sindh province. They were above the age of 18, with diverse economic, social, and geographical (rural and urban) backgrounds. Using a convenience sampling method, we conducted two focus group discussions (FGDs), one with female students and one with male students, all in the last semester of their final year. Along with the FGDs, we conducted 10 interviews, 5 each with male and female students. Again, FGDs and interviews were conducted through Zoom conferencing/meeting software and WhatsApp messenger service. We also carried out an online survey on the impacts of online education on students' mental health during COVID-19, using a random sampling method. Additionally, we prepared a self-administered structured questionnaire and WhatsApped and emailed it to undergraduate students. Filling out the questionnaire implied consent for participation in the survey. Students were asked about their demographic details, such as name, age, gender, residence (rural-urban), and academic session year/level. Fifty students submitted filled survey forms, some with an additional note about their challenges and problems with online learning due to situations beyond their control, such as power cuts, unavailability of Internet connection, and the unaffordability of smartphones and of maintaining the cost of 4G Internet connectivity.

Since we teach in this university, it was convenient for us to contact our colleagues in the Faculty of Natural and Social Sciences and Art and Design to ask them for their cooperation in reaching out to their students. Students also passed on the survey randomly among their colleagues and classmates. All names used for the students quoted herein are pseudonyms.

Findings and Discussion

In order to avoid academic setbacks and the derailing of students' career plans, both private and state-run educational institutions in Pakistan have turned to online learning. With COVID-19 bringing an end to physical classroom learning, online learning ideally should have provided a new way for students and teachers to maintain a sense of normalcy. Yet interactive online learning/teaching became problematic for everyone as the traditional classroom setup moved to the digital "classroom," and the students had to live at home instead of at or near the university. As previously noted, this shift demanded considerable technical skills and, most importantly, device and Internet accessibility. And thereby, online learning, though a necessary step, proved to be highly discriminatory against students who lived in rural areas and the socio-economically poor, resulting in increased mental and psychological anxiety and stress for those students—which, again, we term "Covistress"—on top of their fears around COVID-19. The pre-pandemic physical classroom had smoothly allowed everyone to discuss and participate actively. Many students enrolled in social science fields who had adequate Internet connections preferred online classes because they did not need to expand on formulas or do experimental work. On the other hand, students enrolled in natural science fields (such as Zoology, Botany, Chemistry, Physics, Biotechnology, and Biochemistry, among others) and Computer Science found the transition to digital learning very discouraging, due to the difficulties associated with formulas and technology methods. Lab work was necessary for the natural science subjects; many students protested that there is no substitute for lab work through Zoom, and the university made no attempt to offer this opportunity.

The factors that had the most detrimental effects on students' mental health as a result of the transition to online learning were fatigue, anxiety, and concern, as well as financial shortages, confusion about the future, and coping with constraints on social activities (Sundarasen et al. 2020)—all these issues combined resulted in high degrees of Covistress for these students. For example, Marui expressed that she was overwhelmed and found online education to be questionable in terms of potential prospects. She said:

> *Hamare subject ki nature jo he wo taqreeban laboratorical work pe based he aur hum practical se hi natural science ke subjects ko smjhne ki koshish kerte hain per online classes ki waja se wo cheezen nahi smjh aa rahi jese on-campus classes me knowledge gain kerte thy. Ab to dar*

rehta he ke degree aage ja ke kaam aayegi ya nahi, future ke liye acha socha tha per ab aisa lagta he ke hamari degree ki koi worth nahi. Bohat preshani he, ab to her student depression me he ke jo hum parh rahe hain kiya ye hamare liye future me faidamand hoga ya bas degree leke ghar me beth jaenge.

Authors' translation (Roman Urdu to English):

Our subject is largely dependent on laboratory work. Via practical experiments in the laboratory, we gain an understanding of different topics of natural science. It's challenging for us to grasp these concepts in our online courses in the same manner as we did in our on-campus physical classes. I am unsure whether my degree is useful or not. I was really optimistic about my career, but I am beginning to believe that my degree might be worthless. I am worried, and most students are apprehensive about the issue of online education's ability to prepare them for the future and whether it would ultimately be beneficial or worthless. We may earn a degree but may be unable to find work.

Marui was a 22-year-old final year undergraduate student of Physiology. She explained that much of her coursework was focused on learning through experimentation (lab work), and that she was anxious about the worth of her degree after graduation. According to her, online learning is a formality but in a real sense, students learn nothing about that particular subject, resulting in Marui's and others' extreme uncertainties about their futures.

According to a previous study on US students, undergraduate female students had higher stress and anxiety levels related to COVID-19 than their male counterparts (Aiyer et al. 2020). In concordance with these results, although most of the students in our study reported that they had trouble focusing on academic work due to multiple disruptions, this burden fell especially hard on women. Both Rabail, a female undergraduate student in her second year, and Saira, a 21-year-old female student of chemistry, reported that they usually missed their online classes because of family pressure to do household chores. This was true for most of our female interlocutors and respondents. Even when they were able to take their online classes, they had to deal with the background noise of the household and lack of family support; thus, they also feared examination failure. Such fears and stresses often caused nervousness, anxiety, angst, and continuous headaches. For example, Rabail said:

جڏهن ئي آن لائين تعليم شروع ڪئي وئي آهي ته شاگرد پنهنجو جهجهو وقت ڊ يسڪٽاپ ۽ ليپ ٽاپ اسڪرين تي صرف ڪري رهيا آهن. چو جو انهن انهن وٽ ٻي چوائيس نه آهي. آءٌ پاڻ نظر جو چشمو پاتو آهي ان جي ڪري جومان گھٽو وقت آن لائين ڪلاس تي اسڪرين جي اڳيان گزاريان ٿي جنهن ڪاٿ اکين جي نظر تي اثر پيو آ، اسڪرين جي روشني اکين جي صحت لاءِ بهتر نه آهي. ڪڏهنڪڏهن مان پنهنجي اکين مان پاڻي ۽ د باءُ نمي محسوس ڪندي آهيان. بعد م

تہ ڪمپيوٽر جي سامھون ويھي پڙھڻ ، نوٽ لکڻ ، ايميل چيڪ ڪرڻ ۽ يونيورسٽي جي لرننگ
مينيجمينٽسسٽم تي گھٽي استعمال جي ڪري مون کي مٿي ۾ سور پوندي محسوس ٿيندو آ. آءُ
ٽڪيلٽڪيل ۽ ڪافي پريشان ٿئڻ لڳم. گھر جو ڪم ، ڀائرن،ڀينرن ۽ والدين جو خيال ۽ ڪورونا
۾ پڙھڻ زندگي مشڪل بنائي ڇڏي آ.

Authors' translation (Sindhi to English)

> As learning is shifting from the classroom to the online setup, the
> students are spending much more time in front of desktops and laptop
> screens because they have no other choice. I have started to wear
> optical glasses as the screens are not conducive to long periods of study.
> I sometimes had eye pressure and watery eyes initially, and later suffered
> from headaches as a result of long hours spent in front of the computer
> screen—attending classes, reading notes, doing tasks, and checking
> emails and the university's learning management system—made me
> sick. I was tired and stressed out from juggling my education, household
> tasks, and looking after my siblings and parents.

Shama, age 22, was a female second-year undergraduate studying in the
department of Art and Design. She emphasized that it was extremely
difficult to learn about art and painting through online classes; she felt that
she was gaining little knowledge of the subjects and was merely completing
the course online in order to fulfill her final term. She always questioned
herself around whether she was acquiring knowledge and expertise on her
subject of choice or was squandering her time. She had long desired a career
as an artist, but her feelings have changed. Similarly, Sana, a married, female
Biochemistry student living with others in a small apartment in Hyderabad,
explained that on-site presence, face-to-face teaching, and exchanging ideas
with teachers were the most important sources in gaining knowledge. She
said, "living in a home with many people and having a child has made life
miserable during the lockdown. It has been challenging to balance several
tasks at a time during the pandemic, even more so when movement was
limited and there were a husband and other male family members present
all the time." She continued:

> My husband had hardly ever before exchanged hurtful words with
> me, but since he was all the time at home, we developed a habit of
> speaking to each other about very petty things. My husband often lost
> his temper, which could be because his business was closed and he
> was facing financial issues. This caused us a lot of stress. Besides, there
> was a schedule disruption, a loss of social interaction, and household
> tension—all contributed to mental illness among women during this
> novel COVID-19.

Due to the pandemic, Sana too had mental health problems as a result of juggling several activities with insufficient finances and too many social interactions. As she mentioned, living in a state of lockdown exacerbated her anxiety and moved her into an untenable lifestyle. This state of ongoing stress was particularly relevant among many suffering from psychiatric illnesses such as depression prior to the pandemic, which escalated their problems significantly.

Transformations in social networking as a result of COVID-19 often have a significant impact on an individual's mental health (Elmer, Mepham, and Stadtfeld 2020). The pandemic has harmed various social structures, but our study found that it also has had significant effects on human networking, as one of Sindhi society's most significant values is social relationships. You may be or do whatever you want, but you still retain close social ties with your family members, colleagues, neighbors, friends, and acquaintances. Once the pandemic hit, the dynamics of social relationships shifted dramatically, and many individuals, including students, were unprepared. For Sindhis, "social distancing" was an unfamiliar idea, and it was considered highly impolite to see a friend and not hug. Keeping oneself disassociated and at a distance causes a rupture in societal expectations and values, and has disturbed many people's ethical and moral feelings about social conduct. For instance, Sarwar, a 23-year-old male student who was in his final year of a mathematics major, shared that being at home alone all day with no interaction with his peers contributed to his mental health issues. We discovered that such anguish was more prevalent in final-year students. For example, Aneel is a final year male student of the anthropology department from a remote district called Umarkot. He described that he was staying in a rented apartment in Hyderabad for study purposes during COVID-19 because he could not productively study at home:

> Following the lockdown, I was compelled to return to my hometown, where I encountered several obstacles. [Before I went home], since I had been having difficulty with my studies, my school friends often assisted me with my assignments and research work. They often paid me visits and encouraged me. So [after I returned home], I felt alone and missed my classmates, who were always willing to lend a hand with any academic difficulties. Besides loneliness, the unstable Internet connection and electricity problems made me mentally disturbed. I often heard my classmates saying I did not attend classes due to an inadequate smartphone, poor Internet connection and living remotely.

Aneel felt that he did not belong at home in a world far removed from his prior academic, on-campus life. He explained to us that his friends too were experiencing a variety of difficulties with online learning. They were all struggling, but particularly those who lived in rural areas with limited services and access. They became disturbed and often criticized the

306 Abdul Razaque Channa and Umbreen Soomro

authorities for failing to address their genuine concerns. Aneel added during the FGD that COVID-19 had increased anxiety, worry over not studying properly, and loss of job prospects for those about to graduate.

Students' stress is associated with the negative effects of futile learning practices, which harm their chances of getting a job, consequently creating another source of worry and stress. In addition, anxiety and depression resulting from home confinement stimulated steadily increasing detachment from others. It is well-known that mental disorders tend to arise and expand due to the lack of interpersonal interaction within peer groups (Hasan & Bao 2020). Common psychological symptoms such as emotional disturbances, depression, tension, low mood, irritability, insomnia, frustration, and emotional fatigue (in short, Covistress) have been found in students during COVID-19 (ibid.).

Protests Against Online Classes and Exams

Students from all Pakistani universities protested against online education. They demanded that semester studies should not be continued online. Students outlined their charter that Pakistan's Higher Education Commission (HEC) should offer basic facilities to all students to enroll and study in online classes as easily and successfully as they could in physical classes. The students insisted that they would continue to demonstrate until their demands were met. They used social media to raise their concerns via trends such as #SayNoToOnlineClasses; #HECStopOnlineClasses; #HECFacilitateStudentsFirst; #HECReduceFee. For instance, Fahad, a 22-year-old male pharmacy student, stated that few technical subjects and laboratory courses could be practiced through video streaming. He argued that the majority of students came from remote areas where Internet connectivity was insufficient to attend virtual classes and that many students lacked the financial means to purchase a smartphone or satisfactory and stable Internet. Fahad, along with other classmates, demanded the immediate postponement of distance classes, an end to online examinations, and the allocation of funds for digitalizing the education system, insisting that the necessary technological devices should be accessible to all students unreservedly. And many students asserted that all students should be promoted to the next grade without having to take a final exam. Similarly, Furqan, a 21-year-old male student in his third year in the political science department, narrated, "I walk a few miles to obtain reliable Internet access. The hot weather of Thar, a sandy area, exacerbates the situation. There is insufficient money or transportation to go from my home to the desired place." He grew enraged and insisted that the university and the relevant political authorities must understand the students' on-the-ground realities. Shortly after the student protests, the Higher Education Commission of Pakistan decided to allow universities to follow a hybrid model to be developed around students' concerns. And the federal government decided to allow the reopening of academic institutions, which had been shut down in late March 2020, and in September 2020, after a National Command and Operation Center (NCOC) meeting to examine the scenario.

Dynamics of Remote Rural Areas and Access to Smartphones and the Internet

Rural areas of the country have seen a dramatic decline in power and network connectivity; there is much room for infrastructure development. Teachers and students in villages are becoming more tolerant of digital learning methods, but infrastructural facilities have not yet grown to the level required for effective online learning. For the rural population, the lack of a steady supply of electricity, a shortage of high-speed broadband, and the lack of ability to afford the necessary electronic devices constitute significant obstacles. Generally, few Pakistanis, especially those in rural areas, have access to personal laptops or tablets. Furthermore, data packages and their associated costs can be a significant deterrent for students, especially in online classrooms. Many students either do not have personal computers or have to borrow them for short periods of time; as a result, their learning is restricted. And while there have been some advancements in basic infrastructure, many areas in Pakistan continue to face difficulties in making educational institutions fully digital/online.

Gender Dynamics of Online Learning and Mental Health During the COVID-19 Pandemic

In terms of the gendered context of COVID-19, both male and female students experienced hardship, but, again, women were disproportionately affected. The roles assigned to female students in the home grew exponentially, from study to domestic chores to looking after their babies and caring for their parents and siblings. Prior to the pandemic, such work was limited and they were used to the household chores and study schedules; many lived in dorms or apartments near campus, so they had few household duties. All of that changed during the lockdown, when everyone was instructed to remain at home in order to avoid viral contagion.

In the majority of Pakistani families, men are generally not expected to do domestic work. It is widely considered that household work such as cleaning, cooking, serving food, and washing clothes is the duty of women, and that female students' careers should be associated with caregiving and men's with professions like engineering (Channa et al. 2020). When all stayed at home, many female students, in addition to their class assignments, were also assigned loads of household work, as described by Rabail, Sana, and Shama. Along with this work, female students reported a constant exchange of angry words among family members, especially among male family members, or often men vs women or husband vs wife. These arguments caused a great deal of stress and mentally disturbed married female students.

Sindhi society often considers domestic space as private, secluded and confined (Channa and Tahir 2020). Thus, in complete contrast to life at home, female students feel liberation when they attend university in a conservative society like Pakistan because they get to see the outside world, engage with new people, make new friends, and enjoy social activities with those friends. COVID-19 snatched away this freedom and mobility, which they possessed solely as a result of leaving their family homes to attend the university. It is a widely held belief among female students that the best years of their lives are those spent at university, where they form unbreakable bonds with their peers, and encounter and become acculturated to an entirely new way of life. But the COVID-19 pandemic changed everything. Being restricted to home and having to do multiple household chores had a strongly negative effect on these young women's mental health, causing them tension and anger— Covistress—and potentially redefining their future possibilities. Pakistan's women have long struggled to overcome gender dualism and gender-based divisions of labor (Patel 2010), but the coronavirus pandemic and its ensuing lockdowns have exacerbated the sense among many undergraduate female students that their futures are at risk, that their educations and degrees will not help them obtain decent careers, and that they will end up succumbing to family pressure to marry and live as housewives.

The Making of the "Other": The Haves and Have Nots in the Digital Divide

The COVID-19 pandemic exposed the vulnerabilities of our society, social relationships, and knowledge production hubs. Prior to the pandemic, the Internet, smartphones, tablets, and other multimedia gadgets were hailed as panaceas for a variety of problems and were celebrated as a great innovation of the Western world for solidifying the idea of globalization. These innovations have improved the living conditions of many. Some Pakistanis are wealthy enough to afford tablets, computers, and Internet bundles, yet, again, many others lack the financial means to purchase these essential devices and their needed accompanying Internet packages. As we have noted previously, especially in Pakistan's rural areas, many students struggle to purchase a good smartphone that they can use for their online classes. Yet, we note again that if they do manage to buy one, they often have to walk a mile or more to access the Internet. This situation results in feelings of frustration and resentment from living in an unequal, inequitable, and digitally divided world.

This digital gap has resulted in the emergence of new "Others." For example, one of our respondents, Aneel, explained that he feels alienated from his classmates when they refer to him as the one who uses the inexpensive smartphone and suffers constant Internet disconnections. "They" are the ones who can afford digital tools and suitable space with a seamless Internet connection, while "He" is the one who struggles with his financial constraints and remote location, which has made him an "Other" among his classmates. Pre-pandemic, he had never before experienced being "Otherized," but Covistress due to the difficulties of online education has created a traumatizing and stigmatizing situation for Aneel and many "Others" like him. Experiences like Aneel's shed light on the structural issues underlying human relationships and people's feelings toward one another, highlighting in new ways the social capital of the wealthy and the lack of social capital of the rural poor, and creating mental health problems for these "Others."

Conclusion: Prioritizing Students' Needs

The psychological problems that have accompanied the global spread of the coronavirus have rapidly exacerbated the pandemic's public health burden, which has been linked to an increased incidence of moderate-to-severe levels of stress and anxiety among university students due to the sudden closing of the campuses and the switch to online learning, as we have demonstrated herein. In this still-shocking Covidian time, these increased degrees of anxiety have had subsequent negative academic effects. The coronavirus pandemic has caused university students in Pakistan to confront the multifaceted problematic aspects of Pakistani culture and thereby to experience anger, indignation, despair, and mental pain and depression, which we have termed "Covistress." The challenges faced by students at this particular university, as elsewhere, included financial constraints resulting in a dearth of digital devices; limited skills for using technological equipment; lack of appropriate spatial arrangements at home; pressure to engage in household or farming activities instead of in their studies; spotty electricity that limits their Internet access and often long-distance walks to access their online classes; low quality of those classes as compared to on-campus classes; social isolation if they lived alone; fear of asking questions to instructors via the Zoom platform; fear for their future careers; fear of contracting COVID-19; knowing someone who had contracted it; and awareness of the high rate of viral spread in Pakistan. The pandemic also exposed the digital divide, reinforced rigid gender norms, multiplied student women's work, and widened the divide between the haves and have-nots, creating a new "Other." All these factors had adverse impacts on students' mental health, social lives, and education due to Covistress, as most likely did poor sleeping and food habits and lack of physical activity for those living alone (Verma and Moawd 2020). Numerous students actually lost confidence in their studies and abandoned them, at least temporarily. Lack of in-person, eye-to-eye communication and nonverbal interpersonal presence erode the bond between teaching and learning.

As a direct result of the transition to online learning, university students have been experiencing psychological disturbances that include lower enthusiasm for their studies, increased needs to study individually, and potentially higher rates of failing exams. Our study results have revealed many of the causes of the negative mental health effects of the transition to online learning; however, much more needs to be known about the symptoms that students are experiencing and what measures can be taken to mitigate their negative effects. Priorities should consider instructional disruptions, variations to habitual coping mechanisms, and approaches taken by learning institutions to minimize negative academic and psychosocial consequences. As we continue to come to grips with the ongoing realities of the COVID-19 pandemic, we need to take steps to support students to reduce their Covistress—the strains on mental health associated with this time of unprecedented anxiety and uncertainty. In addition to ensuring that all students have effective electronic devices and stable Internet connectivity, there is a huge need for therapeutic programs that include counseling sessions in which students are taught new skills for handling stress more efficiently. The health and safety of university students, who represent many possible futures for Pakistan, should be a top priority.

References

Aiyer, A., Surani, S., Gill, Y., Iyer, R., and Surani, Z. 2020. Mental health impact of Covid-19 on students in the USA: A cross-sectional web-based survey. *Journal of Depression and Anxiety* 9(5): 1–9.

Channa, A.R., Channa, K.H., and Tahir, T.B. 2020. Gendered discourse of Pakistani parents regarding professional choices for their children. *Progressive Research Journal of Arts and Humanities (PRJAH)* 2(2): 55–64. https://doi.org/10.51872/prjah.vol2.Iss2.38.

Channa, A.R., and Tahir, T.B. 2020. Be a man, do not cry like a woman: Analyzing gender dynamics in Pakistan. *Liberal Arts and Social Sciences International Journal (LASSIJ)* 4(2): 361–371. https://doi.org/10.47264/idea.lassij/4.2.28.

Elmer, T., Mepham, K., and Stadtfeld, C. 2020. Students under lockdown: Comparisons of students' social networks and mental health before and during the COVID-19 crisis in Switzerland. (V. Capraro, Ed.) *PLoS ONE* 7(15): 1–20.

Hasan, N., and Bao, Y. 2020. Impact of "e-Learning crack-up" perception on psychological distress among college students during COVID-19 pandemic: A mediating role of "fear of academic year loss". *Children and Youth Services Review* 118(105355): 2–9. doi: 10.1016/j.childyouth.2020.105355. Epub 2020 Aug 12. PMID: 32834276; PMCID: PMC7422835.

Husky, M.M., Kovess-Masfety, V., and Swendsen, J.D. 2020. Stress and anxiety among university students in France during Covid-19 mandatory confinement. *Comprehensive Psychiatry* 102(152191): 1–3. https://doi.org/10.1016/j.comppsych.2020.152191.

Mishra, L., Gupta, T., and Shree, A. 2020. Online teaching-learning in higher education during lockdown period of COVID-19 pandemic. *International Journal of Educational Research Open* 1–8.

Patel, R. 2010. *Gender Equality and Women's Empowerment in Pakistan*. Oxford: Oxford University Press.

Sahu, P. 2020. Closure of universities due to coronavirus disease 2019 (COVID-19): Impact on education and mental health of students and academic staff. *Cureus* 12(4): e7541.

Sundarasen, S., Chinna, K., Kamaludin, K., Nurunnabi, M., Gul, B.M., Heba, K.B., et al. 2020. Psychological impact of COVID-19 and lockdown among university students in Malaysia: Implications and policy recommendations. *International Journal of Environmental Research and Public Health* 17(17): 6206.

Verma, A., and Moawd, S.A. 2020. The impact of Covid-19 on mental health in allied health undergraduate students during lockdown phase: An observational study. *Psychology and Psychological Research International Journal* 5(3): 1–9.

Conclusions
Global Negotiations Around COVID-19

Inayat Ali and Robbie Davis-Floyd

Our book—a contribution to what we are calling "Covidian anthropology"—began with a description of the origins of the coronavirus, which was first discovered as early as the 1960s, the process of its current naming, and a brief description of its global impacts. Our chapters have elaborated on these impacts and have centered on sociocultural constructions of and negotiations around COVID-19 at individual, local, sociocultural, national, and global levels. In these Conclusions, we will summarize their key findings in sections dealing with each of the four parts of this volume, and will conclude with some provoking thoughts about possible futures.

Part I. Autoethnographic Reflections on Negotiating the Coronavirus Pandemic

We commenced Part I with editor Inayat Ali's autoethnographic conversations with himself—"I" and "You"—in which he described his experiences during his self-isolation with a probable coronavirus infection. He took this opportunity to reflect on his early lessons in anthropology about Malinowski's theory of functionalism in contrast to Radcliffe-Brown's theory of structural functionalism, and on his later deep engagements with critical medical anthropology's more holistic approach to syndemic disparities. His self-reflections illustrate his intellectual growth in the field as well as the emotional coping mechanisms he developed to deal with his fears and his self-isolation. They also encompass his sudden understanding of the cultural wisdom behind a strong traditional norm that he grew up following throughout his childhood in a small village in Pakistan's Sindh Province—not wearing shoes in bed because they allow a *Balla* (snake) to climb onto the bed and bite. The pandemic and his self-reflections enabled him to unpack the deeper meaning of this sociocultural prohibition—to understand the *Ballā* as a metaphor for actual micro-organisms, such as viruses, that can be carried on shoes and cause illnesses; hence those potentially contaminated shoes should be removed before going to bed. As Ali demonstrates, in a theme that carries throughout our chapters, *there is often profound meaning and solid science behind seemingly irrational cultural customs and taboos.*

DOI: 10.4324/9781003187462-25

In Chapter 2, Rachel Irwin provided autoethnographic reflections on Sweden and its international media coverage during the coronavirus pandemic. Sweden was highlighted in international media, including social media, for having an "open society" relative to other high-income countries, meaning that the Swedish government neither imposed a lockdown nor demanded compliance with restrictive measures. Instead, it chose to rely on "individual responsibility" for following preventive measures, informally enforced by strong social pressure to do so. Some media outlets framed the Swedish approach to the pandemic as "deviant," while others lauded it as "preserving civil liberties." In both cases, contestations appeared, and misinformation and even disinformation characterized much of the polarized coverage. Irwin's anthropological "fieldsite" was the 24/7 news cycle. She chose to research the media coverage of Sweden's COVID-19 responses because she was alarmed by the vitriol that she was reading, which did not reflect the reality she was living. In the international media, Swedish "culture" was regularly invoked as an explanation for the country's "open" (as opposed to "locked down") approach. Yet the media's definitions of "Swedishness" focused on superficial and stereotypical markers of identity and were often discussed by commentators who had little connection to the country.

Irwin showed that the results of Sweden's informally enforced preventive policies have been neutral; Sweden's numbers of COVID-19 cases and mortalities fall in the middle of those achieved by other European nations. Yet unlike in other countries that did impose strict lockdowns, Sweden's economy continued to thrive—although, as Irwin stresses, this was not the primary reason for Sweden's more relaxed policies, which instead had much to do with Sweden's constitutional prohibitions on imposing lockdowns and restricting people's movements. Thus, Sweden's Covidian approach reflected a national commitment to stay true to its foundational principles. Irwin herself became engaged with the media, writing articles and blogs and giving televised interviews to try to refute the media stereotyping of Sweden's approach as "disastrous" and "irresponsible" and to present a more balanced picture. She saliently pointed out that, although "the anthropologist as culture-broker" is an outdated model, if anthropologists do not engage with media, then "others"—some of whom speak with authority in the absence of experience—will define, use, and abuse the concept of "culture." Irwin concluded that while anthropologists are no longer culture-brokers, we (anthropologists) do have a responsibility to be *context*-brokers helping people to negotiate meaning, particularly in times of crises. And indeed, a recurrent theme in many of our chapters is *media mis- and disinformation*, the troubles they cause, and how anthropologists can help, as Irwin did for Sweden and as we will further discuss below.

In Chapter 3, Kate Senior, Richard Chenhall, and Fran Edmonds autoethnographically described their loss and longing for the field that resulted from indefinite travel bans between many states in Australia. For the first time in 23 years, Kate was unable to visit the Aboriginal *Ngukurr* community where she had been conducting ethnographic research, and more importantly to her, where she has three generations of friends and people whom she calls family, and who call her the same. These authors note that the process of separation and grieving for the field has prompted discussion about "the end of fieldwork," and whether it is possible to *be* an anthropologist when the field itself becomes physically inaccessible. Yet as they showed, they did ultimately find a creative way to conduct "fieldwork from home"—by analyzing archived material related to Ngukurr to re-capture stories that had been lost, and thereby to return these stories to the community as important pieces of their cultural heritage. We note that their creativity in this endeavor illustrates the flexibility of anthropology in general: once you have the tools, you can apply them to any topic and in any place.

Part II. Conceptualizing and Negotiating the Pandemic Across Professions, Cultures, and Countries

Moving on from the autoethnographies of Part I, our chapters in Parts II–IV presented ethnographic research. In Chapter 4 on negotiating COVID-19 in Kenya, author Violet Barasa focused on stigma, noting the endless media reports about doctors and nurses refusing to attend patients with high temperatures and community members actually publicly lynching one man who was considered to be a "super-spreader"—even though he did not have the disease. She also criticized the heavy-handedness with which the government has dealt with civilians accused of breaking curfew rules. Using both public and individual accounts, Barasa analyzed Kenya's official response to the coronavirus pandemic, demonstrating how its lockdowns, quarantines, and punitive attitude have negatively affected people's healthcare-seeking behaviors. She explored how rumors, lay theories of viral transmission, rampant misinformation, and insufficient testing complexify people's abilities and willingness to access healthcare in this low-resource setting.

Barasa also provided a poignant account of her own mother's struggles with chronic comorbidities and how she had been turned away numerous times from the health facility that she previously frequented as a high blood pressure (HBP) patient, either because the clinicians were afraid that her HBP reading was a symptom of COVID-19 or there were simply no healthcare personnel at the hospital—perhaps too afraid to come to work. Thus she had to manage her symptoms at home using over-the-counter-medication, which left her health in worse condition—as is also true for many others with chronic conditions. Barasa demonsrated that the stigma surrounding COVID-19 in Kenya, fueled by rumors and misinformation, has led to many symptomatic people choosing to keep news of their illness private due to the risk of *any* kind of illness being associated with the coronavirus; as one person put it on their social media feed, "as soon as people see you cough, they say you have the disease." Barasa's work clearly demonstrates the intense dangers Kenyan people face when they are coded as COVID+, even if they are not, and reveals the global need for increased health literacy, most especially in low-resource countries but also in high-resource countries, where rumors and conspiracy theories continue to abound, as illustrated in the Introduction to this volume and in many of its chapters.

Chapter 5, co-authored by Kim Gutschow and Robbie Davis-Floyd, examined how US obstetricians, midwives, doulas, and labor and delivery nurses have negotiated the dangers of COVID-19 by adapting their practices according to ever-changing scientific information and ever-emerging policies and protocols. Gutschow and Davis-Floyd showed how hospital-based practitioners struggled with the COVID-based protocols allowing only one support person in the labor room, as they were keenly aware that many women want both their partner and their doula to be present, and suffer psychological distress when they are forced to choose between them. Sadly, as these authors showed, some hospital protocols still demand separating COVID+ mothers from their newborns at birth, despite the fact that evidence shows extremely low rates of mother-to-baby transmission, and that those separated from their newborns at birth nevertheless leave the hospital with those newborns two days later (unless they are too ill). As these authors demonstrated, other hospitals and practitioners have discontinued this irrational and harmful practice with relief.

Meanwhile, as Gutschow and Davis-Floyd described, as childbearers flee hospital contagion by seeking to give birth in homes and freestanding birth centers, midwives and the few holistic obstetricians in the USA who attend out-of-hospital births have been struggling with massively increased demands for their care. Given that, under normal circumstances, only around 2% of US births are planned to take place outside of hospitals under midwifery care, these holistic practitioners noted that an ideological commitment to out-of-hospital birth is a generally necessary factor in its success. Choosing out-of-hospital (OOH) birth simply out of fear of hospital contagion often results in hospital transfers, as women need to give birth where they truly feel safest. Primary lessons learned by their maternity care provider respondents included the fundamental importance of clear treatment protocols for all childbearers under pandemic conditions, and of the need for more out-of-hospital maternity care providers to meet the rising demands for their services. Gutschow and Davis-Floyd strongly argued for the *decentralization* of maternity care in all countries to meet the need for flexible, on-the-ground care provision—especially during pandemics and other disasters, but also during more normal times, as the vast majority of childbearers want care in their communities. In low-resource countries, these authors argued that such decentralization should translate into government support for the world's remaining traditional midwives (see Ali et al. 2021; Ombere 2021; Graham and Davis-Floyd 2021).

In Chapter 6, Mayarí Hengstermann addressed the issues of health literacy (HL) and information fatigue in relation to understanding people's beliefs and behaviors as they navigate COVID-19 in Germany. She explored the challenges of oversimplifying this complex phenomenon to make it more understandable, which left gaps in which misinformation is spread and lack of trust is generated, opening a window where absurd ideas concerning COVID-19 coexist—and often compete with—scientific and biomedical healthcare and knowledge—even in this high-resource country where health literacy could be expected to be widespread. Ironically, other chapter authors recommend just this sort of information simplicity for reaching people with low HL, creating a sort of Covidian Catch-22. Noting that people's perceptions of COVID-19 and of the preventive measures against it shape their actions, Hengstermann described the strong protests against these measures taken by an alt-right group, whose members stormed the Parliament building, resulting in a government clampdown against large gatherings and the institution of even stronger preventive measures. We call attention to Hengstermann's useful identification of the "prevention paradox," in which mixed and contradictory messages intended to encourage people to use preventive measures have the opposite effect.

As Hengstermann made clear, many Germans consider the information concerning COVID-19 too technical, unreliable, contradictory, inconclusive, or insufficient to act upon—the prevention paradox—which directly adversely impacted adopting the preventive health measures and in turn is now negatively affecting the inclination to get vaccinated. The obvious solutions, as Hengstermann suggested, are for the authorities—the government and the scientists—to agree on messages before they are published and to make sure that they are clear, well-explained, responsive to people's primary questions and concerns, directly relevant to people's everyday lifeworlds, and within their health literacy levels. We strongly suggest that such clear and relevant guidelines should be applied globally, and that governments and educational institutions should work to increase the health literacy of their populations to better prepare them for improving health in ordinary or extraordinary times, such as future epidemics or pandemics.

In Chapter 7 on Switzerland, Nolwenn Bühler, Melody Pralong, Célia Burnand, Cloé Rawlinson, Semira Gonseth Nusslé, Valérie D'Acremont, Murielle Bochud, and Patrick Bodenmann demonstrated how, as in Sweden (Chapter 2), the principle of "individual responsibility"—which lies at the core of Swiss values, along with a "culture of consensus" and of "social solidarity"—was adopted in health authorities' and medical experts' public communications, which favored transparency and acknowledging the multiple uncertainties of the pandemic, and appealed to individuals' common sense. This emphasis on individual responsibility placed a large burden on every Swiss citizen to comply with preventive measures in order to protect—to "care for"—others, and was internalized as a *moral* responsibility embedded in logics of blame and guilt.

According to Bühler and colleagues, in Switzerland's French-speaking context, the term *gestes-barrière*—"barrier gestures"—became widely used. These *gestes-barrière* consist of hygiene and distancing measures, such as sneezing in the elbow, washing hands regularly, stopping handshaking, and maintaining a two-meter distance between individuals. (Revealing international inconsistency, other countries required only a one-meter distance.) Bühler and colleagues analyzed these barrier gestures as boundaries, both material and symbolic, that are made and negotiated in practices. Barrier gestures separate the inside from the outside, the safe spaces and relations from the risky ones. Their mass and willing implementation in Switzerland—and its "flexible lockdowns"—relied on the core Swiss value on individual responsibility to care for others, putting others' needs above one's own. Yet, as these authors showed, the issue of vaccination has generated cracks in the Swiss edifice of social solidarity, as a part of the population seems reluctant to get vaccinated. They are happy to care for others by following the preventive measures, yet less willing to put themselves at what they perceive as the personal risk of, for example, vaccine side-effects. Thus, Switzerland, as is also the case in many other countries, may not be able to achieve herd immunity through mass vaccination.

In Chapter 8, Katarzyna E. Król and Małgorzata Rajtar explored the Covidian experiences of people, mostly children, with rare diseases in Poland, who are at heightened risk of severe illness if they become infected by SARS Cov-2. Surprisingly and paradoxically, these authors found that such supposedly more vulnerable people were better prepared for the exigencies of the pandemic than their healthier counterparts because they had already been practicing daily hygienic vigilance and often isolation from their peers, so did not have to change their habits in any significant ways. The authors suggested that this situation reverses the power dynamics: rather than being the recipients of biomedical interventions and the objects of biomedical recommendations, these patients and their caregivers already possess cultivated know-how and skills that are vital for surviving the pandemic—a phenomenon the authors called "positive vulnerabilities." As they already acknowledge uncertainty and vulnerability as normal parts of life, persons with rare metabolic disorders are well-positioned to employ their already established resilience practices to help them through the dangers posed by the coronavirus pandemic.

In Chapter 9, co-authors Tatiana O. Novikova, Dmitry G. Pirogov, Tatyana V. Malikova, and Georgiy A. Murza-Der chose a transitional moment in time—the end of March 2020—after the virus had started to spread in Russia and before lockdowns were imposed—to analyze public awareness of COVID-19 in Russia during that time and people's self-reflective readiness to deal with social restrictions. At that point, social restrictions were only recommended, not enforced. These authors sought to learn, early on in the pandemic, whether or not the Russian people were ready for the necessary changes, and whether or not they relied on objective information about COVID-19 or tended to believe in "myths." They studied 1,108 people from diverse backgrounds, dividing them into three groups based on age. They found age differences in information use—younger people tended to rely more on social media, middle-aged people on online mass media, and older people on print media. Their younger respondents were the most frustrated by the restriction of freedoms and were more likely to share their fears and anxieties around COVID-19 than their older ones. All respondents became warier of people with pronounced symptoms of respiratory diseases and generally avoided tactile contact with them. The authors noted some medical pluralism among their respondents: the older ones were more likely to use home remedies, such as drinking tea infused with ginger and lemon and eating garlic and onions to provide protection against COVID-19. Even that early on in the pandemic, which the authors, following Hans Selye, called the early "alarm phase" of the crisis, their respondents became more likely to avoid public places, to use public transport more rarely, to avoid leaving their homes except in cases of emergency, and to restrict their contacts with their loved ones more often. Respondents in all groups reported a high level of subjective willingness to follow almost all restrictions; nevertheless, some were not so willing, in what Novikova and colleagues termed "Covidian dissidence," which often included refusals to wear masks and keep social/physical distance. The older respondents were more likely to work remotely from home due to concerns about office contagion. While reporting multiple expectations of negative effects from coronaviral spread, Novikova and colleagues also reported a surprising number of expected positive effects: these included more leisure time; more time for self-reflection; increased attention to health care, hygiene, and personal relationships; increased budget-planning skills; and increases in "knowledge and experience." All respondents were the least prepared for restrictions on their movements, such as the bans on leaving home, on traveling to other parts of the country, and curfew imposition. According to these authors: "Many of our respondents at that time had not yet accepted that the world had changed."

In Chapter 10, author Danuta Penkala-Gawęcka addressed "Controversies and Negotiations around Biomedical Treatments and Traditional Asian Medicines." She first focused on the quest for drugs to fight COVID-19 that began in biomedical research just after the first announcements of the epidemics, and on the search for non-biomedical treatments, especially those stemming from various types of traditional medical systems. She highlighted the strengthening of these Asian systems during the pandemic and described some of the controversies around the use of their treatments that stem from major differences in biomedical and traditional medical epistemologies involving the causes and cures of illness and disease.

Penkala-Gawęcka also highlighted the role of mediatization in the spread of information about the pandemic in close connection with "biocommunicability," understood as multiple ways of production, circulation and reception of health knowledge that can generate uncertainty and fear—which, as previously noted, contribute to the circulation of rumors and conspiracy theories. She saliently noted that UN Secretary-General António Guterres has called this dissemination a "pandemic of misinformation." She stresses the term "infodemic," meaning the proliferation of information during an epidemic, both accurate and inaccurate, and WHO's efforts via its "Myth Busters" initiative to combat the inaccuracies of the infodemic, as acting on misinformation, such as to drink bleach or excessive amounts of alcohol to ward off or cure COVID-19, can and has cost lives. We reiterate here Penkala-Gawęcka's salient quote from Partington (2020): "Like the virus itself, the infodemic seems to call for vaccination."

Penkala-Gawęcka also showed how biomedical professionals have sought to use antiviral pharmaceuticals and other drugs developed for other diseases off-label to treat COVID-19 patients and how, in these attempts, one can observe successive waves of hope and disappointment. She specifically detailed the use and testing of the drug so widely recommended by then-US President Donald Trump—hydroxychloroquine—which had been primarily used for treating autoimmune diseases and which, as Penkala-Gawęcka explained, has been shown to be ineffective in the treatment of coronavirus-infected people. She also explained in detail the curative possibilities of the allopathic drug amantadine, which does show promise yet requires further testing in randomized controlled trials (RCTs) that have been designed but, as of December 2021, are yet to be completed.

As Penkala-Gawęcka noted, the biomedical gold standard of the RCT often cannot apply to the testing of traditional medicine remedies and cures, as the traditional medical systems she discussed employ highly individualized treatment methods that generally cannot be standardized enough for RTCs. She showed that China, proud of its system of traditional Chinese medicine, endorsed its use for COVID-19 patients and how its practitioners have been creating hybridized models combining allopathic and traditional treatments. In contrast, she showed that India has a more problematic relationship with traditional and "complementary" medical systems, acronymized there as AYUSH—Ayurveda, Yoga, Unani, Siddha, Sowa Rigpa (Tibetan medicine) and Homeopathy. She described the longstanding antagonisms between AYUSH and the hegemonic biomedical system, which is seen as the main obstacle to using the potential of AYUSH and other traditional medicines to fight COVID-19 in India. Penkala-Gawęcka emphasized that, as a result of the urgent need to treat COVID+ people, in some medically pluralistic regions of Asia, "traditional medical systems have been strengthened, and new and positive negotiations and collaborations with biomedical practitioners have been established," despite their ongoing disputes and controversies. Penkala-Gawęcka noted that India's Prime Minister, Narendara Modi, did meet with representatives of the AYUSH sector in March 2020, urging them to start evidence-based research on traditional remedies, and that the AYUSH Ministry has followed suit where possible. We look forward to the results of this research, and we add here the point made in Chapter 15 that *just as medical systems like Ayurveda and Unani-Tib can be "alternative" or "complementary" to biomedicine, so biomedicine can be "alternative" or "complementary" to other medical systems.*

In a change of pace, and in recognition of the "economic pandemic" (see Introduction), Chapter 11, by Santirianingrum Soebandhi, Kristiningsih, and Ira Darmawanti, addressed how small-to-medium enterprises (SMEs) have been negotiating the COVID-19 pandemic in Indonesia as consumer shopping in physical stores has given way to online shopping—given that public spaces have a high potential for viral transmission. Large-scale social restrictions implemented by the Indonesian government have led to a decline in sales and to the closure of many offline SMEs. As elsewhere, those Indonesian SMEs that have survived and even thrived have had to move to digital platforms—a strategy supported by research asserting that SMEs that take advantage of e-commerce can actually increase their productivity and income during the pandemic. These authors demonstrated that even SMEs that cannot sell their products online, such as barbershops and hair and nail salons, have creatively adapted by offering services in people's homes, and provide other examples of creative online adaptations.

Part III. Culturally Constructing and Negotiating COVID-19 in South Asia

The chapters in Part III of this volume focus on South Asia, beginning in Chapter 12 with the surprising and inspiring ways in which Sri Lanka has successfully negotiated COVID-19. In this chapter, authors Tharaka Ananda and Inayat Ali point out that a culture can include resistance features that enable its members to successfully negotiate sudden biocultural challenges such as pandemics. During the coronavirus pandemic, it became evident that whereas technologically advanced countries could not effectively control the outbreak, some low-resource nations with no advanced medical systems have managed to negotiate a successful controlling process due to their longstanding cultural systems, which include various traits that worked successfully in controlling viral spread and preventing further outbreaks.

Noting that these countries include Bhutan (see Chapter 13), Taiwan, Vietnam, Micronesia, Samoa, the Solomon Islands, and Vanuatu, and stating that Sri Lanka is one such country, Ananda and Ali investigated the influential "resistance traits" of Sri Lankan culture that helped to negotiate and control the COVID-19 outbreak. While acknowledging that Sri Lanka is a multicultural and multiethnic country, Ananda and Ali focused on Sinhalese Buddhist cultural practices, as they represent the majority. They examined the effects on pandemic preparedness of multiple relevant factors, including specific Sinhalese traditional cultural practices and customs; Buddhism and its belief system, which includes traits such as flexibility, "middle path" observance, and others; and the Indigenous medical system, called *Hela wedakama* (among other names), which has over 3000 years of history and incorporates immune system-enhancing traditional health practices long designed to be performed in pandemic situations. In conjunction with an all-important Sri Lankan shared cultural history, Ananda and Ali included in their analysis of cultural traits that served the country well in negotiating the pandemic: traditional medicine; rites of passage; traditional foods and beverages; family kinship systems, which include respect and obedience to elders; self-sustainability (most Sri Lankans have not become addicted to overconsumption and are satisfied with what they have); collectivity and collective endurance; integrity; knowledge sharing; traditional greeting practices that do not involve touching; strong mental stability that includes health and balance; and endurance during crises such as the 30-year Civil War, the 1989 riot, numerous earthquakes, and others. Ananda and Ali show how these strong cultural traits have acted as resistance factors against the spread of COVID-19 and will continue to do so in Sri Lanka in future crises and public health emergencies.

This chapter on Sri Lanka provides a strong demonstration of how historical cultural practices can prepare a society for a pandemic; it reminds us greatly of the Andaman Islanders and how their historical societal memory told them how to survive the giant tsunami of 2004 that killed millions. Those who had boats simply went far out to sea to allow the wave to rise and pass under them, while those on land headed far inland. In contrast, those Islander groups who had been Christianized had lost the societal memory about how to survive a tsunami; as a result, many drowned (see Davis-Floyd and Laughlin 2022). In this story, we can read the positive effects of long-term memories encoded in some societies that provide a template for how to deal with disasters. And we trust, as we further discuss below, that our global collective societal memories of the coronavirus pandemic will—or at least should—serve us in good stead during future biocultural global crises.

In Chapter 13 on Bhutan, authors Mary Grace A. Pelayo, Ian Christopher N. Rocha, and Jigme Yoezer present the case of a tiny country—wedged between the two giant countries of India and China, both of which have suffered major and ongoing waves of COVID-19—that successfully managed to halt coronaviral spread among its people and also engaged in a highly successful vaccination campaign, with majority coverage by June 2021. The authors explained that the factors involved in Bhutan's remarkable success include social cohesiveness and profound respect for the King and other national leaders, and most especially *a strong pre-pandemic preparedness for a pandemic*. In 2018, the Bhutanese government began working with WHO and other organizations to generate emergency preparedness, presciently constructing tents to serve as quarantining facilities for people with respiratory illnesses, which thus were there and ready to receive and treat the COVID-19 patients that eventually came flowing in for a time. The country's first case of COVID-19, officially identified on March 6, 2020, was a male tourist who had likely contracted COVID-19 in India. Within hours of his diagnosis, his contacts had been traced and quarantined, and so it went with all other diagnosed cases until viral spread was effectively stopped. As of June 2021, Bhutan had a total of only 1,724 confirmed cases and just 1 fatality. As with Sri Lanka, as described above, specific cultural traits facilitated Bhutan's successful negotiations with COVID-19.

For example, once vaccinations were available, rather than simply administering them immediately, the government took its deeply religious culture into account. Government officials consulted with the leaders of the Buddhist monks, who picked the most auspicious day and time for vaccine administration to begin—which the government honored, despite having to wait for an inauspicious month to pass. And the vaccination program was preceded by a three-day, nationally televised religious ceremony during which a mantra believed to stave off disease was chanted. This ceremony and deep trust in the country's leadership led to high vaccine uptake; by November 2021, 76% of the population, including children between 12–17 years of age, had been fully vaccinated (www.bts.bt/news) —very close to the 80% vaccination rate needed to achieve full herd immunity nationwide. Among all the countries addressed in our volume, Bhutan stands out as a success story that others should seek to emulate—again, most especially in terms of its extensive pre-pandemic preparedness for a pandemic—a lesson we hope all the nations of the world will put into effect. Another Bhutanese lesson that should be widely exported has been the *clarity and consistency of the government's messages* to its people—something most other governments have been unable to achieve, as especially shown in Hengesterman's chapter on Germany and its government's confusing and obfuscating messages.

In Chapter 14 on "Negotiating India" during the Covidian crisis, author Suman Chakrabarty showed us the devastating effects, primarily in urban areas, of the second wave of COVID-19 that resulted from the development in India of a new and deadlier viral strain called B.1617. Chakrabarty described India's "culture of negotiation" and how it has been working in the Covidian context at multiple levels. National-level negotiations included working with China to rectify India's severe lack of PPE (personal protective equipment) and essential medical equipment, such as ventilators. Indian states negotiate with each other and with the national government around supplies of testing kits and other medical equipment, the duration of lockdown, the selection of targeted containment zones, and the online formal education system and its evaluation process. At local levels, citizens negotiate compliance with the formal preventive measures; many choose not to comply.

At the micro-level, Chakrabarty devoted considerable attention to the members of India's so-called "Scheduled Tribes." Surprisingly, the members of such tribes have suffered more from the economic effects of the pandemic than from its physical effects, as COVID-19 has not spread widely among these groups, likely due to their remoteness and lack of contact with outsiders. The author illustrated how such tribal groups have relied both on religious ceremonies and on their own Indigenous medical systems to protect themselves from contagion. Chakrabarty also showed how landless and migratory laborers, unable to negotiate paid work leaves, had to compromise their physical and mental health to keep on working to feed their families. Also suffering were job seekers who, due to the pandemic, experienced either salary cuts or discharge from their previous jobs. From March to April 2020, as Chakrabarty noted, Indians' salaries were cut by 47%, in the economic pandemic generated by the coronavirus pandemic. Despite an enormous coronavirus relief package delivered by the national government, many in India remain in a state of economic precarity—with no end in sight, as by May 2021, the Indian government had managed to vaccinate only 12% of the population and was suffering a vaccine shortage. Yet as of October 17, 2021, India had fully vaccinated around 31% (291 million) of its eligible population, and 707 million had received their first dose (see: Covid vaccine: India administers more than one billion Covid jabs—BBC News). Nevertheless, it is unlikely that the coronavirus will be contained in India any time soon, as vaccine resistance is high, and rumors are flying around about its dangers.

In Chapter 15, Inayat Ali and Sudipta Das Gupta presented perceptions and practices around COVID-19 in Bangladesh. Situating the outbreak within Bangladesh's sociocultural, economic, political, and historical contexts, these authors described the politics surrounding COVID-19 at local and governmental levels and stressed the importance of local knowledges, attitudes, perceptions, and practices in combatting or ignoring the pandemic. Based on a survey taken by 45 Bangladeshi respondents from a diverse variety of backgrounds, they addressed the primary themes that emerged from their respondents—their perceptions, beliefs, and behaviors around preventive measures, vaccines and vaccination, personal experiences of COVID-19, and when and how this pandemic might end. Ali and Gupta showed that around 64% of their respondents were not satisfied with the government's efforts to deal with this pandemic, as is also the case in many other countries—as shown in most other chapters in this volume. This mistrust must be situated within Bangladesh's historical political systems, in which governments have not been elected but rather have been selected by the military. The government's lifting of the first lockdown was called "extremely irresponsible" and even "suicidal" by the opposition political parties, who accused the government of trying to create herd immunity by encouraging everyone to catch—and thereby become immune to—COVID-19, which was of course not the government's goal, which was to stimulate its hard-hit economy.

Ali and Gupta also demonstrated how lay perceptions changed as the pandemic spread. Resultantly, most of their respondents view COVID-19 as a dangerous disease, often due to their first-hand experiences of either contracting the virus themselves or knowing someone who had. This also led 80% of respondents, including the people around them, to observe the preventive measures; the remainder of their respondents followed no preventive measures, in part because the people around them did not and group pressure can be felt very strongly. Regarding vaccination, most of their respondents consider the COVID-19 vaccine to be safe, and even want to pay money to get vaccinated—yet, paradoxically, had made no effort to receive the vaccine. Around 44% think that people in their community would not accept this vaccine, mainly due to a "lack of education and knowledge" and doubts about its effectiveness. 40% of respondents think that a vaccine is not the only solution to this pandemic and that people should also take preventive measures. However, 26% believe that vaccination is a permanent solution to the dilemma of how the pandemic can end. Nonetheless, some respondents thought that only supernatural authority would bring the pandemic to an end, and so put their faith and trust in Allah. Briefly, this chapter presents a useful case study on how an emergent infectious disease has been negotiated at various levels.

Part IV. Negotiating COVID-19 in Pakistan: Cultural Conceptions and Pandemic Responses

The chapters in Part IV take Pakistan as a case study, examining its multifaceted responses to the coronavirus pandemic. Pakistan recorded its first case of COVID-19 on February 26, 2020, started observing lockdown from March 24, 2020, and ended the official lockdown in August 2020 (see Ali et al. 2020). Despite lockdown, two of the most significant religious festivals—*Eid ul Fitr* and *Eid al-Adha*—along with the observance of the holy month of Ramazan (as it is called in Pakistan), occurred during this time and became major hotspots for viral spread.

As our chapters have shown, COVID-19 is not just a biomedically defined disease; it is also a multifaceted set of social constructs that vary among regions. In Chapter 16, authors Sara Akram and Rao Nadeem Alam investigated such social constructions of COVID-19 in Pakistan's Punjab province, showing that the coronavirus's biomedical construction as a potentially deadly disease is contested by local constructions of COVID-19, such as the belief that Allah predetermines everyone's time of death. Rejecting the government-enforced complete lockdown from March to May 2020, religious leaders encouraged people to continue their congregational prayers at mosques. (One of their 353 respondents insisted that "A virus cannot enter sacred places.") And many laypeople have continued to congregate, arrange marriages, and perform religious festivals, thereby "demonstrating a lack of the necessary knowledge about viral spread and the existing mistrust between the government and the people," as Akram and Alam show. Noting that "viral spread cannot be stopped until local perceptions and levels of awareness are fully understood and taken into account," these authors illustrate such local perceptions, including the rumors and conspiracy theories that abound in Pakistan and that fill local people with fear and resultant unwillingness to follow the government-instituted standard operating procedures (SOPs). They saliently noted the consequences via a US infectious expert's statement: "When you extend your hand, you are extending a bioweapon." One of their respondents, a government official, affirmed that "Extending a hand is equal to having a bomb in the other hand that would explode if you shake hands, and the person would die."

Akram and Alam noted that the majority of their interlocutors, most of whom lived in cities and had relatively high health literacy, did state that they currently avoid handshaking and hugging, while their rural interlocutors did not. The influences of culture and tradition are strong: most of their interlocutors, including many city-dwellers with high health literacy, chose nevertheless to attend, for example, funerals, to avoid the cultural stigma resulting from not showing up at these culturally significant ceremonies. Even at the peak of viral spread in 2020, 42% of their respondents continued visiting their relatives and friends, ignoring physical distancing. Many who wore masks in public were stigmatized as "cowards"; most ignored that stigma, yet 29% of their interlocutors had been negatively affected by being labeled a coward. As these authors stated, "During pandemic times, clearly, many cultural customs can be downright dangerous, causing every Pakistani who believes that COVID-19 is real to have to choose between two dangers: that of not following custom and perhaps getting sick, and that of breaking custom to avoid contagion and suffering negative cultural consequences." Additionally, they doubt that vaccination will prove to be the solution in Pakistan, as people's generic mistrust in their government and suspicions of vaccines in general will likely keep vaccine uptake unsustainably low.

In Chapter 17, authors Inayat Ali, Salma Sadique, and Shahbaz Ali demonstrated the local perspectives on COVID-19 that have appeared in the rural areas of Pakistan's Sindh province. Focusing on a small town of that province, these authors found that many there believe that the disease is either a "political game" played by the government to obtain more foreign aid and to control its people, or a "supernatural test" brought by Allah—or by Hindu gods and goddesses—to test people's faith and punish them for their bad deeds. Consequently, local people either ignore preventive measures or employ only supernatural ones. To appease Allah or other supernatural beings, depending on whether they are Muslim or Hindu, they perform prayers and rituals; for example, the Indigenous Hindu *Bāgrrī* community has used cow urine for such rituals, considering it to be a potent cure (a particular type of cow urine is often used in Ayurveda; it is known to have anti-bacterial and anti-oxidant properties). Some have also conceptualized the pandemic as a "Western conspiracy" to control Muslims. Consequently, not only have they avoided following preventive measures, but have even started refusing the polio vaccine, conceiving it as a "Western" product just like COVID-19—even though the virus that causes this disease originated in China—so they imagine that the polio vaccine may contain the same or a similar virus. (This is one of the many reasons why polio remains a significant danger both in Pakistan and in its neighboring country, Afghanistan (see Ali 2020; Ali, Sadique, and Ali 2021).) These perceptions and practices reveal various levels of mistrust and scales of negotiations between the local and the national, between the local and the global, and between the culturally conceived natural and supernatural worlds. And, as these authors show, local people's distrust of vaccination in general is likely to translate to low vaccine uptake once a COVID-19 vaccine is widely available in Pakistan, again revealing how local perceptions can negatively influence healthcare behaviors. As of November 10, 2021, only 50% of Pakistan's population had received at least one vaccine dose (see: 50% of Pakistan's population partially vaccinated against Covid-19: Asad Umar – SAMAA).

Returning to the topic of consumer behavior described for Indonesia in Chapter 11, in Chapter 18, authors Tayyaba Rafique Makhdoom, Sanaullah Jamali, and Maria Tufail Memon investigated changes in consumers' shopping behaviors after the March 2020 outbreak of COVID-19 in Pakistan. Due to lockdowns, which by June 2021 were still ongoing in that country in certain targeted large cities, consumers in Pakistan (and worldwide) were compelled to renegotiate their shopping habits and buy online rather than going to brick-and-mortar stores. These authors described how demographic factors, income, and employment status affected buying behavior during the COVID 19 outbreak in Pakistan, showing that the primary products their survey respondents bought online, as in Indonesia, were clothing and accessories, followed by food deliveries. Makhdoom and colleagues noted that Pakistanis tend to think economically, as price was usually the deciding factor in whether or not to purchase an item. They concluded by showing that Pakistanis in general still prefer shopping in physical stores, and thus extensive online shopping in Pakistan may well not become a long-term practice.

In Chapter 19, Abdul Razaque Channa and Umbreen Soomro described how Pakistani undergraduate students dealt with the closure of the University of Sindh, Jamshoro, the subsequent move to online classes, and its negative effects on these students' mental health. Those university students staying at or near the university had to return home to live with their families, where, especially in rural areas, they encountered multiple difficulties in attending their online classes. These included lack of a quiet and private space to study and frequently interrupted Internet connectivity, which led many of them to have to walk for a mile or more in suffocating heat to reach a place where they could connect. Many who had been doing well in their physical classes began to fall behind, and due to what these authors refer red to as "the digital divide," a new "Other" was created—that "Other" was from a humble background, could not afford the needed devices and connectivity packages, and so was divided from and "othered" by those who could. Yet the burden of what these authors term "Covistress" fell most disproportionately on the female students, who had idealized their futures as professional women and enjoyed much freer lives on campus but, once forced back home by the government's preventive measures, were expected to perform housework and childcare in addition to their studies. Resultantly, these young women worried that they might have to give up their dreams of a professional career and end up as housewives—a future they had gone to university precisely to avoid.

Channa and Soomro noted a climbing scale of young students facing mental health issues due to Covistress; significant sources of this stress came from struggling to adapt to online classes, exam anxiety, family disputes, and career holdups. Recommending creating counseling sessions for students' psychological care, the authors argued that ignoring students' Covistress and the mental health issues it causes may trigger severe problems in the future, while successfully negotiating them can produce significant benefits for the students—who represent many possible futures for Pakistan, and whose needs should therefore be prioritized.

Looking Ahead: A Cure for COVID-19, and Vaccination Acceptance or Refusal?

Viruses can infect anyone, yet their effects are disproportionate. Thus the pandemic has highlighted systemic inequalities among those who are exposed to or who contract COVID-19 and how those people cope. For example, as shown in Chapter 7, the wealthy who have a great deal of space to live in during quarantine cope well, while at-risk groups of low socioeconomic status contract the virus more frequently and have a much harder time in dealing with their illness while trying to continue to feed their families. These are some of the specific biosocial circumstances that make people more or less vulnerable. Our chapters have demonstrated these differences within and between countries, such as being able to afford mass testing or providing economic relief packages to those who most need them. The pandemic has exposed and multiplied the existing disparities. Employing the concept of "syndemics" (synergistic epidemics), one can see how biosocial conditions and relationships have shaped COVID-19 processes and practices, including contagion, through political-economic, structural, and environmental factors (Singer and Rylko-Bauer 2020; Ali, Sadique, and Ali 2020). These disparities will significantly affect vaccine uptake, as many people in many countries will refuse the vaccine, and many countries and individuals will not have equal access to it (Ali, Ali, and Iqbal 2021).

As we write these Conclusions in December 2021, the new variant of COVID-19 called "Omicron" is infecting many people around the world. Thus we now ask an as yet unanswerable question: How might this pandemic be brought to an end? Should an effective cure for COVID-19 become widely available, either from allopathic biomedicine or a "complementary" medical system, this question could become moot. Should it not, it would be comforting to assume that, once sufficient vaccines are available, mass inoculation will end the global pandemic via creating herd immunity. Yet that hopeful scenario may well not come to pass. Most of our chapter authors describe vaccine resistance or refusal in their respective countries, high and low resource alike. For example, as noted above for Chapter 7 on Switzerland, the vaccination issue could cause a "crack in the edifice" of Swiss solidarity. "Anti-vaxx" movements have long existed in many high-resource countries, often fueled by rumors and conspiracy theories, while various forms of these—as illustrated in our Introduction—are also found in many low-resource countries, particularly among the rural poor. As our chapters have shown, some cultural environments, such as those of Bhutan and Sri Lanka, are conducive to high vaccine uptake, whereas others are not. It is quite likely that those anti-vaxxers who oppose the MMR (measles, mumps, and rubella) vaccine—among others—will also oppose the COVID vaccines. It is equally likely that those in Pakistan (and in other low-resource countries) who oppose vaccination in general as a "Western plot" and a "conspiracy against Muslims" will oppose the COVID-19 vaccines for the same reasons (see Ali 2020; Ali, Sadique, and Ali 2021)—and also because, as shown in Chapter 19, many rural Pakistanis do not even believe that COVID-19 is real, so why would one bother to be vaccinated against this "fake" disease?

And so, we further ask, will the cultural conceptions and beliefs around COVID vaccines result in uptakes of insufficient numbers to create herd immunity in some or many countries? What factors will help—or impede—people's vaccine uptakes? How will these factors vary by culture and country? What socio-cultural, economic, and (geo-)political factors will come into play to affect vaccine accessibility, affordability, and acceptability? The unequal distribution of the COVID-19 vaccine at the global level has already been criticized and called "vaccination apartheid" (see Aginam 2021) as high-income countries have piled on the vaccine; while low-income countries wait to receive a "free-of-cost" vaccine. According to Aginam (2021) and others, the Omicron variant is a result of these unequal vaccine distributions, because when the countries of the Global South are denied sufficient supplies of vaccines, opportunities are created in un-vaccinated people "for the virus to mutate into easily transmissible vaccine-resistant variants" (ibid., p. 1). How can anthropologists help? And how can the media help? Thus far, as shown in Chapter 8, the media have tended to sensationalize deaths that seem to be related to having received a vaccine; what roles might the media instead play in increasing health literacy and therefore vaccine uptake?

As is clear in our writings, we are strongly supportive of universal vaccine uptake and do not share in the multiple reasons people find to refuse it. Yet at the same time, we argue for the appropriate consideration of all contexts that cultivate vaccine refusals, and we respect the use of "complementary" medical systems to prevent or to treat the symptoms of COVID-19 and the medical pluralisms that allow these non-biomedical, integrative medical systems to survive and thrive in many countries—as addressed in some of our chapters. No one medical knowledge system has all the answers; thus it makes sense for all these systems to be complementary *to each other*, without hegemonizing biomedicine, and to co-engage in finding effective treatments for COVID-19.

A common theme running throughout our chapters is the dis- and misinformation spread by the media and the multiple harms this spreading has caused; an equally common theme is that truthful, clear, and comprehensible information on COVID-related restrictions, and on COVID-19 itself, could reduce the intense stresses of fear and anxiety by reducing ambiguity and uncertainty. Here we point to the excellent suggestion made by the authors of Chapter 16 that understanding local attitudes, beliefs, and practices and their underlying rationales could greatly help health officials in any country to present science-based strategies for preventing infection in culturally appropriate and acceptable ways. For example, just as treatments for COVID-19 have been hybridized in China, where both traditional Chinese medicine and biomedicine are jointly employed (see Chapter 10), for Pakistan (and many other countries), government protocols could become hybrids of biomedical recommendations and locally believed in preventive measures, such as drinking green tea, head shaving, and performing rituals and prayers—harmless practices that carry great psychological benefits—while noting that the beneficial effects of such home remedies or large-scale ceremonies would be greatly enhanced by also wearing masks, hand-sanitizing, and physical distancing. In such ways, and from needed anthropological perspectives, *government SOPs could be presented as a package that includes local remedies and honors local beliefs.* Certainly, anthropologists could help with such endeavors. Health officials could also work to de-stigmatize COVID-infected people in Pakistan, Kenya, and other countries where stigmatization is prevalent through public relations campaigns that correlate COVID-19 with other potentially deadly and infectious diseases, such as polio, which do require prevention efforts and treatment but do not carry a stigma.

Vaccine production and its patent rights encourage some countries and stakeholders to control the production, price, and distribution of vaccines. This hegemonic control creates a conducive environment for exploiting low-income countries. We suggest that the production and dissemination of effective vaccines should be without any restrictions, so that every country and every individual in the world can be vaccinated without charge. Yet we are also aware that it is likely to take at least 3–5 more years before enough vaccines can be made available in all countries, and that the lowest resource countries of Sub Saharan Africa will likely be the last to receive sufficient doses to achieve herd immunity (Belluz 2021). This, combined with ongoing vaccine refusals, makes it clear that the coronavirus pandemic will constitute a plague on humanity for years to come.

Now we ask, if and when it ever does end, what will be the pandemic's long-term consequences for social behavior? It has been noted in many countries that rates of colds, flu, and other infectious disease transmissions are down as a result of the preventive measures taken against coronavirus transmission. Will we immediately revert to former greeting patterns such as handshaking, hugging, and kissing? Or will physical distancing, mask wearing, and frequent handwashing become socially and individually ingrained? (Pre-pandemic, mask wearing was already common in the densely populated cities of, for example, Japan.) We venture a guess here that the results will be mixed. We can imagine that handshaking as a greeting ritual can be relatively easily given up: as noted in Chapter 16, infectious disease expert Gregory Poland called the hand a "bioweapon" and also called handshaking an "outmoded custom" that should cease to exist. Perhaps we should all adopt the Japanese custom of bowing in greetings and farewells; it indicates respect and friendliness, as handshaking does. Or can we follow the folding of hands in greeting others, as people do in India? Many in the USA are now settling for an "elbow bump" along with a warm smile. Kissing on both cheeks, as was the custom in many countries, can likely also disappear as a cultural norm. Yet speaking personally, we ourselves are practically desperate to go back to hugging those whom we care about deeply. Hugs are both expressions of love and generators of much-needed endorphins; we miss them and hope to return to them as soon as possible!

Thus we must also ask, will the world learn valuable lessons from COVID-19 that can be put to practical use in future pandemics, or forget what it took to cope with this disease and simply carry on with our lives, as people did after the gradual dying out of the Great Influenza pandemic of 1918–1920? That global pandemic, along with the lesser and much more recent SARS, MERS, Ebola, and Zika epidemics, should have taught the whole world, and especially national governments, to develop and maintain pandemic preparedness; the global failure to learn that lesson left the world—again excepting Bhutan—unprepared for the coronavirus pandemic. Have we finally learned that *we must always be prepared for pandemics*?

We suggest that some of the most essential lessons to be learned from this present pandemic involve the permanent establishment of mechanisms for early disease detection, rapid and early transmission prevention measures, and the implementation of disease testing and tracking protocols that should be in place in every country to stop the next pandemic before it becomes one. Had such systems already been in place, as they were in Bhutan, the coronavirus pandemic itself could have been stopped early on, as indeed it was in that small kingdom. *Every new infectious disease that emerges should be treated as a potential pandemic until proven otherwise.*

In conclusion, we point to the onrushing Climate Crisis. As ocean levels rise and millions are displaced and forced to live in closer quarters, and as animals are displaced and forced to live in closer proximity to humans, the likelihood that "new" and deadly viruses will make themselves known increases exponentially, as does the need for global pandemic preparedness. How can we use the social and economic upheavals brought on by the coronavirus pandemic to help us mitigate the effects of climate change? As we rebuild our economies, will we turn to green energy to create more jobs and put people back to work in energy-efficient ways, thereby mitigating the Climate Crisis and helping to prevent it from turning into the predicted Climate Catastrophe? It is our hope that the findings described in the chapters in this volume may be of use in that endeavor. And what changes will occur once the pandemic is over (if it ever is) certainly will constitute rich subject matters for researchers in multiple disciplines. We expect much to be done within the subfield of medical anthropology that in this volume we have called *Covidian anthropology*.

References

Ali, I. 2020. *Constructing and Negotiating Measles: The Case of Sindh Province of Pakistan*. (PhD Thesis). Vienna: University of Vienna.

Ali, I. 2021. Rituals of containment: Many pandemics, body politics, and social dramas during COVID-19 in Pakistan. *Frontiers in Sociology* 6: 83. https://doi.org/10.3389/fsoc.2021.648149

Ali, I., Ali, S., and Iqbal, S. 2021. COVID-19 vaccination: Concerns about its accessibility, affordability, and acceptability. *Frontiers in Medicine* 8: 647294. doi:10.3389/fmed.2021.647294

Ali, I., Sadique, S., and Ali, S. 2020. COVID-19 significantly affects maternal health: A rapid-response investigation from Pakistan. *Frontiers Global Womens Health* 1: 591809.

Ali, I., Sadique, S., and Ali, S. 2021. COVID-19 and vaccination campaigns as "Western plots" in Pakistan: Government policies, (geo-) politics, local perceptions, and beliefs. *Frontiers in Sociology* 6: 82.

Aginam, O. 2021. *Omicron is a product of vaccine apartheid*. Kuala Lumpur, Malaysia: International Institute of Global Health. https://iigh.unu.edu/news/news/omicron-is-a-product-of-vaccine-apartheid.html (accessed December 31, 2021).

Beluz, J. 2021. Poorer Countries Might Not Get Vaccinated until 2023. Vox. India and poorer countries may wait years for Covid-19 vaccines as rich countries hoard them – Vox; accessed June 14, 2021.

Davis-Floyd, R., and Laughlin, C.D. 2016. *The Power of Ritual*. Brisbane, Australia: Daily Grail Press.

Graham, S., and Davis-Floyd, R. 2021. Indigenous midwives and the biomedical system among the Karamojong of Uganda: Introducing the Partnership Paradigm. *Frontiers in Sociology* 6: 670551. doi:10.3389/fsoc.2021.670551

Ombere, S.O. 2021. Access to maternal health services during the COVID-19 pandemic: Experiences of indigent mothers and health care providers in Kilifi County, Kenya. *Frontiers in Sociology* 6: 613042. doi:10.3389/Fsoc.2021.613042

Partington, G. 2020. Infodemic. *Polyphony*, April 29. https://thepolyphony.org/2020/04/29/infodemic/?utm_source=rss&utm_medium=rss&utm_campaign=infodemic (accessed May 20, 2020).

Singer, M., and Rylko-Bauer, B. 2020. The syndemics and structural violence of the COVID pandemic: Anthropological insights on a crisis. *Open Anthropological Research* 1(1): 7–32.

Index

Australia 3–5, 42–55, 313
Austria 3–5, 15, 104

Ballā 18, 312
Bangladesh 3, 6, 205, 232–43,
    246–8, 323
barrier gestures 4, 5, 110–2, 317;
    see also gestes-barrière
Bhutan 3, 4, 6, 19, 191, 205–14, 278,
    320–2, 328, 330
bioweapon 269, 325, 330
Buddha 195–7, 198, 201; anti-Buddha
    17; new Buddha 17–8
Buddhism 195, 197–8, 201–2, 205, 212,
    244, 320

China 1, 3, 8, 13, 17, 31, 61, 64, 95–6,
    158, 163–4, 181, 205–7, 219, 224,
    237–9, 277, 319, 321–2, 326, 329
construction/constructions 4, 6, 21, 50,
    176–8, 181, 219, 223, 255–6, 266,
    312, 324
context-brokers 3, 39, 313
coronaviral 3, 191, 206, 308, 313, 318,
    321, 332
Covidian: adaptation 267;
    anthropology 3, 13, 312, 331;
    approach 313; catch-22 316;
    concerns 209; conditions 182;
    context 156, 322; crisis 221, 322;
    dissidence 140, 318; experiences 317;
    movement 140; negotiating attitudes
    224 (see also negotiation); present 9;
    situation 23; social norms 33; times
    182, 309; vignettes 256
Covistress 3, 299–309, 327
cow urine 7, 276, 325
culture: culture 2–6, 8, 9, 21, 28, 30,
    34–6, 39, 49, 50–3, 179, 196, 206,
211, 218, 267, 313, 325–8: Buddhist
    culture 4, 192, 203; culture brokers
    3, 35–9, 313 (see also context-
    brokers); construction of culture 50
    (see also culture); culture of blame
    221; culture of consensus 110–14,
    316, 320; culture of negotiation 219,
    227, 322 (see also negotiations);
    culture making 52; Indigenous
    culture 51; Ngukurr material culture
    49; Pakistan's culture 281 (see also
    Pakistani culture); political culture
    191; popular culture 96; religious
    culture 322; Russian culture 142–7;
    Sri Lankan culture 191–2, 202;
    Sinhalese culture 198; Swedish
    culture 28, 34; 313

Delta 1
disparities 36, 83, 227, 232–9,
    242, 259, 278, 312, 327; see also
    structural and inequities

ethnography 30, 45, 49: archival
    49; autoethnography 14–15, 24;
    cyber-ethnography 3, 256; internet
    ethnography 30

fieldwork 3, 13, 20, 21, 30, 42–9,
    55, 217, 271, 301, 314; and end of
    fieldwork 3, 42, 55, 314
functionalism 21, 312
funerals 260–1, 325

Germany 3, 5, 94–7, 99, 102–6, 110, 316
gestes-barrière 5, 110–12, 115–17, 120,
    317; see also barrier gestures
god/gods 20, 199, 201, 219, 223–4,
    260–3, 265–6, 275–7, 325; and

goddesses 199, 219, 223, 227, 276, 325; *Chakha* 223; *Khasuli* 223; and Mātta 276

health literacy 3, 5, 9, 63, 65, 69, 71–2, 94–5, 97–9, 102–8, 151–3, 213, 240–1, 249, 260, 315–6, 325, 328
health-seeking behaviors 61–2, 66–8
herd immunity 4, 27, 32–7, 97, 120, 208–9, 234, 247, 267, 317, 322–3, 328, 329
Hindu/Hinduism 195–7, 223, 276–7, 325; and Hindus 233–6
hugs/hugging 259, 260, 325–9, 330

India 3, 4, 6, 165–6, 194–6, 205, 206, 208, 216–27, 235, 238–9, 276, 283–4, 286, 295, 319, 321–4, 330
Indonesia 3–5, 172–83, 295, 320, 326
inequities/inequity 111, 114, 117; *see also* structural and disparities
infodemic 2, 97, 156, 166, 217, 319; *see also* misinformation pandemic; conspiracy theories 2, 4, 6, 7, 9, 32, 70, 107, 156, 158, 237–8, 256, 270–3, 277, 315–19, 325–8; misconceptions 70–2, 156; misinformation 5, 29, 31–6, 62–3, 70–2, 78, 97, 100, 142–56, 217, 221–2, 233–9, 313–28; rumors 2, 4, 6, 7, 9, 32, 36, 62, 70, 107, 156, 158, 175, 226, 237–8, 256, 270–3, 277, 314–15, 319, 323–5, 328
Islam 35, 238

Kenya 3, 5, 61–72, 314, 329
kinship 50, 191, 201–2, 225, 321
kissing on the cheek 330
Kula Ring 20, 22

Maternity care 4, 5, 76, 78, 80–1, 83, 88–90, 315
medicine: alternative/complementary 3, 162, 239, 247, 320; ayurveda 165–6, 196, 238, 247, 319, 320, 325; AYUSH 165–6, 319; and biomedicine 3, 128, 162, 165–7, 238–9, 247, 320–9; traditional Asian medicines/ T&CM/TCM 155, 162–6, 318; traditional medicine 3, 162–5, 167, 191–2, 205, 223, 319; telehealth/ telemedicine 81, 86, 235; and Siddha 156, 165–6, 319; and Sowa Rigpa

164, 165, 319; and Unani/Unani-Tib 165, 238, 247, 319, 320; and Yoga 165–6, 319
moral: moral activity 115; moral burden 122; moral common sense 34; moral duty 120; moral economy 111–18, 120; moral feelings 305; moral implications 115; moral and logistical dilemma 116; moral responsibility 114–15, 117, 121, 316; moral sentiments 115–17; moral and practical negotiations 116; moral work 116
Muslim/Muslims 6, 175, 195, 219, 220, 233–6, 238, 243, 261–3, 271–2, 274, 325, 328

negotiation/negotiations 1, 2, 4–6, 9, 14, 83, 106, 115–16, 139, 155–6, 162–6, 191–3, 217–25, 227, 312–19, 322–6; *see also* culture of negotiation
new normals 2, 284

Oedipus complex theory 21
Omicron 2, 327

Pakistan 3, 6, 15, 20–3, 70, 212, 242–7, 253–9, 261–2, 270–2, 275–7, 278, 281–6, 295–6, 299–302, 306–10, 312, 324–9
pandemic: multiple pandemics 2; publication pandemic 1; economic pandemic 2, 5, 174, 216–23; social pandemic 2, 216; structural pandemic 2, 116; emotional/psychological pandemic 2, 116; political pandemic 2, 217; misinformation pandemic 2, 217; *see also* infodemic
Papua New Guinea 13, 18–23
Poland 3, 5, 125, 127, 129, 131–2, 134, 156, 160–1, 259, 317, 330
preventive measures 5, 6, 32–6, 94–102, 105–7, 112–14, 118, 139, 149, 156, 174, 192–4, 197–9, 202, 213, 220–5, 232–3, 236–8, 240–1, 243–8, 255, 276–8, 299, 313–17, 322–5, 327–9; handshake/handshaking 112, 259–65, 317, 325, 330; isolation/self-isolation 2, 13–18, 23–4, 42, 50, 55, 65–7, 82, 95–7, 99, 117, 125–8, 130–4, 139, 145–8, 150–3, 174, 192–7, 199–202, 242, 270–5, 283, 309, 312–17; and mask/masks 2, 8, 15–16, 23, 36–7, 69, 79–81, 84–6, 96–7, 99, 100–6,

112–13, 118, 146, 153, 178–9, 183, 222, 225, 235, 240–1, 246–9, 262–4, 274–5, 278–9, 318, 325, 329; and personal protective equipment (PPE) 36, 78–80, 86, 145–6, 218, 322; and physical distance/distancing 2, 23, 33, 36–7, 66, 69, 99, 104, 113–18, 175, 181, 201, 222–5, 233–5, 240–2, 259–66, 270, 274–5, 278–9, 299, 318, 325–9; and preventive paradox 4, 98, 102, 107–8, 316; and self-quarantine 5, 17–18, 97, 274, 283; and social distancing 2, 69, 81–2, 96–7, 101, 112–13, 128, 131–2, 146, 153, 181, 241, 259, 305; and standard operating procedures (SOPs) 255–6, 259, 261, 264–7, 281, 295, 299, 325, 329; and quarantine 2, 13, 17, 45, 54, 61–8, 71, 99, 116, 139, 193, 200, 208–10, 237–8, 242, 270–4, 283, 314, 327

refusal/refusals 153, 255, 278, 318
religion/religious 35, 43, 70, 96, 174–5, 195–7, 205–6, 210–16, 218–19, 223–5, 227, 233–8, 241, 255–6, 260–7, 271–7, 281, 322–4
ritual/rituals 6, 9, 48, 87, 96, 191–2, 198–203, 221–4, 233, 260–6, 276–9, 281, 325–30; and rituals of containment 199, 221, 233
Russia 3, 5, 139–4, 147, 149, 151, 237, 317

socialization 191, 202
Sri Lanka 3, 4, 6, 191–9, 201–3, 320–2, 328
stigmatization 2, 3, 5, 6, 63–4, 66–7, 148, 220–5, 278, 329; and stigma 6, 8, 61–72, 224, 266, 277, 314, 325
structural: structural violence 22; structural disparities 3, 23, 259 (*see also* disparities and inequities); structural inequities 114; structural issues 35, 72, 309; structural ring 22; structural vulnerabilities 9
structural functionalism 21, 312
Sweden 3–5, 27–9, 31–9, 63, 110, 158, 313, 316
Switzerland 3–5, 22, 110–15, 117, 119–22, 316–17, 328

United States/USA 3, 5, 8, 22, 126, 159, 181, 208, 259, 277, 299

vaccination 6, 96–9, 120–1, 133, 156, 174–5, 182, 193–4, 208–13, 217, 225–6, 232–6, 244–8, 267, 272, 317–19, 321–8; and vaccination apartheid 328; and vaccine refusal 4, 99, 272, 327–9 (*see also* refusal/refusals); vaccine resistance 272, 323–8; and vaccination suicide 272 (*see also* vaccination)

Western plot 6, 272, 328

For Product Safety Concerns and Information please contact our EU
representative GPSR@taylorandfrancis.com
Taylor & Francis Verlag GmbH, Kaufingerstraße 24, 80331 München, Germany

www.ingramcontent.com/pod-product-compliance
Lightning Source LLC
Chambersburg PA
CBHW052118230326
41598CB00080B/3847